Dr Bailey
Room 540

Reye's Syndrome II

Proceedings of the International Conference on
Reye's Syndrome, Halifax, Nova Scotia, Canada
June, 1978

SPONSORED BY

The National Institute of Neurological and
Communicative Disorders and Stroke,
National Institute of Health, Public Health Service,
Bethesda, Maryland, USA

National Health Research Directorate of the
Department of National Health and Welfare
Agency of Canada

Medical Research Council of Canada

National Reye's Syndrome Foundation,
Bryan, Ohio, USA

National Reye's Syndrome Foundation,
Dexter, Michigan, USA

The Robert Katz Medical Research Foundation,
Highland Park, Illinois, USA

The Izaak Walton Killam Hospital for Children
and the Faculty of Medicine, Dalhousie University,
Halifax, Nova Scotia, Canada

GRUNE & STRATTON RAPID MANUSCRIPT REPRODUCTION

Reye's Syndrome II

Edited by

John F. S. Crocker, M.D.

Department of Pediatrics
The Izaak Walton Killam Hospital for Children
and Dalhousie University
Halifax, Nova Scotia, Canada

With

Philip C. Bagnell
Spencer H. Lee
Rudolph L. Ozere
Kenneth W. Renton
Kenneth R. Rozee

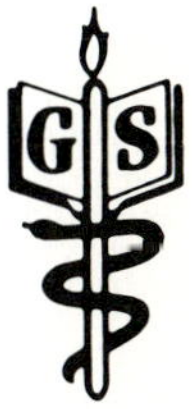

GRUNE & STRATTON
A Subsidiary of Harcourt Brace Jovanovich, Publishers
New York   San Francisco   London

Grune & Stratton, Inc.
111 Fifth Avenue
New York, New York 10003

Distributed in the United Kingdom by
Academic Press, Inc. (London) Ltd.
24/28 Oval Road, London NW1

Library of Congress Catalog Number 78-26355
International Standard Book Number 0-8089-1178-3
Printed in the United States of America

Contents

Acknowledgments

The Editors of this volume would like to thank Sharon Digout for her outstanding contribution to the editorial work of this book; Dr. Richard Goldbloom, Chairman of the Department of Pediatrics, Dalhousie Medical School; and Francine Gaudet, Public Relations Director, I. W. K. Hospital for Children, for their encouragement and comments; Catherine Imrie, Sue Moreira, and Elsie Manuel for their patience with the secretarial work involved in the Conference and in this book; and Beverly Carlsen for her volunteered time and assistance.

Foreword

It is now 15 years since Dr. Douglas Reye at the Royal Alexandra Hospital in Perth, Australia, first described in 21 children the syndrome that bears his name. There is little to add to his original description of a syndrome preceded by a viral infection, possibly synergistic with a toxin, and characterized by a fatty liver, cerebral edema, and a high mortality (17 out of his 21 cases died). In the intervening decade and a half we have learned more about the details of the syndrome and have realized that it is both widespread around the world and more prevalent than originally suspected. The contributions to this volume come from the proceedings of the First International Conference on Reye's Syndrome held in Halifax, Nova Scotia, Canada, June 22 and 23, 1978. The conference was sponsored by the Faculty of Medicine, Dalhousie University; the Izaak Walton Killam Hospital for Children in Halifax; the Medical Research Council of Canada; the National Health Research Directorate of the Department of National Health and Welfare of Canada; the National Institute of Neurological and Communicative Disorders and Stroke of the U.S. Public Health Service in the U.S. Department of Health, Education and Welfare; the National Reye's Syndrome Foundation in the United States in Bryan, Ohio, and Dexter, Michigan; and the Robert Katz Medical Research Foundation. The conference brought together more than 150 participants from around the world who represented virtually all the centers or groups concerned with the study of this syndrome.

As the papers in this volume attest, there is a definite association of acute viral infections—particularly influenza B, varicella, upper respiratory infections and gastrointestinal (diarrheal) diseases—as prodromes to the development of Reye's syndrome. The epidemiological data are very clear, but they also implicate other factors, in particular, genetic susceptibility and exposure to some toxic agent. Thus, the causes of the syndrome are multifactorial in nature, and in the United States it is most typically a winter illness of white upper-class children living in suburban areas.

The ultrastructural changes in liver and brain are highly characteristic, with accumulation of fat droplets in hepatocytes, swelling and internal disorganization and pleomorphism of mitochondria in both hepatocytes and neurons, swelling of cerebral astrocytes and neuronal endoplasmic reticulum, and formation of myelin blebs (very much like those seen experimentally in hexachlorophene or alkyl tin intoxication). The mitochondrial changes appear to be highly characteristic and of diagnostic value (e.g., in a liver biopsy). Thus, the manifestations of the syndrome are those of a multisystem disease.

There is much circumstantial evidence to implicate various toxins as a necessary component in the pathogenesis of the syndrome, and many of the conference papers address this aspect at the experimental as well as the clinical level. Some exogenous toxic agents such as the polyethoxylate emulsifiers or detergents used in pesticide formulations or aflatoxin contaminants of crops are rather strong candidates, but the possibilities of endogenous toxins have also been raised. As the organizers of the conference have emphasized, there remains much to be done in this area. Precisely what are the interactions among virus, toxic chemicals, and host tissues? How does one study the toxin problem when the thousands of pesticides formulations on the market can be so readily withdrawn or reformulated and when many such toxins disappear from body organs so rapidly following exposure? In this context, how many types of Reye's syndrome are there? Clearly there is need for more collaborative studies involving virologists, chemists, pharmacologists, epidemiologists, and clinicians—just the sort of interdisciplinary mix present at the conference.

Data from clinical centers with the most extensive experience with Reye's syndrome indicate general agreement on effective clinical management. There is no doubt that early diagnosis and prompt institution of intensive supportive care in an experienced hospital setting are the key features of successful clinical management. The level of coma is inversely proportional to the survival rate and to the minimization of neurological sequelae. Thus, with early optimal management, survival rates now run well over 80 percent, with neurological sequelae in only 10 percent or less of survivors, except in infants under one year of age where the percentage of brain-damaged survivors may reach 40 to 50 percent.

Reye's syndrome is unquestionably a complex disorder, confronting the clinical and the laboratory researchers alike with some very tough challenges. It is multifactorial in nature and multisystem in involvement. The numbers of cases are small, albeit major clinical emergencies; but careful studies of the syndrome and elucidation of the problems it presents are likely to contribute in a major way to the advancement of our knowledge about interactions among viral infections, various toxins, hepatic function, and cerebral function. These published proceedings of the Halifax conference suggest that there are numerous groups of investigators already sufficiently involved and interested to ensure continued research and progress.

Donald B. Tower, M.D., Ph.D.
Director
National Institute of Neurological
and Communicative Disorders and Stroke

Contributors

Peter Ahmann, M.D., Emory University School of Medicine and Henrietta Egleston Hospital for Children, Atlanta, Georgia, USA

Farouk M. Ali, M.D., Emory University School of Medicine and Henrietta Egleston Hospital for Children, Atlanta, Georgia, USA

*June R. Aprille, Ph.D., Department of Biology, Tufts University, Medford, Massachusetts, USA

Gregory K. Asimakis Jr., Ph.D., Department of Biology, Tufts University, Medford, Massachusetts, USA

Philip C. Bagnell, M.D., Department of Pediatrics, The Izaak Walton Killam Hospital for Children and Dalhousie University, Halifax, Nova Scotia, Canada

Joseph V. Baublis, M.D., Ph.D., University Hospital, University of Michigan Medical Center, Ann Arbor, Michigan, USA

William E. Bell, M.D., University of Iowa Hospitals and Clinics, Iowa City, Iowa, USA

Kevin Bove, M.D., Childrens Hospital Research Foundation, Cincinnati, Ohio, USA

Daniel B. Caplan, M.D., Emory University School of Medicine and Henrietta Egleston Hospital for Children, Atlanta, Georgia, USA

Guy A. Carter, M.D., University of Iowa, College of Medicine, Iowa City, Iowa, USA

E. Chaves-Carballo, M.D., University of Iowa, College of Medicine, Iowa City, Iowa, USA

*A. R. Colon, M.D., Department of Pediatrics, Georgetown University Hospital, Washington, D.C., USA

J. Craenen, M.D., Ohio State University, College of Medicine, Children's Hospital, Department of Pediatrics, Columbus, Ohio, USA

John F. S. Crocker, M.D., Department of Pediatrics, The Izaak Walton Killam Hospital for Children and Dalhousie University, Halifax, Nova Scotia, Canada

Larry E. Davis, M.D., Department of Neurology, University of New Mexico School of Medicine and the Veteran's Administration Hospital, Albuquerque, New Mexico, USA

*Kamnual Dhiensiri, M.D., Khon Kaen Hospital, Khon Kaen, Thailand

---

*Invited Speakers

T. E. Duff, M.D., University Hospital, University of Michigan Medical Center, Ann Arbor, Michigan, USA

I. Dvorackova, M.D., Department of Pathology, Faculty Hospital, Hradec, Kralove, Czechoslovakia

W. D. Engle, M.D., University Hospital, University of Michigan Medical Center, Ann Arbor, Michigan, USA

Bahjat A. Faraj, M.D., Emory University School of Medicine and Henrietta Egleston Hospital for Children, Atlanta, Georgia, USA

Rosa B. Fuksman de Cherjovsky, M.D., Polioclinico Mariano R. Castex-Servicio de Anatomia Patologica San Martin-Pcia de Buenos Aires, Argentina

Ronald E. Gates, M.D., University of Tennessee, Center for Health Sciences, Memphis, Tennessee, USA

M. C. Gelfand, M.D., Georgetown University Hospital, Washington, D.C., USA

Steven L. Giannotta, M.D., University Hospital, University of Michigan Medical Center, Ann Arbor, Michigan, USA

D. Harper, D.O., Ohio State University, College of Medicine, Childrens Hospital, Department of Pediatrics, Columbus, Ohio, USA

*Michael A. W. Hattwick, M.D., Division of Health Examination Statistics, Department of Health, Education and Welfare, Bethesda, Maryland, USA

Ralph Haynes, M.D., Ohio State University, College of Medicine, Childrens Hospital, Department of Pediatrics, Columbus, Ohio, USA

Milo D. Hilty, M.D., Ohio State University, College of Medicine, Childrens Hospital, Department of Pediatrics, Columbus, Ohio, USA

R. Hochberger, D.O., Ohio State University, College of Medicine, Childrens Hospital, Department of Pediatrics, Columbus, Ohio, USA

Jonathon W. Hopkins, M.D., University of Michigan Medical Center, Ann Arbor, Michigan, USA

*Otto Hutzinger, Ph.D., Laboratory of Environmental Chemistry, University of Amsterdam, Amsterdam, The Netherlands

N. Iyngkaran, M.D., Faculty of Medicine and University Hospital, University of Malaya, Kuala Lumpur, Malaysia

J. S. Juggi, M.D., Department of Physiology, Faculty of Medicine and University Hospital, University of Malaya, Kuala Lumpur, Malaysia

Ellen S. Kang, M.D., University of Tennessee, Center for Health Sciences, Memphis, Tennessee, USA

Patrick G. Kealey, M.D., University of Iowa Hospitals and Clinics, Iowa City, Iowa, USA

R. C. Kelsch, M.D., University Hospital, University of Michigan Medical Center, Ann Arbor, Michigan, USA

Benny Kerzner, M.D., Ohio State University, College of Medicine, Childrens Hospital, Columbus, Ohio, USA

Glenn W. Kindt, M.D., University of Michigan Medical Center, Ann Arbor, Michigan, USA

K. Koranyi, M.D., Ohio State University, College of Medicine, Childrens Hospital, Department of Pediatrics, Columbus, Ohio, USA

Mario Kornfeld, M.D., University of New Mexico, School of Medicine and the Veteran's Administration Hospital, Albuquerque, New Mexico, USA

Mary Laltoo, M.Sc., Department of Microbiology, Dalhousie University, Halifax, Nova Scotia, Canada

Spencer H. S. Lee, Ph.D., Department of Microbiology, Dalhousie University, Halifax, Nova Scotia, Canada

Suwat Lertsookprasert, M.D., Khon Kaen Hospital, Khon Kaen, Thailand

Michael Letarte, M.D., Hospital St. Justine, Montreal, Quebec, Canada

Roger M. Loria, M.D., Medical College of Virginia, Richmond, Virginia, USA

Faye A. Luscombe, M.P.H., University of Michigan, Ann Arbor, Michigan, USA

*Gordon E. Madge, M.D., Medical College of Virginia, Richmond, Virginia, USA

James S. Marks, M.D., Center for Disease Control, Viral Disease Division, Bureau of Epidemiology, Atlanta, Georgia, USA

Merle Mason, Ph.D., University of Michigan, Ann Arbor, Michigan, USA

A. James McAdams, M.D., Childrens Hospital Research Foundation, Cincinnati, Ohio, USA

Hugo J. McClung, M.D., Ohio State University, College of Medicine, Childrens Hospital, Department of Pediatrics, Columbus, Ohio, USA

Robert L. McLaurin, M.D., Childrens Hospital Research Foundation, Cincinnati, Ohio, USA

Arnold H. Menezes, M.D., University of Iowa Hospitals and Clinics, Iowa City, Iowa, USA

Arnold S. Monto, M.D., University of Michigan, Ann Arbor, Michigan, USA

David M. Morens, M.D., Center for Disease Control, Viral Disease Division, Bureau of Epidemiology, Atlanta, Georgia, USA

*Claude L. Morin, M.D., M.Sc., Division of Gastroenterology, Hospital St. Justine, Montreal, Quebec, Canada

David B. Nelson, M.D., Center for Disease Control, Viral Disease Division, Bureau of Epidemiology, Atlanta, Georgia, USA

Stephen L. Newman, M.D., Emory University School of Medicine and Henrietta Egleston Hospital for Children, Atlanta, Georgia, USA

Shojiro Okada, M.D., Department of Pediatrics, School of Medicine, Kurume, Japan

Rudolph L. Ozere, M.D., Department of Pediatrics, Dalhousie University and the Izaak Walton Killam Hospital for Children, Halifax, Nova Scotia, Canada

*Jacqueline S. Partin, M.S., Childrens Hospital Research Foundation, Cincinnati, Ohio, USA

*John C. Partin, M.D., Childrens Hospital Research Foundation, Cincinnati, Ohio, USA

*J. Dennis Pollack, Ph.D., Ohio State University and The Children's Hospital Research Foundation, Columbus, Ohio, USA

K. Prathap, M.D., Faculty of Medicine and University Hospital, University of Malaya, Kuala Lumpur, Malaysia

C. Proks, M.D., Department of Pathology, Faculty Hospital, Hradec, Kravlove, Czechoslovakia

Ijaz A. Qureshi, Ph.D., Hospital St. Justine, Montreal, Quebec, Canada

Charles B. Reiner, M.D., Ohio State University, College of Medicine, Childrens Hospital, Columbus, Ohio, USA

Kenneth W. Renton, Ph.D., Department of Pharmacology, Dalhousie University, Halifax, Nova Scotia, Canada

Judith W. Rittenhouse, Ph.D., Department of Biological Chemistry, University of Michigan, Ann Arbor, Michigan, USA

R. Roberts, M.D., Ohio State University, College of Medicine, Children's Hospital, Department of Pediatrics, Columbus, Ohio, USA

Carolyn A. Romshe, M.D., Ohio State University, College of Medicine, Columbus Childrens Hospital, Columbus, Ohio, USA

N. M. Rosenberg, D.O., University of Michigan Medical Center, Ann Arbor, Michigan, USA

Kenneth R. Rozee, Ph.D., Department of Microbiology, Dalhousie University and the Victoria General Hospital, Halifax, Nova Scotia, Canada

*Frederick L. Ruben, M.D., Infectious Disease Unit, Montefiore Hospital, Pittsburgh, Pennsylvania, USA

*Stephen Safe, Ph.D., Department of Chemistry, University of Guelph, Guelph, Ontario, Canada

Rona Beth Sayetta, M.S., Division of Health Examination Statistics, Department of Health, Education and Welfare, Bethesda, Maryland, USA

Lawrence Schonberger, M.D., Center for Disease Control, Viral Disease Division, Bureau of Epidemiology, Atlanta, Georgia, USA

*William K. Schubert, M.D., Childrens Hospital Research Foundation, University of Cincinnati, Cincinnati, Ohio, USA

Earl S. Sherard, Jr., M.D., Ohio State University, College of Medicine, Childrens Hospital, Colulmbus, Ohio, USA

Arnold Silverman, M.D., University of Colorado Medical Center and Denver General Hospital, Denver, Colorado, USA

Poonsiri Sinavatana, M.D., Khon Kaen Hospital, Khon Kaen, Thailand

Clive C. Solomons, Ph.D., University of Colorado Medical Center and Denver General Hospital, Denver, Colorado, USA

John Z. Sullivan-Bolyai, M.D., M.P.H., Center for Disease Control, Bureau of Epidemiology, Atlanta, Georgia, USA

Dugald A. Taylor, Ph.D., Department of Pathology, Dalhousie University, Halifax, Nova Scotia, Canada

*M. Michael Thaler, M.D., School of Medicine, University of California, San Francisco, California, USA

P. Tokarski, M.D., Ohio State University, Childrens Hospital, Columbus, Ohio, USA

Donald B. Tower, M.D., Ph.D., National Institute of Neurological and Communicative Disorders and Stroke, National Institute of Health, Bethesda, Maryland, USA

R. P. Tucker, M.D., University Hospital, University of Michigan Medical Center, Ann Arbor, Michigan, USA

Michel Weber, M.D., Division of Gastroenterology, Hospital St. Justine, Montreal, Quebec, Canada

R. Weeks, Ph.D., University Hospital, University of Michigan Medical Center, Ann Arbor, Michigan, USA

J. F. Winchester, M.B., Department of Pediatrics, Georgetown University Hospital, Washington, D.C., USA

Toru Yamada, M.D., University of Iowa Hospitals and Clinics, Iowa City, Iowa, USA

Masashi Yamamoto, M.D., Department of Pediatrics, School of Medicine, Kurume, Japan

Fumio Yamashita, M.D., Department of Pediatrics, School of Medicine, Kurume, Japan

Ichiro Yoshida, M.D., Department of Pediatrics, School of Medicine, Kurume, Japan

Makoto Yoshino, M.D., Department of Pediatrics, School of Medicine, Kurume, Japan

SECTION   I

EPIDEMIOLOGY AND ETIOLOGY

THE INCIDENCE AND ETIOLOGY OF REYE'S SYNDROME
IN EASTERN CANADA

J.F.S. Crocker, M.D. and R.L. Ozere, M.D.

In 1963, Dr. Douglas Reye reported the clinical
and pathological features of 21 children admitted to
the Royal Alexandra Hospital for Children from New South
Wales between March 1951 and March 1962.(1). These children appeared to have had an illness which he and his
colleagues believed represented a distinct clinical pathological entity and referred to it as fatty degeneration of the viscera of unknown cause. The outstanding
clinical features were profoundly disturbed consciousness, fever, convulsions, vomiting, disturbed respiratory rhythm, altered muscle tone, and altered reflexes.
The onset was associated with cough, rhinorrhea, sore
throat or earache. There was often hypoglycemia and a
low cerebral spinal fluid (CSF) glucose, serum glutamic
oxalaic acid (SGOT) and serum glutamic pyruvic transaminase (SGPT) levels were increased in each of the 7
patients in whom they were measured. Seventeen of the
children died and, at necropsy, remarkably uniform pathological changes were found. To the unaided, these
were expressed as cerebral swelling, a slightly enlarged firm and uniformly bright yellow liver, and with
pallor and slight widening of the renal cortex.

Numerous reports of other cases followed from
Great Britain, New Zealand, Czechoslovakia, South Afri-
ca, Belgium, United States, Thailand,Argentina, Japan
and Canada. Interestingly, recent correspondence from
Dr. D.M.O. Becroft, New Zealand, shows that although
they had an "epidemic" of Reye's syndromes in the late
50's and early 60's, the disease has disappeared with-

in the past seven years (2). The appearance of Reye's
syndrome as well as its disappearance may be a great
epidemiological clue if one were able to scrutinize the
possible changes in New Zealand life in this time. The
estimated incidence of Reye's syndrome by the Center
for Disease Control (CDC) between December 15 and June
30, 1974 was 0.58:100,000 children (below 18 years of
age).(3). The dates showing the highest incidence in
this period also showed a high incidence of Influenza B.
Our interest in Reye's syndrome began seven years ago,
when a clustering of cases occurred in one area of the
Maritime Provinces of Canada (Figure 1) over a short

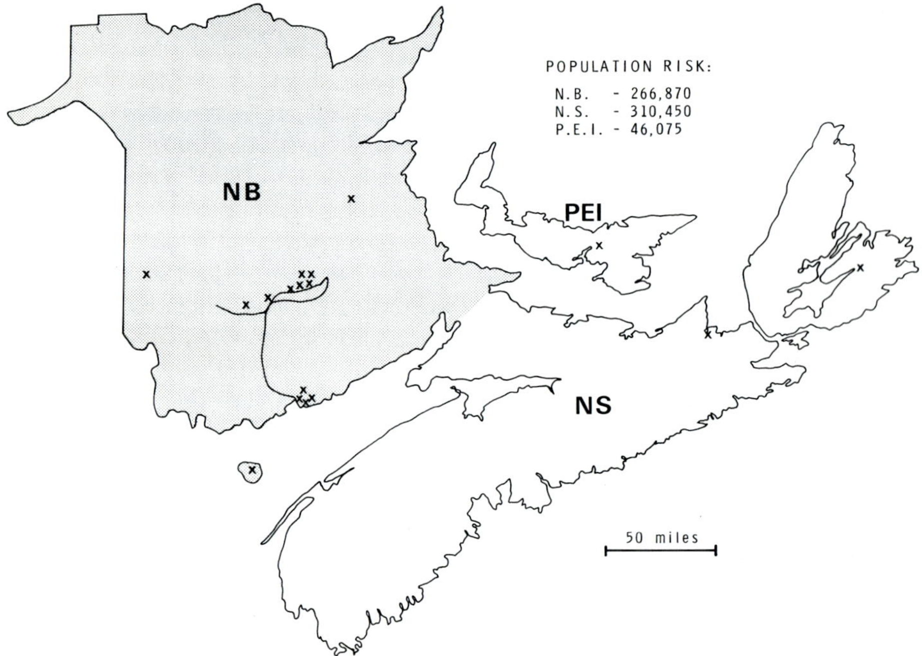

Fig.1. Incidence of Reye's syndrome in Canada's
Maritime Provinces. Each case is indicated by an X.
Shaded area indicates the province conducting yearly
aerial spray programs. *(Chemosphere 7-565-1978)*.

interval period, giving an incidence figure one and
one-half times the incidence reported by CDC.

    Efforts at establishing an etiological basis for
Reye's syndrome have been recently centered around pro-

ponents of three basic features: (1) an intrinsic or extrinsic toxin (2) having a priming effect (to react abnormally to specific groups of viruses, particularly Influenza A and B, varicella and, less commonly, respiratory viral infections, mumps, etc.) (3) on a susceptible host.

Of potential importance in considering a virustoxin interaction hypothesis for the etiology of Reye's syndrome was the work of Friend and Trainer. These workers showed that, if young mallard ducks were pre-exposed to polychlorinated biphenyl (PCB's) and then to duck hepatitis virus, they developed a fatty visceromegaly and a non-specific encephalopathy (4). Our cases of Reye's syndrome lived contiguous to a large forest spray program, where several millions of acres of forest land were sprayed at least once a year for twenty-five years with a pesticide formulation. We were aware that children were particularly prone to pesticide toxicity (5) and we were always impressed that the encephalopathic component of Reye's syndrome was more important than the liver disease, the mortality from the disease being due to the cerebral disfunction.

Red cell (AChE) and plasma cholinesterase (PChE) may be depressed following exposure to organocarbomate and organophosphate pesticides, and these enzymes are related structurally to the cholinesterases of the functionary neuron (6). This led us to study cholinesterase levels in children with Reye's syndrome by the pH stat radiometer method (7). Table 1 reviews this data and illustrates the decreased plasma and red cell changes in cholinesterase. This may reflect only contact with an agent capable of inducing depression and not necessarily play any patho-physiological role in the disease itself. Plasma cholinesterase is also known to be depressed with liver cell damage and thus depressed levels may only reflect the degree of metabolic liver change. Our results are different from those of Pollack (8) and may reflect a different patient population.

Safe and Hutzinger will outline later in this book our attempts to isolate environmental chemicals from tissue of cases of Reye's syndrome. Aflatoxin assays on four of our cases were performed through the coöperation

TABLE 1.

REYE'S SYNDROME CASES IN EASTERN CANADA:

RED CELL AND PLASMA CHOLINESTERASE

Pt. Age	Stage	PChE	AChE
7	3	0.94 (2.26* ± 0.13)**	7.0 (9.5* ± 0.13)**
6	3	1.78 (2.26 ± 0.13)	9.2 (9.5 ± 0.13)
11	3	1.90 (2.10 ± 0.17)	11.8 (9.5 ± 0.11)
11	3	1.24 (2.10 ± 0.17)	6.6 (9.5 ± 0.11)
4	2	1.12 (2.50 ± 0.13)	8.8 (9.5 ± 0.13)
7	4	1.15 (2.26 ± 0.13)	0 (9.5 ± 0.13)
12	4	0.64 (2.10 ± 0.17)	6.3 (9.5 ± 0.11)
6	4	1.11 (2.26 ± 0.13)	5.9 (9.5 ± 0.13)
12	4	1.56 (2.10 ± 0.17)	12.3 (9.5 ± 0.11)
6	4	0.26 (2.50 ± 0.13)	9.6 (9.5 ± 0.13)
4	4	1.12 (2.5 ± 0.13)	7.6 (9.5 ± 0.13)
14	4	1.00 (2.3 ± 0.15)	8.2 (10.0 ± 0.15)

*Mean   **Standard error

PChE and AChE values from Eastern Canada indicate that only one out of twelve plasma cholinesterase levels were normal, while eight out of twelve red cell cholinesterase levels were depressed. Higher than normal values of red cell cholinesterase can be seen in cases where "rebounding" of the enzyme activity occurs after previous depression.

of Dr. J. Harwig,Health Protection Branch, Health and Welfare,Canada. Aflatoxin was not detected in the tissues of these patients.

We have also attempted to develop an animal model of Reye's syndrome to test the hypothesis that it is biologically possible for chemicals to alter the response of a human host to viral infections which are normally relatively benign.

Swiss white mice (Biobreeding,Ottawa) from an outbred strain (ICR) were mated in our laboratories and allowed to deliver their young. Dermal exposure of the chemical was begun at two hours of age, to allow the usual attrition of runts in the litters. Chemicals were applied to a standard area of the abdomen, and dosages were based on known medium lethal dose,LD50 (9) and our own trials of toxic dermal dosage. The painting concentrations chosen were well below the lethal range. All groups of mice were studied simultaneously.

The following chemicals in a corn oil base were applied: (1) corn oil (2) pure DDT (3) commercial fenitrothion (which contains the emulsifiers and the solvent) (4) DDT plus the commercial fenitrothion (5) DDT plus 3.8 percent pure fenitrothion (equivalent to DDT plus commercial fenitrothion without emulsifiers and solvent) and (6) emulsifiers and solvent. The emulsifiers used were Toximul MP8 (Chas.Tennant & Co. of Canada Ltd., Toronto, Ontario 1972 Lot), Atlox 3409 (Atlas Chemical Industry Ltd.,Brantford, Ontario), and the solvent was Aerotex 3470,(Texaco of Canada.)

Contact with chemical was daily from second day of life to day 12. The virus EMC (encephalomyocarditis) was injected on day fourteen of life.

The encephalomyocarditis virus (EMC) used was supplied as primary mouse-kidney cell yield by the National Institute for Medical Research, London. Stock virus titer was between 10^6 and 10^7 medium tissue culture infections doses (TCID$_{50}$) per milliliter. The dose of virus innoculated subcutaneously was 0.05 ml of 0.5 $\log_{10}$ dilutions of this virus pool in phosphate buffered saline.

The initially tested pesticides in our experiments consisted of a commercial formulation of insecticides plus solvents and emulsifiers. The question then arose as to whether these carriers of the insecticide could be responsible for the viral chemical interaction observed. The results of these experiments are shown graphically in Figure 2, indicating that emulsifying agents were responsible for altering the host response to a sublethal dose of virus.

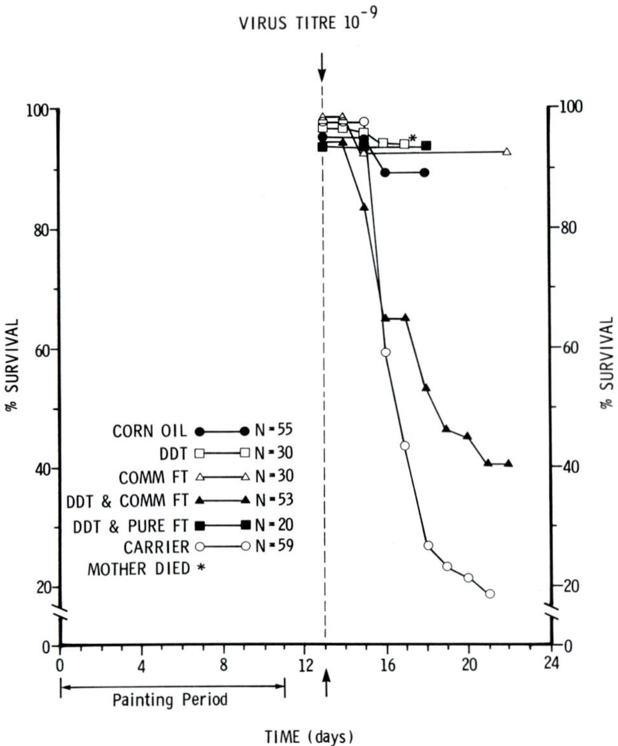

Fig.2. Survival curves of newborn mice. Zero time on abscissa is 24 hours of age. Painting period is contact exposure to chemical and combinations. The ordinate on the left side of each graph is the percentage of animals alive at 24 hours of age. The ordinate on the right side of each graph is the percentage of animals alive after virus exposure. The median dose of virus dilution (10^{-9}) of a stock containing 10^6 to 10^7 TCID/ml was chosen for calculation of confidence limits.

The estimates of the probabilities of survival were calculated by the Kaplan and Meier (10) (1958) "product-limit" method. Approximate standard errors and 95% confidence limits were then determined for each total group at the time of the viral injections (day 13) and for each subgroup receiving the 10^{-9} dilution of stock virus 6 days later (day 19).

Young mice were observed for symptoms, although we studied mainly the lethality of the viral/chemical interaction. Most deaths occurred within five days after viral exposure in animals exposed to a mixture of solvent and emulsifier and then injected with EMC virus.

Pathological evaluation of the brain by light microscopy showed no gross morphological changes, such as inflammatory reaction or necrotic areas. The liver morphology also showed no signs of inflammatory reaction or areas of gross cellular distortion. Histological evaluation was done for the most part on animals that survived the experiment, since autolysis distorted the results in the animals dying before fresh tissue could be obtained. Frozen sections stained for lipids (oil-red-O) varied from normal to a fine fat-droplet dispersion as previously noted (11).

This animal work, we felt, illustrated that certain insecticide carriers may have effect on its young animals' ability to respond to a benign dose of virus.

The emulsifying agents used in pesticide formulations may be used in immense quantities in other applications besides forest spray operations. However, forest spray programs may be unique, in that they use millions of gallons of formulations in a short period of time.

The animal experiments utilized 45,000 young mice over a three-year period and required the calculation of LD_{50}'s for each chemical tested, and individual control for each batch of virus. This led to the development of *in vitro* techniques which are less costly and more sensitive. Rozee et al and Taylor et al later in this book outline their work in this area with both monolayer cultures and organ culture of human and animal origin.

Attempts to reproduce our work in mice in a larger animal led us to look at the Hormel Pigmee Pig as a model. Exposing two-week-old piglets by tube feeding to the chemicals, and later injecting the animals with pig polio virus, showed a trend to increased incidence of paralysis and death in the emulsifier-exposed group(12). (Figure 3). Unfortunately, large numbers were not available in this set of experiments to give us as clear-cut a conclusion as we would like.

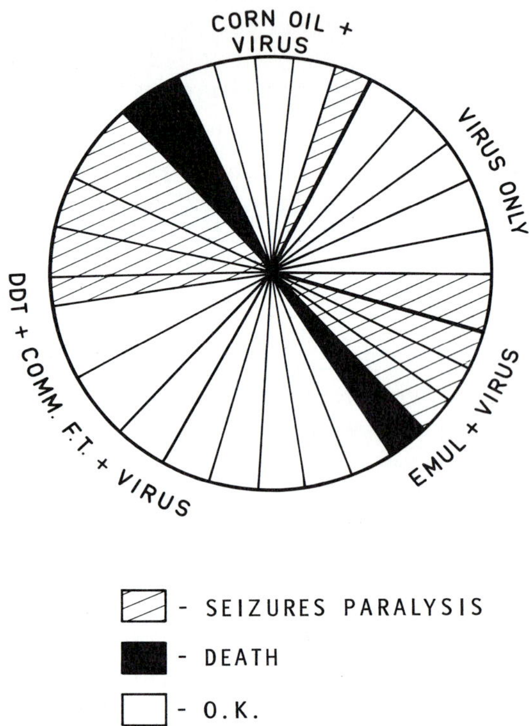

Fig.3. A graphic representation of an experiment in which Hormel piglets were tube fed chemicals from the second day of life to the thirteenth day of life (7 feedings in all). Virus was administered on day 15 of life.(*Chemosphere 7- 549-1978*).

The theory that Reye's syndrome is a reaction to environmental toxins and a virus in a susceptible host now links into epidemiological work. The difficulties in working out such theories is that it is unlikely to

be a single toxin or virus, and thus the research is
bound to be very expensive. The chemical structures capable of interacting with certain virus, the structure
and nature of the viruses involved, and the intracellular changes that allow such an interaction to occur,
will be the thrust of much future work. It is only at-
tainable with coöperative and collaborative work by
many laboratories. As researchers and/or physicians,we
work on probabilities and often our concepts change
drastically as these probabilities change. There is a
great probability that, with international research collaboration and interest by governments to seek an answer to Reye's syndrome, the etiology and control could
be found. The answer, however, may not be a pleasant
one for our modern society.

ACKNOWLEDGEMENT

The authors wish to express their thanks to the
physicians who supplied clinical samples for this work,
which is supported by Grants from the Medical Research
Council of Canada, and The Province of New Brunswick,
Canada.

REFERENCES

1. Reye,R.D.K., Morgan,G., and Baral,J. 1963. Enceph-
    alopathy and Fatty Degeneration of the Viscera: a
    Disease Entity in Childhood. *Lancet ii:*749.

2. Becroft, D.M.O. Personal communication.

3. Corey,L.R.J.,Rubin,R.J.,Hattwick,M.A.W.,Noble,G.R.
    and Cassidy,E. 1976. A Nationwide Outbreak of Reye
    Syndrome.*Am. J. Med. 61:*615-625.

4. Friend,M.,Trainor,D.O. 1970. Polychlorinated bi-
    phenyl:Interaction with Duck Hepatitis Virus. *Sci-
    ence 1970,* 1314.

5. Taylor,W.J.R.,Mason,H.M. 1971. Pesticide Poisoning
    in Chickens. *Drug Therapy (November).*

6. Herz,F., Kaplan,E. 1973. A Review: Human Erytrocyte
    Acetylcholinesterase. *Pediat.Res.7:*204-214.

7. Ecobichon,D.J.,Stephens,D.S. 1975. Perinatal De-
    velopment of Human Blood Esterases.*Clin.Phar.and
    Ther. 1*:41-47.

8. Pollack,J.D.,Hughes,J.H.,Hamparian,V.V.,Burech,D.
    1978. An Interaction of Chemicals and Viruses and
    Their Role in Reye's Syndrome.*Chemosphere 7*:551.

9. Sunshine,I. 1969. Physical,Toxicological and Ana-
    lytical Data. *Chemical Rubber Co.,Cleveland,Ohio.*

10. Kaplan,E.L., Meier,P. 1958. *J.Am.Stat.Assoc.53*:457.

11. Crocker,J.F.S.,Rozee,K.R.,Ozere,R.L.,Digout,S.C.,
    Hutzinger,O. 1974. Insecticide and Viral Inter-
    action as a Cause of Fatty Visceral Changes and
    Encephalopathy in the Mouse. *Lancet (July 6)*:22-24.

12. Crocker,J.,Digout,S.,Bagnell,P.,Lee,S.,Rozee,K.,
    Safe,S. 1978. Viral Interaction with Pesticide
    Emulsifiers *in vivo*.*Chemosphere 7*:549.

TIME TRENDS OF REYE'S SYNDROME
BASED ON NATIONAL STATISTICS

Michael A. W. Hattwick, M. D.
and Rona Beth Sayetta, M. S.

INTRODUCTION

The fascinating disease to which this conference
is devoted, Reye's syndrome, probably has a multiple
etiology. This paper reviews what has been learned so
far of its associations with antecedent viral-like conditions and with demographic and environmental variables.
It then describes national time trends in disease mortality due to Reye's syndrome.

Statistics on Reye's syndrome have been difficult
to collect and classify by existing data system mechanisms at the national level, other than the special
disease surveillance activities conducted by the Center
for Disease Control (CDC) in Atlanta, Georgia. Because
this syndrome did not receive widespread attention until
Reye (1), Johnson (2), and others (3) described it in
1963, there is as yet no consensus of opinion about the
importance of modifying the International Classification
of Diseases in order to permit precise medical coding
of this particular clinicopathologic entity. In addition, because Reye's syndrome involves more than one
organ system (consisting of an acute encephalopathy
coupled with fatty degeneration of the liver and other
viscera), there is no agreed-upon rubric in ICDA-8 that
has been used exclusively to encode medical or cause-
of-death data for this disease. As a result, this paper
highlights time trends in the occurrence of mortality
from Reye's syndrome on the basis of the best national
data that are available at the present time from the

13

National Center for Health Statistics. These data reflect total U.S. deaths due to Reye's syndrome and to certain other or unspecified diseases of brain, but as can be shown, cases of Reye's may in fact comprise the bulk of the figures.

Time Trends in CDC Data and Epidemiological Studies. Table 1 displays CDC data on the total cases of Reye's syndrome reported in the United States by year from 1962 to 1978. Influenza outbreaks are shown for the same period of time. The strong relationship seen between these two data sets suggest the need for further evaluation of influenza B and other viruses as necessary antecedent conditions in the causation of Reye's syndrome.

The largest outbreak of Reye's syndrome yet recognized occurred in the United States in 1974. During this epidemic, the Bureau of Epidemiology at the Center for Disease Control conducted two careful studies to ascertain the incidence of Reye's syndrome and its relationship to influenza B and other possible etiologies. The first study was a randomized point-prevalence survey of 1,041 school children in Kalamazoo County, Michigan, who experienced simultaneous outbreaks of influenza B and Reye's syndrome in 1974 (4). The second study describes the nationwide epidemic of Reye's syndrome which occurred between February and March 1974 and was found epidemiologically to be associated with a widespread influenza B outbreak (5). The data for this paper were gathered prospectively through a nationwide surveillance system for Reye's syndrome initiated by the CDC in 1973. Some very interesting findings have emerged from these studies about the disease.

Figure 1 (5) shows the number of cases of Reye's syndrome that were reported for the total United States by week from December 15, 1976 to June 30, 1974. The cases clearly cluster in February and March 1974 during the peak of the influenza epidemic which also occurred in February and March. Figure 2 bears out this pattern as seen in the distribution of reported Reye's cases by their date of hospital admission. Figure 2 also cate-

TABLE 1.   Reported Cases of Reye's Syndrome and Influenza Epidemics,
                          United States, 1962-1978

Jan.-Mar. of Calendar Year	Reye's Cases Reported [1]	Influenza Epidemics by Severity [2]
1962	16	Minor B, No A
1963	NR	No B, Major A
1964	NR	No B, No A
1965	NR	No B, Minor A
1966	NR	No B, Moderate A
1967	11	Minor B, No A
1968	17	Minor B, Major A
1969	41	Major B, Major A
1970	13	No B, Moderate A
1971	83	Major B, No A
1972	30	No B, Moderate A
1973	32	Minor B, Moderate A
1974	379	Major B, No A
1975	NR	No B, No A
1976	NR	No B, Moderate A
1977	259	Major B, No A
1978	100	No B, Major A

NR = Not Reported to CDC

Sources: 1) Corey [5] and U.S. Department of Health, Education and
             Welfare, Public Health Service, Center for Disease
             Control, Atlanta, Georgia (Unpublished data).

          2) CDC Influenza-Respiratory Disease Surveillance Reports, various
             publication dates [7], and U.S. Department of Health, Education
             and Welfare, Public Health Service, Center for Disease Control,
             Immunization Division, Bureau of State Services, Atlanta,
             Georgia (Unpublished data).

gorizes cases by type of antecedent illness: upper respiratory illness, confirmed influenza B, varicella, or
gastrointestinal illness.

    Antecedent viral-like illnesses were noted in most
cases of Reye's syndrome for whom specimen cultures for
viral isolation or serologic tests were done (5).
Influenza B or varicella were the major agents found
(Fig. 2). A few patients were found to have double
viral infections (5). As Figure 3 shows, an upper respiratory infection was the most frequent antecedent

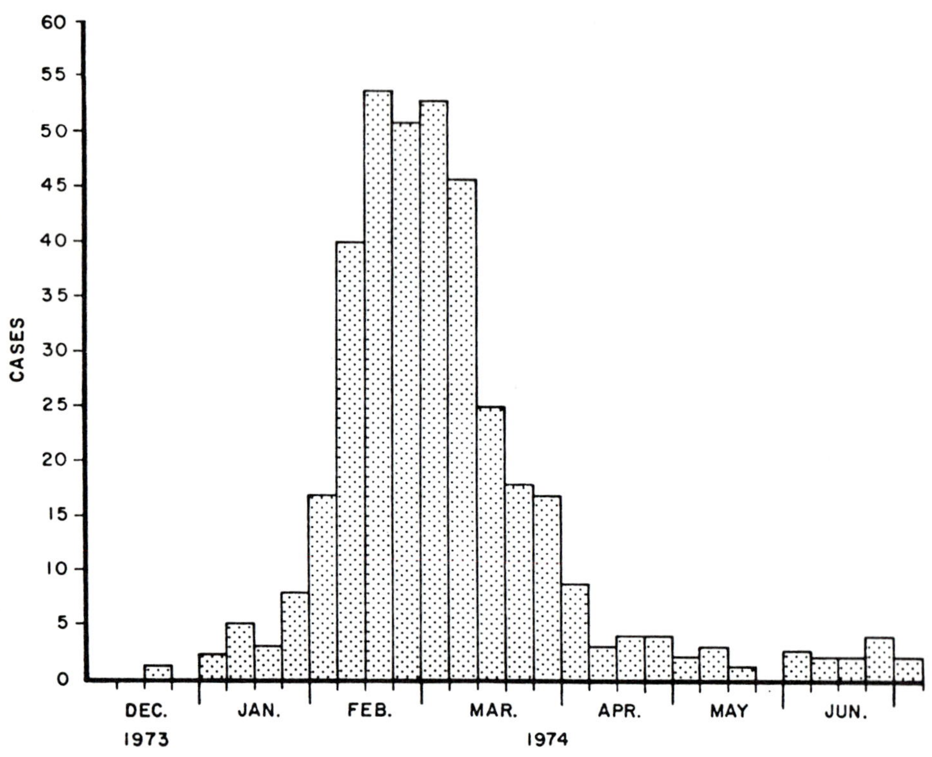

Source: Corey [5]

condition among Reye's patients who died. Of those
with confirmed viral infections, influenza B and varicella prodromes occurred in significant numbers of
cases. A few patients' courses of illness were characterized by gastrointestinal prodromes such as cramps,
diarrhea, nausea and vomiting, possibly ascribable to
an enterovirus (5). The same patterns were found in
the data derived from Reye's syndrome patients who
were hospitalized for their disease (Fig. 2). Temporal
and geographic clustering of Reye's cases did not occur
for patients with antecedent viral infections other than
the four types just mentioned; and the sporadic cases
of Reye's tended to be associated with varicella and
other viral agents in younger children, rather than
with the influenza B virus (5).

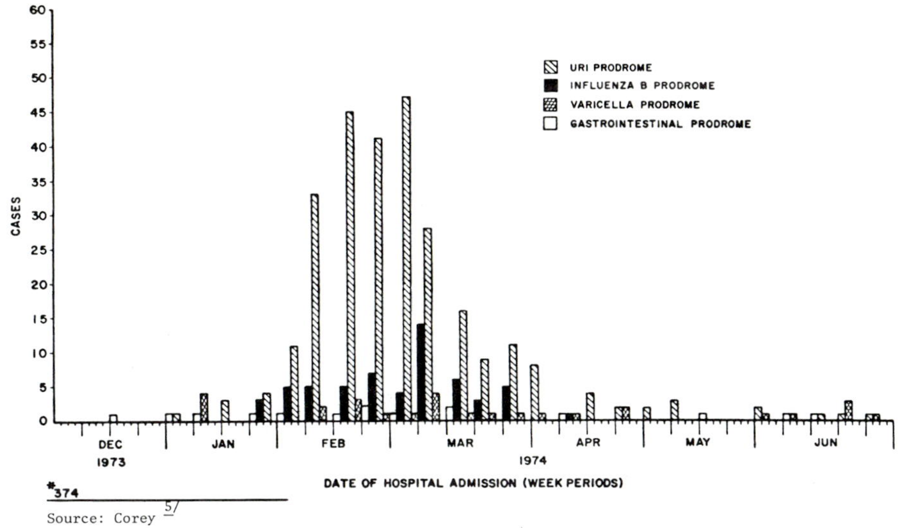

*374

Source: Corey [5]

Fig. 3 REYE'S SYNDROME CASES* BY AGE, UNITED STATES, DECEMBER 15, 1973 - JUNE 30, 1974

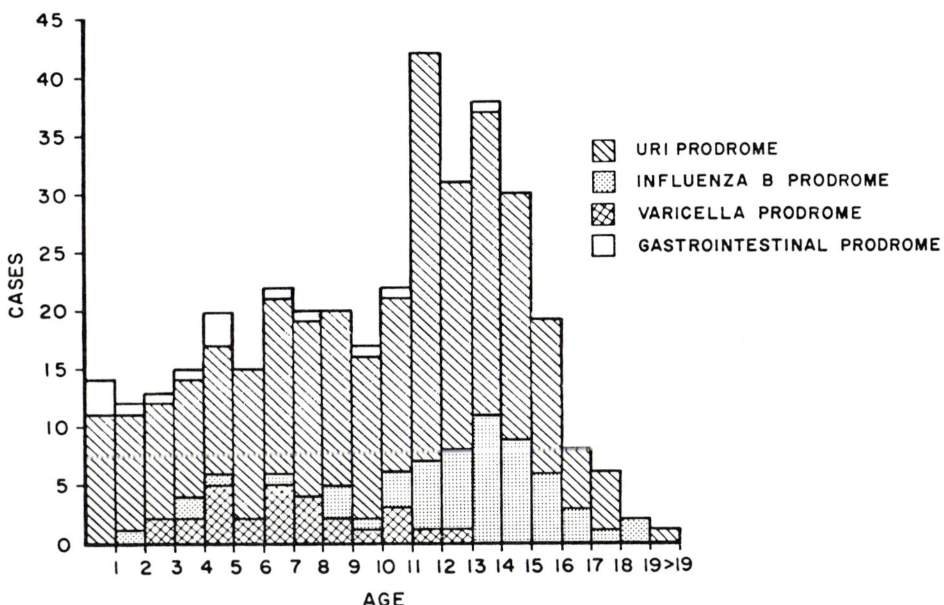

Source: Corey [5]

Recent vaccinations were not found to be related to development of the syndrome. In fact, no Reye's patient had a history of recent influenza vaccination (5).

Reye's syndrome following influenza has a predilection for older children and young adolescents, in contrast to the illness following varicella, where children 10 or under are most often affected. Figure 3 above shows a distribution of cases by age during the epidemic in the winter of 1974 (5). Peak incidences of the disease occurred in ages 11 to 14, accounting for 37% of all patients. The median age for all Reye's syndrome patients was 11, with only 4% of the cases occurring in those over age 16. Ages ranged from 3 months to 28 years, although there was only a single outlying patient above age 18. Note the different age distribution for influenza- and varicella-associated cases.

The 379 Reye's syndrome deaths reported in the epidemic were nearly evenly distributed between males and females (47% and 53%, respectively). Table 2 shows that the overall case fatality rate for both sexes was 41% (5). There were no statistical differences among the case fatality rates computed for specific age groups, or by type of prodrome (5).

Table 2

Mortality Data on Reye's Syndrome Patients
United States, 1974

	Survived	Died	Total
Male	107 (60%)	72 (40%)	179 (47%)
Female	115 (58%)	85 (42%)	200 (53%)
Total	222 (59%)	157 (41%)	379

Source: Corey [5]

Data on racial and ethnic affiliation were available for 224 cases in the 1974 epidemic (nearly three-fifths of the reported total). Of these, 95% were white, only 4% were black, and 1% each were American Indian or of Asian extraction (5). This under-represents non-whites, an observation that deserves more extensive evaluation.

The geographic distribution of cases of Reye's syndrome is particularly interesting for the support it lends to two different hypotheses about the etiology of the disease. A clustering of cases was found in rural areas, where Reye's syndrome occurred 3 to 4 times more frequently than in urban areas (Table 3).

Table 3

Distribution of Reye's Syndrome Cases by Home Address
Michigan, New York, Pennsylvania, December 1973 – June 1974

	Rural	Other Urban	Urbanized
Total Population <18	3,096,854	1,175,378	8,659,498
Total White Population <18	3,047,349	1,119,483	7,008,489
No. Cases Reye's Syndrome	56	5	50 (31 suburban)
Cases/100,000 Population <18	1.80	.42	.58
Cases/100,000 White Population <18	1.83	.44	.71

Source: Corey [5]

An additional clustering was found in urbanized areas that are described as "urban fringe" or suburban (4). The incidence rate for Reye's syndrome in urban fringe areas (not shown in this table) was 1.65 times that for central cities (0.81 cases per 100,000 population less than age 18 vs. 0.49 per 100,000, respectively). This predominantly rural-suburban distribution of cases was also found when incidence rates specific for the white population only were calculated (4).

The Kalamazoo, Michigan study (4) indicated that influenza B attack rates for urban and rural locales did not differ, so a higher attack rate of influenza B in rural areas is probably not the explanation for the greater concentration of cases there. It has been proposed that some environmental factor as yet unidentified may be responsible for the urban-rural pattern seen in observed cases.

The other reason for great interest in the geographic distribution of Reye's syndrome is that examination of the state-by-state morbidity due to this disease (Fig.4) reveals a striking correlation with the

Fig. 4   INCIDENCE OF REYE'S SNDROME BY STATE, DEC. 15 - JUNE 30, 1974

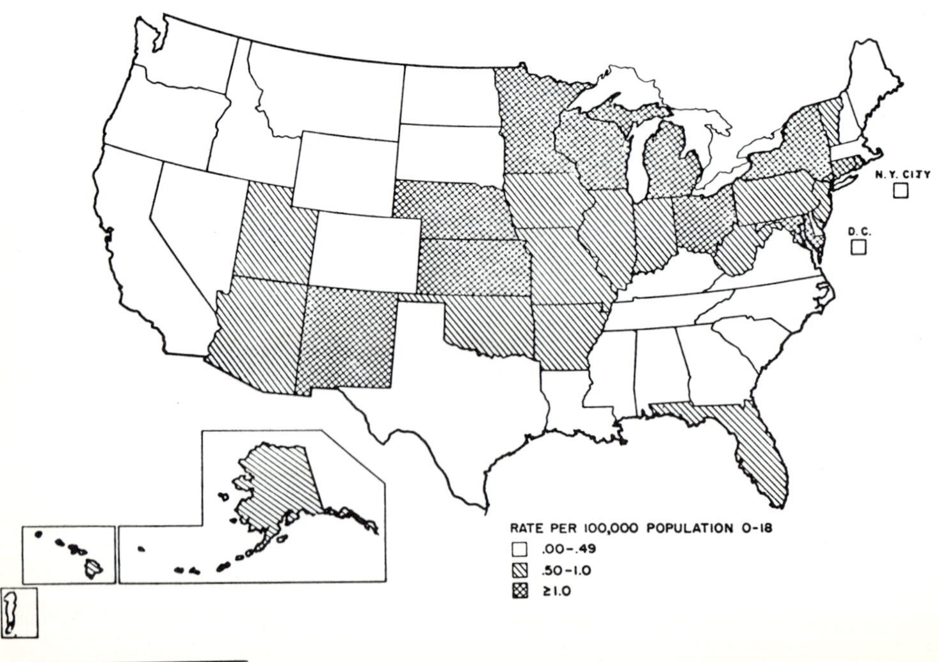

state-by-state incidence of reported influenza B outbreaks in early 1974 (Fig. 5). Influenza B and other
viral-like illnesses have been studied further to ascertain their geographic and temporal relationships to
Reye's syndrome.

Fig. 5   STATES REPORTING INFLUENZA B OUTBREAKS FROM DECEMBER 1, 1973
          TO MARCH 1, 1974

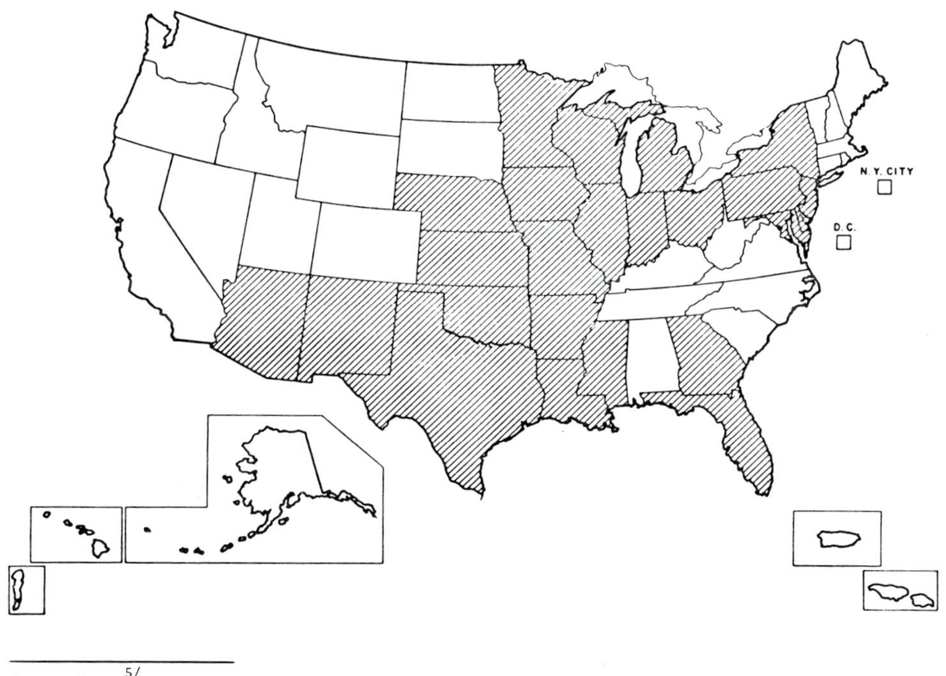

Source: Corey [5/]

A small-area study of the relationships between
data from influenza surveillance activities and cases
of Reye's in Cook County, Illinois, from December 1,
1973 to March 16, 1974, showed a very close correlation
between the two (Fig.6) (5).

Fig. 6 RELATIONSHIP BETWEEN INFLUENZA SURVEILLANCE AND INCIDENCE OF REYE'S SYNDROME, COOK COUNTY ILLINOIS, DECEMBER I — MARCH 16, 1974

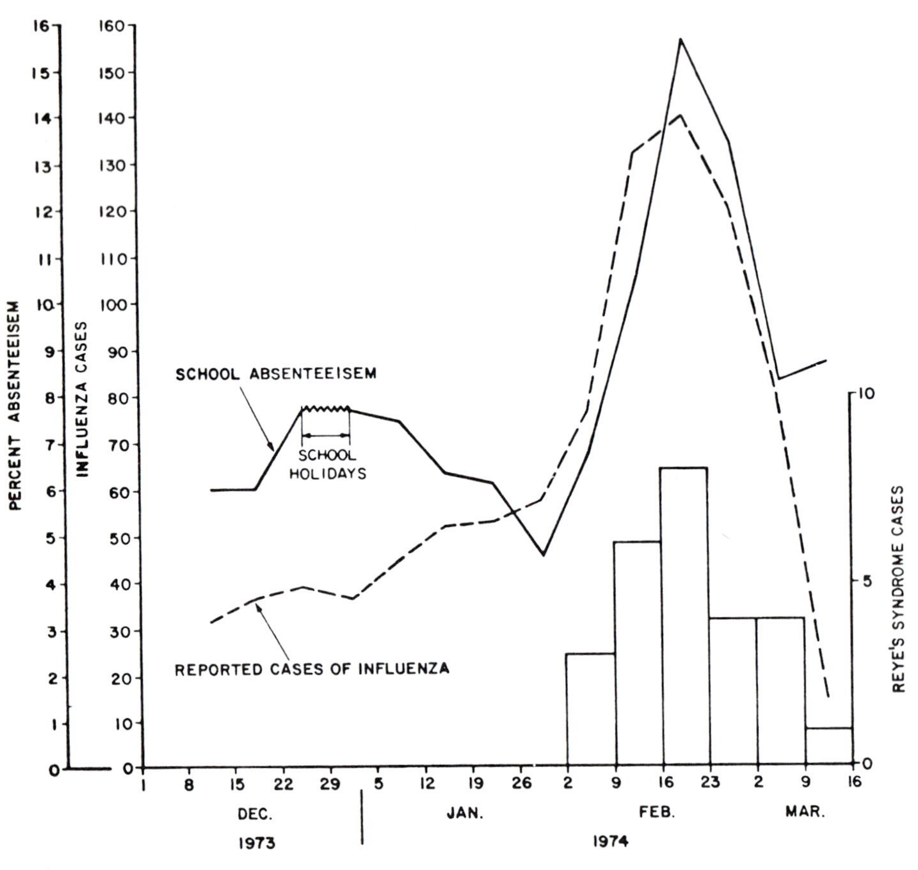

Source: Corey $\underline{5/}$

The curve of Reye's is displaced slightly to the right when superimposed on that for influenza, indicating about a 2-week time lag between the incidence patterns of the two diseases. Broader-based regional studies for the Northeastern, Mid-Atlantic and Midwestern States for the 1974 epidemic period, as well as for the United States as a whole, allow us to segregate the differential effects of influenza A and influenza B. Figure 7

(5) indicates that it is the influenza B strain which shows by far the stronger correlation with Reye's syn-

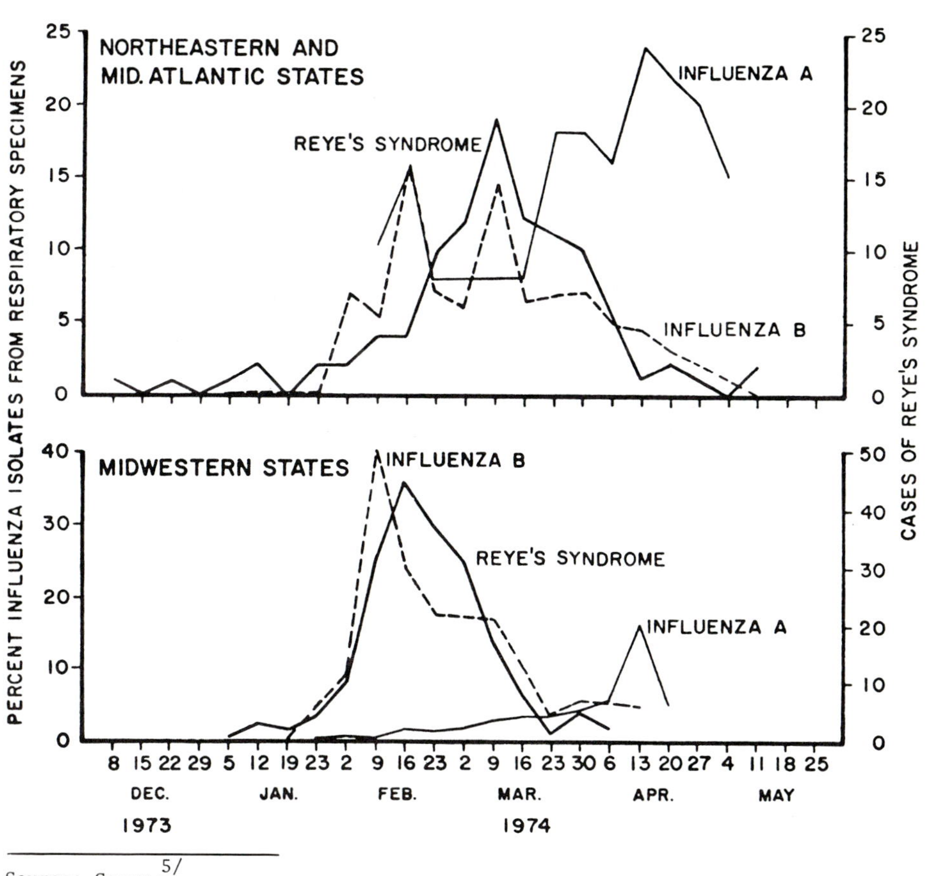

Fig. 9 REPORTED CASES OF REYE'S SYNDROME AND INFLUENZA ISOLATES IN 2 REGIONS, DECEMBER 1, 1973 - MAY 25, 1974

Source: Corey [5/]

drome. A three-week lag between the peak activity of influenza B and the peak incidence of Reye's was noted in these studies (Fig.8). (5).

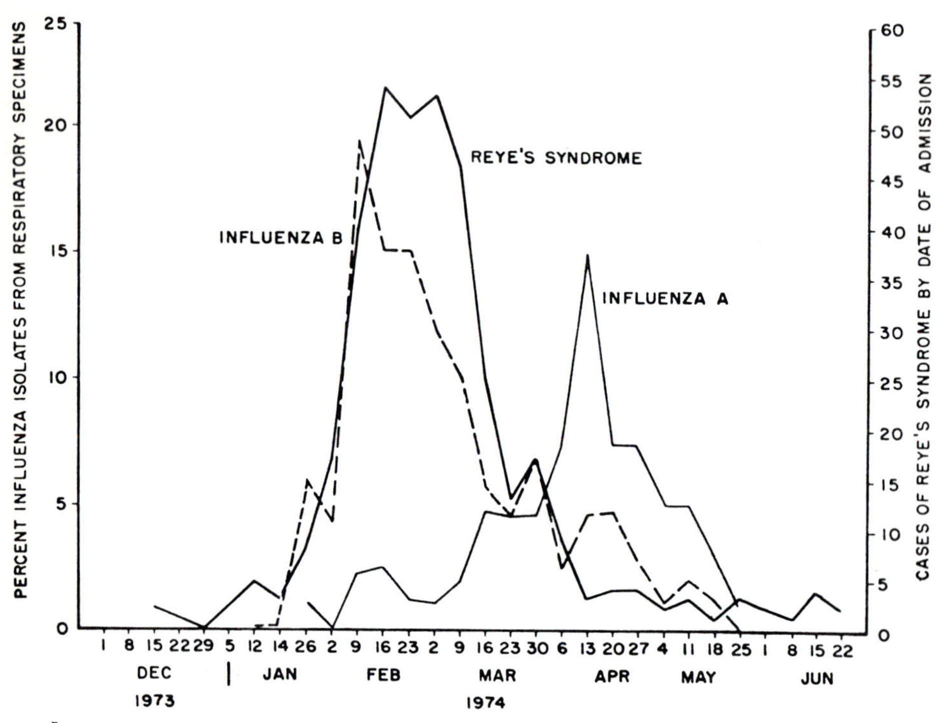

Source: Corey $\underline{5/}$

National Mortality Data from NCHS

The new information available from U.S. national
mortality statistics corroborates the earlier findings
of the Center for Disease Control that have just been
described with respect to: disease incidence; age, sex,
and race patterns of its distribution; and correlation
with outbreaks of influenza B.

Table 4 shows the annual mortality due to ICDA
Code 347.9, a category which includes other and unspecified diseases of brain as well as Reye's syndrome,

TABLE 4. U.S. Total Annual Mortality Due to Other and Unspecified Diseases of Brain (ICDA Code :*347.9) by Age, 1968-1976

Year	Total All Ages [1]	Total Under Age 30 [2]	Under 1 Year	1-4 Years	5-9 Years	10-14 Years	15-19 Years	20-24 Years	25-29 Years	30+ Years
Total, 1968-1976	17,216	6,459	1,665	1,733	927	677	636	453	368	10,757
1968	1,423	542	164	162	63	45	40	35	33	881
1969	1,484	636	179	175	95	54	61	41	31	848
1970	1,654	661	202	164	94	54	70	47	30	993
1971	1,741	710	180	195	104	76	71	44	40	1,031
1972	1,872	704	180	184	100	76	80	52	32	1,168
1973	2,071	760	179	228	122	81	61	45	44	1,311
1974	2,388	908	197	205	147	134	100	67	58	1,480
1975	2,266	791	188	217	113	74	89	62	48	1,475
1976	2,317	747	196	203	89	83	64	60	52	1,570

*The fourth digit was added in the U.S. adaptation of the Eighth Revision of the International Classification of Diseases.

Source: 1) U.S. Department of Health, Education and Welfare, National Center for Health Statistics [6]

2) U.S. Department of Health, Education and Welfare, Public Health Service, Health Resources Administration, National Center for Health Statistics, Division of Vital Statistics, Hyattsville, Maryland (Unpublished data)

by year from 1968 through 1976 (6). Although this is a
very non-specific grouping, the peak incidence of
disease-related deaths among children aged 5 to 19 can
be seen in the epidemic year of 1974. The age distribution for those persons under age 30 who died from
this cause in 1974 peaks in the early childhood years
and trails off by late adolescence, similarly to the
earlier CDC findings. Although the exact death rates
for Reye's or the various other viral encephalopathies
in childhood are not available from current NCHS data,
it can be estimated from the figures in Table 4 above
that, among children aged 5 to 19, about 30% of deaths

in this category may be due to Reye's syndrome during epidemic years.* The mixture of several disease entities in the one category, "Other and unspecified diseases of brain," makes more detailed analysis difficult at present. However, NCHS since 1968 has coded multiple causes of death on computer tape, and it should be possible to examine further the relationships between specified diagnoses, Reye's syndrome among them, using national data.

Table 5 shows sex and race differentials in these mortality statistics (6). The sex distribution for this cause of death among persons under age 30 did not differ markedly in the epidemic year 1974 as compared to the other years. The findings by race category shown in the table again indicate an increase for whites, consistent with earlier data in revealing an excess of whites relative to the incidence in blacks and other groups.

TABLE 5. U.S. Total Annual Mortality Due to Other and Unspecified Diseases of Brain (ICDA Code *347.9) for Persons Under Age 30, by Sex and Race, 1968-1976

Year	Total No. of Deaths	Total Percent		Sex Categories					Race Categories			
				Total No. of Males	Total No. of Females	Percent Males	Percent Females		Total No. of Whites	Total No. of Others	Percent Whites	Percent All Others
Total, 1968-1976	6,459	100.0										
1968	542	100.0		286	256	52.8	47.2		417	125	76.9	23.1
1969	636	100.0		367	269	57.7	42.3		504	132	79.2	20.8
1970	661	100.0		363	298	54.9	45.1		535	126	80.9	19.1
1971	710	100.0		406	324	55.6	44.4		586	144	80.3	19.7
1972	704	100.0		362	342	51.4	48.6		566	138	80.4	19.6
1973	760	100.0		415	345	54.6	45.4		599	161	78.8	21.2
1974	908	100.0		505	403	55.6	44.4		717	191	79.0	21.0
1975	791	100.0		460	331	58.2	41.8		649	142	82.0	18.0
1976	747	100.0		417	330	55.8	44.2		597	150	79.9	20.1

*The fourth digit was added in the U.S. adaptation of the Eighth Revision of the International Classification of Diseases.

Source: U.S. Department of Health, Education and Welfare, Public Health Service, Health Resources Administration, National Center for Health Statistics, Division of Vital Statistics, Hyattsville, Maryland (Unpublished data).

* Computed as follows: the number of excess deaths over the 1973-1975 average, expressed as a percentage of actual deaths in 1974.

TABLE 6. Frequency and Percentage Distributions of Total U.S. Monthly Mortality Due to Other and Unspecified Diseases of Brain (ICDA Code *347.9), 1968–1976

Year	Total[1)	Jan	Feb	Mar	Apr	May	June	July	Aug	Sept	Oct	Nov	Dec
		Total U.S. Deaths due to code 347.9											
1968	1,423	137	111	110	113	131	99	109	112	116	113	133	139
1969	1,484	131	125	118	126	137	105	140	123	124	127	105	123
1970	1,654	147	130	117	117	120	137	141	138	160	173	142	132
1971	1,741	167	129	168	138	132	151	140	132	166	146	130	142
1972	1,872	206	160	152	136	142	150	154	160	136	158	156	162
1973	2,071	194	170	161	160	175	167	194	159	188	173	151	179
1974	2,388	204	238	215	203	186	185	210	188	184	198	172	205
1975	2,266	210	195	175	165	208	150	201	187	201	189	191	194
1976	2,317	184	201	213	216	192	168	169	177	158	194	206	239
		Percent of Total U.S. Deaths due to Code 347.9											
1968	100.0	9.6	7.8	7.7	7.9	9.2	7.0	7.7	7.9	8.2	7.9	9.3	9.8
1969	100.0	8.8	8.4	8.0	8.5	9.2	7.1	9.4	8.3	8.4	8.6	7.1	8.3
1970	100.0	8.9	7.9	7.1	7.1	7.3	8.3	8.5	8.3	9.7	10.5	8.6	8.0
1971	100.0	9.6	7.4	9.6	7.9	7.6	8.7	8.0	7.6	9.5	8.4	7.5	8.2
1972	100.0	11.0	8.5	8.1	7.3	7.6	8.0	8.2	8.5	7.3	8.4	8.3	8.7
1973	100.0	9.4	8.2	7.8	7.7	8.5	8.1	9.4	7.7	9.1	8.4	7.3	8.6
1974	100.0	8.5	10.0	9.0	8.5	7.8	7.7	8.8	7.9	7.7	8.3	7.2	8.6
1975	100.0	9.3	8.6	7.7	7.3	9.2	6.6	8.9	8.3	8.9	8.3	8.4	8.6
1976	100.0	7.9	8.7	9.2	9.3	8.3	7.3	7.3	7.6	6.8	8.4	8.9	10.3

*The fourth digit was added in the U.S. adaptation of the Eighth Revision of the International Classification of Diseases.

Sources: 1) U.S. Department of Health, Education and Welfare, National Center for Health Statistics [6/]

2) U.S. Department of Health, Education and Welfare, Public Health Service, Health Resources Administration, National Center for Health Statistics, Division of Vital Statistics, Hyattsville, Maryland (Unpublished data).

Table 6 provides a more detailed look at the distribution of U.S. mortality from other and unspecified diseases of brain, looking at total deaths by month from 1968 to 1976. Excess deaths during the epidemic months in the first half of 1974 stand out prominently and give weight to the contention that a major proportion of the deaths from this cause in this time period were due to Reye's syndrome. Figure 9 graphs these U.S. total deaths by month (6) against the weekly incidence of influenza B for the same period of time (5) to illustrate the close correlation between these curves and to underscore the assumption that a significant part of these deaths are probably due to Reye's.

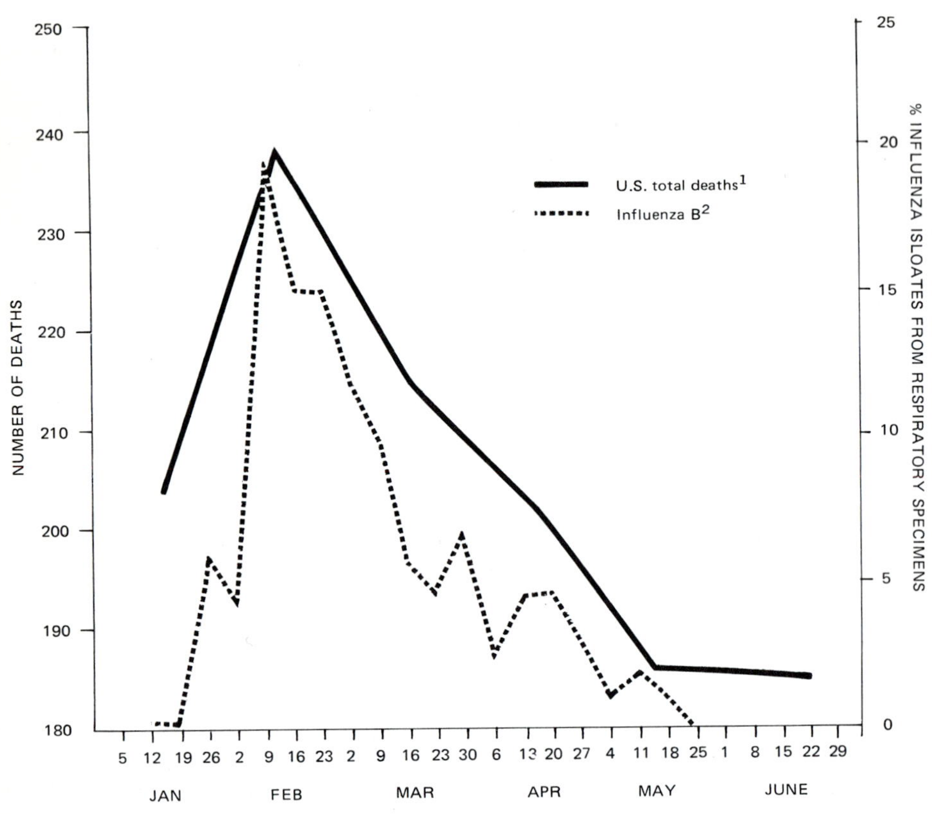

*The fourth digit was added in the U.S. adaptation of the Eighth Revision of the <u>International Classification of Diseases</u>.

**Regularly Reporting, WHO Cooperating Labs.

Sources: 1) U.S. Department of Health, Education and Welfare, Public Health Service, Health Resources Administration, National Center for Health Statistics, Division of Vital Statistics, Hyattsville, Maryland (Unpublished data).

2) Corey [5/]

28

Conclusion

Based on the above studies, the overall morbidity rate for Reye's syndrome following influenza B is estimated to be between 30.4 and 57.8 cases of the disease per 100,000 cases of influenza B (4) depending on the level of antibody titer accepted as indicating a definitive attack rate (Table 7). Assuming a case fatality rate of 41% as was documented by the Center for Disease Control in its nationwide surveillance program (5), the rate of influenza B-associated mor-

TABLE 7. Morbidity and Mortality Rates of Reye's Syndrome and Encephalitis Associated with Selected Viral Prodromes

Reportable Disease/Viral Prodrome	Morbidity Rate Per 100,000 Cases With The Viral Prodrome	Case Fatality Rate (%)	Estimated Mortality Rate Per 100,000 Cases With The Viral Prodrome
Reye's syndrome/influenza	30.4-57.8 [1/]	41 [1/]	12-24
Reye's syndrome/varicella	17.1 [2/]	41 [1/]	7
Encephalitis/measles	80.6 [2/]	15 [3/]	12
Encephalitis/varicella	31.7 [2/]	5-25 [5/]	2-8

Sources: [1/] Corey [5/]

[2/] Corey [4/]

[3/] Hoeprich [8/], pp. 829, 869

tality due to Reye's syndrome is estimated to be in the range of 12 to 24 cases per 100,000 influenza B patients. The incidence rate for Reye's associated with a varicella prodrome has been estimated at 17.1 cases per 100,000 corresponding to a Reye's syndrome mortality rate of 7 cases per 100,000 patients with varicella. One may conclude from these figures that the incidence of Reye's syndrome is not so rare as was formerly thought, particularly in the wake of influenza B epidemics. Table 7 shows morbidity rates for measles- and varicella-associated encephalitis as well, for comparison.

As a growing subject of international concern, Reye's syndrome certainly warrants our continuing best efforts to understand its etiology and to interrupt the causal chain involved in this disease.

REFERENCES

1.   Reye,R.D.K.,Morgan,G. 1963. Encephalopathy and fatty degeneration of the viscera: a disease entity in childhood. *Lancet 2:*749.

2.   Johnson,G.M.,Scurletis,T.D.,Carroll,N.B. 1963.A study of sixteen fatal cases of encephalitis-like disease in North Carolina children. *N.C.M.J.24:* 464.

3.   Brain,W.R.,Hunter,D. 1963. Encephalopathy and fatty degeneration of the viscera. *Lancet 1:*881.

4.   Corey,L. et al. Influenza B - associated Reye's syndrome incidence in Michigan and potential for prevention. Bureau of Epidemiology,CDC, Public Health Service,U.S.Dept.of Health,Education and Welfare,Atlanta,Georgia (to be published).

5.   Corey,L. et al. A nationwide outbreak of Reye's syndrome..its epidemiologic relationship to influenza B. Bureau of Epidemiology, CDC,Public Health Service,U.S.Dept. of Health,Education and Welfare,Atlanta,Georgia (to be published).

6.   U.S. Department of Health, Education and Welfare, Public Health Service,Health Resources Administration, National Center for Health Statistics. <u>Vital Statistics of the U.S.</u> Series. Rockville,Maryland. (various publication dates).

7.   U.S. Department of Health, Education and Welfare, Public Health Service,Center for Disease Control, <u>Influenza-Respiratory Disease Surveillance Report</u> Series. Atlanta,Georgia.(various publication dates).

8.   Hoeprich,P.D.,ed. Infectious Diseases, Hagerstown, Maryland: Harper and Row,Publishers,Inc.,c.1972.

DISCUSSION

J.C. Partin   -   I just wanted to ask about the age
               composition of the influenza isolate curves.
               Is that curve composed primarily of adults,
               or are those curves selected for the under-
               18 age group?

M.A.W. Hattwick- Influenza isolate surveillance is
               what we call a mercy sample. It is any spe-
               cimen the Center for Disease Control infor-
               mation has collected from about 60 partici-
               pating Laboratories throughout the United
               States, and all isolates are reported.There
               is some preponderance of younger age groups
               so this kind of national data does not lend
               itself well to trying to make statements
               about the incidence of Influenza B infec-
               tion by age group. We did, however, look at
               age specific attack rates based on serolog-
               ical studies in Kalamazoo, Michigan.

D.B. Tower   -   Most of the neurological disorders we
               see every day are hidden somewhere in the
               international classification for disease,
               and the new classifications are even worse
               than the previous ones.

M.A.W. Hattwick- I'd like to add to that. This is not
               a common disease and the statisticians and
               other people who design these classifica-
               tions don't design them for people who are
               interested in uncommon diseases.

F.L. Ruben   You mention the low incidence of
               Reye's syndrome in black people. I seem to
               have the impression that the low incidence
               in the black population is related to the
               fact that they aren't living in the subur-
               ban rural areas in the parts of the country
               where Reye's syndrome is occurring. Do you
               have any more information on that?

M.A.W. Hattwick -   The observation came because we
          looked in Michigan and found a low incidence
          in black children and at unequal distribu-
          tion. In that area black populations are pre-
          dominantly urban. If it takes a particular
          infection and exposure to some rural toxin,
          and black children aren't in the rural area,
          that would explain the observation.

REYE SYNDROME: AN EPIDEMIOLOGIC ASSESSMENT
BASED ON NATIONAL SURVEILLANCE 1977-1978
AND A POPULATION BASED STUDY IN OHIO 1973-1977

David B. Nelson, M.D., John Z.Sullivan-Bolyai,M.D.,
M.P.H., James S.Marks, M.D., David M. Morens, M.D.,
Lawrence Schonberger, M.D., and the Ohio State De-
partment of Health Reye's Syndrome Investigation
Group*

Since its description by Reye et al (1) in Australia in 1963 and Johnson et al (2) in 1963 in the United
States, over 1,000 cases of Reye   syndrome have been
reported to the Center for Disease Control (CDC). In
spite of this large number of cases, much of the epidemiology is still not understood. The relationship
of Reye   syndrome to viral illnesses, particularly influenza B, has been well documented (3,4). Several investigators (5,6,7) have described the age, race and
geographic features of Reye   syndrome, stressing the
preponderance of cases occurring in suburban-rural
areas and the generally few black patients with Reye
syndrome. These epidemiological data, however,lack two
essential elements: (1) No continuing prospective surveillance has been maintained for longer than 6 months
and (2) very few data in the literature are population
based; therefore, true attacks rates are generally not
available. The data presented here are based on a
prospective 16-month surveillance period extending from
December 1976 through to April 1978 and on a retrospective population-based study in Ohio in the years 1973-
1977.

*Deane Johnson, Frank Holtzhauer,Frank Bright,
Taylor Kramer, and Thomad J. Halpin

METHOD:

Surveillance. The CDC has maintained surveillance
for Reye syndrome for the years 1977 and 1978 throughout the United States. Cases are reported to the CDC
by state and territorial epidemiologists, hospitals,
and private physicians on standard case-investigation
forms. A case is defined as acute onset of non-
inflammatory encephalopathy with (1) microvesicular
fatty metamorphosis of the liver diagnosed by biopsy or
autopsy, or (2) a threefold or greater rise in serum
glutamic oxaloacetic transaminase (SGOT), serum glutamic pyruvic transaminase (SGPT), or serum ammonia (NH_3).
If cerebral spinal fluid is obtained, it must have
$\leq$ 8 leukocytes/mm^3. These surveillance studies are
based on 259 cases in 1977 and 93 cases through April
1978.
Ohio Retrospective Study. Incidence data were obtained through a 5-year retrospective study done in
Ohio. All hospitals in the state with more than 40
pediatric beds were canvassed for patients with Reye
syndrome admitted to these institutions in 1973-1977.
In addition, pediatric centers in neighboring states
were queried for possible cases of Reye syndrome in
Ohio residents. These cases were reviewed by 2 of the
authors (JSB, JM). A case definition for this study is
the same as the case definition used for surveillance.
For the years 1973-1977, 190 cases were identified and
are the basis of the incidence data in this discussion.

RESULTS

Temporal Distribution. Figure 1 shows the months
of onset for cases of Reye syndrome from December 1976
through April 1978 in the United States. While 1977
was an epidemic year for influenza B, only 15 isolates
were reported in 1978 (12). The peak in the epidemic
curve for the onset of cases of Reye syndrome correlates with the peaks of isolates of influenza B virus
in 1977 and influenza A virus in 1978.
Composite graphs from Ohio for 1973-1977 show the
temporal relationship of Reye syndrome to the anteced-

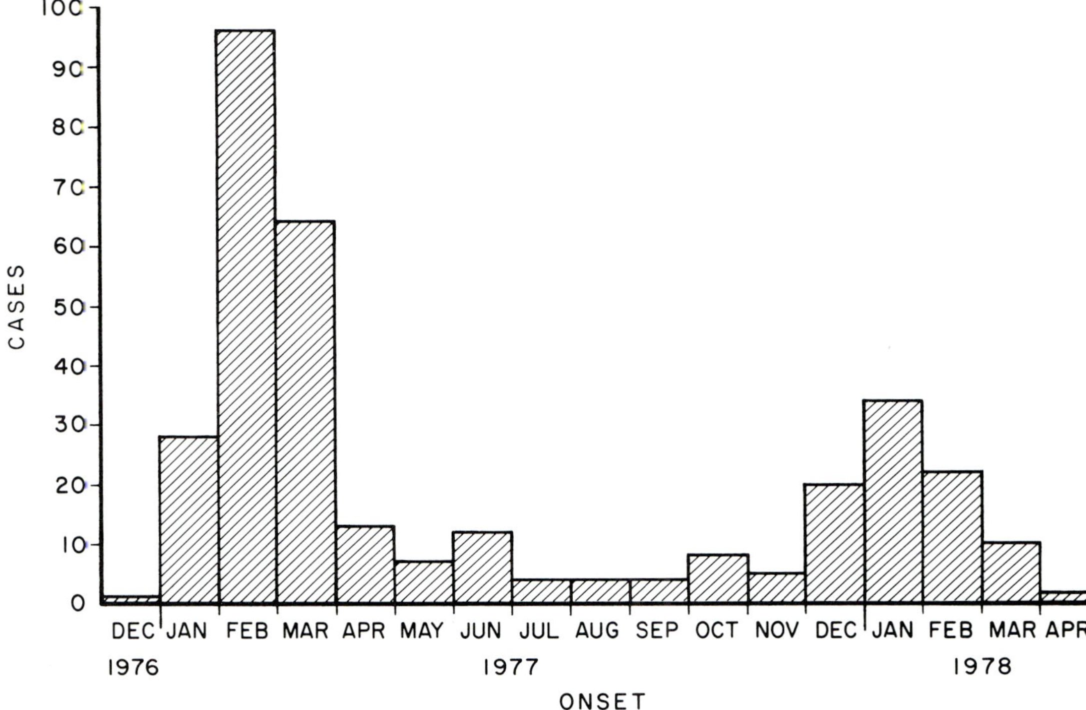

Figure 1.   Reye syndrome cases, by month of onset, United States
December 1976 - April 1978

35

ent illness (Figures 2,3 and 4). During periods when
influenza B was epidemic, cases of Reye syndrome clustered in February and March, the peak months for cases
of influenza B (13,14).Varicella-associated cases occurred in the early spring, typically the season for varicella (8,10).While Reye syndrome cases associated with
non-influenza respiratory illness peaked in the fall
and winter, they clustered in time less than varicella
or influenza B, and cases were present from early fall
to late spring.

Figure 2.   Cases of Reye Syndrome after respiratory ill-
            ness, by month of onset of antecedent illness,
            influenza B periods*, Ohio, 1973-1977

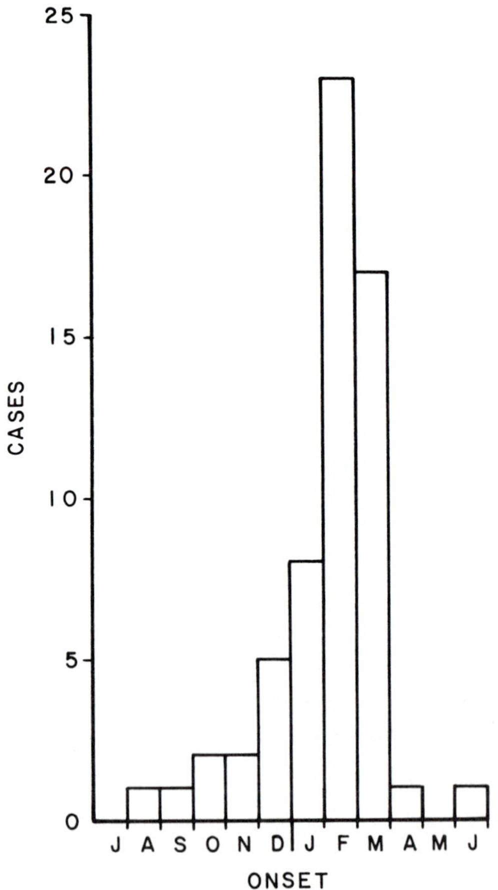

Figure 3. Cases of Reye syndrome after varicella,
           by month of onset of varicella,
           Ohio, 1973 - 1977

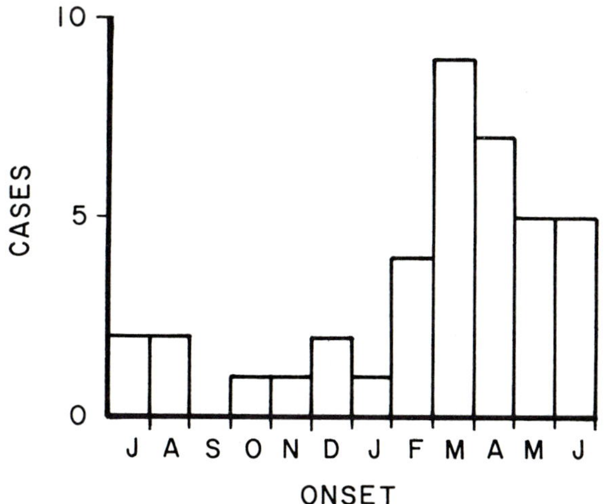

Figure 4. Cases of Reye syndrome after respiratory ill-
           ness, by month of onset of antecedent illness,
           non-influenza B periods*, Ohio, 1973-1977

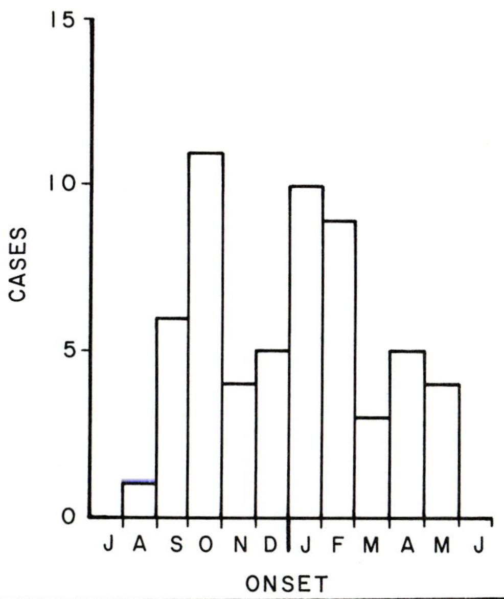

*January 1973 - June 1973
 July 1974 - June 1976
 July 1977 - December 1977

Attack rates for influenza B and non-influenza B periods in Ohio are given in Table 1. Except for the high attack rate during months when influenza B was epidemic, attack rates tended to be higher in nonepidemic years for influenza B. Except for the influenza B period, the differences were not statistically significant. Overall, the mean annual attack rate for Reye syndrome in Ohio for 1973-1977 was 0.89 cases per 100,000 population less than 18 years of age.

TABLE 1

Rate of Non-Varicella Associated Reye Syndrome, By 3-Month Periods, Influenza B and Non-Influenza B** Epidemiologic Years, Ohio, 1973-1977*

	24-Month Influenza B Period		36-Month Non-Influenza B Period	
Months	Patients	Rate***	Patients	Rate***
July-Sept	6	0.35	9	0.35
Oct-Dec	9	0.53	22	0.86
Jan-March	62	3.64	27	1.06
April-June	3	0.18	13	0.51

*July 1973-June 1974 and July 1976-June 1977
**January 1973-June 1973, July 1974-June 1976, and July 1977-December 1977
***Persons aged 0-17, Ohio, 1975, US Bureau of Census Estimate

Geographic Distribution. Table 2 shows the geographic distribution of cases of Reye syndrome by race for 1973-1977 in Ohio. Attack rates are given by standard metropolitan statistical area (SMSA) and non-SMSA area. Overall, the attack rate was higher in urban areas than in rural areas, with the highest attack rate being in the urban non-central city. The lowest attack rate was in rural areas within an SMSA. This is in contrast to non-SMSA rural areas where the attack rate was relatively high. These trends were the same regardless of the antecedent illness and were also consistent when controlled for the racial characteristics

TABLE 2

*Reye Syndrome, Rates by Race and Geographic
Distribution, for the Population Less Than 18
Years of Age, Ohio, 1973-1977*

Location	Black		White		All Races	
	No.	Rate*	No.	Rate*	No.	Rate*
Total Urban						
SMSA***	14	0.77	128	1.33	144**	1.26
Central City SMSA	9	0.57	40	1.01	49	0.88
Urban, Non-Central City SMSA	5	2.22	88	1.56	95**	1.62
Total Rural	0	0	32	0.83	32	0.77
Rural SMSA	0	0	12	0.46	12	0.44
Rural Non-SMSA	0	0	20	1.43	20	1.40
Urban, Non-SMSA	0	0	12	0.39	12	0.39

*Cases per year per 100,000 persons aged 0-17 years,
 1970 Census, Ohio

**Includes 1 person of unknown race and 1 of
 "other" race

***An SMSA is defined as a county or group of contiguous
 counties containing at least one city of 50,000 or
 more inhabitants. Areas are included in an SMSA if
 they are considered to be socially and economically
 integrated with the central city. An SMSA is divided
 into three parts: the central city (inside the city
 limits), the urban non-central city (the heavily populated areas directly adjacent to large cities), and
 rural areas that are economically or socially tied
 to the central city. Non-SMSA areas include rural
 areas and smaller urban centers of less than 50,000
 population (11).

of the various geographic areas.

   Age Distribution. The age distribution for Reye
syndrome cases not related to varicella in 1977 and
1978 for the United States is shown in Table 3.The peak
age was higher in the influenza B epidemic year of 1977
but the mean age was the same in both years (8.2 years).
The peak age for persons with varicella-associated Reye
syndrome cases appeared to be consistent from year to
year,with the majority of cases occurring in the group
aged 5-9 years.

TABLE   3

*Non-Varicella Associated Reye Syndrome
Cases by Age,United States, 1977 - 1978*

Age	1977 No.	1977 %	1978 No.	1978 %
<1	17	8	5	6
1-4	36	16	9	12
5-9	66	30	33	43
10-14	91	41	20	26
>15	11	5	10	13
Total	221	100	77	100

   The age-specific attack rates in Ohio for 1973-77
had a distribution similar to that of the United States.
Case-fatality ratios for this period in Ohio were approximately the same for all age groups, about 20%.
   Sex. Sex-specific attack rates in Ohio were slightly higher for females, 1.17/100,000, than for males,
0.87/100,000;this is statistically significant(p<.05).
However,there was no statistical difference in the
case-fatality ratios between the two groups.
   Race. Six percent of persons with Reye syndrome
reported nationwide in 1977 and 1978 were black.Forty
percent of black patients with Reye syndrome were under
1 year of age. Only 4% of the non-black patients with
Reye Syndrome were under 1 year of age. This is statistically significant (p<.001).

This observed difference in age distribution for black and white patients with Reye syndrome was also seen in Ohio (Table 4). Blacks less than 1 year of age had the highest age-specific attack rate regardless of prodromal illness. This difference is statistically significant (p<.001). Overall, however, the attack rate was less for blacks than for whites, 0.7 per 100,000 black population less than 18 years of age compared with 1.04 per 100,000 white population under 18 years of age. This difference is not statistically significant. Black and white patients were similar in temporal, geographic, prodromal, and sex characteristics, differing only in their age distribution. No difference in case-fatality ratios was present between whites and blacks.

TABLE 4

Reye Syndrome, Rates by Race and Age,
Ohio, 1973-1977

Age	White No.*	White Rate**	Black No.*	Black Rate**
<1	5	0.61	5	4.88
1-4	35	1.07	4	1.05
5-9	70	1.48	3	0.54
10-14	57	1.14	2	0.33
15-17	7	0.25	0	0
Total	174	1.04***	14	0.70***

*Excludes 12-year-old of unknown race and 3-year-old of "other" race
**Cases per year per 100,000 persons, Ohio, 1970 Census
***Age adjusted to 1970 Ohio population, all races

Socioeconomic Status. Table 5 shows socioeconomic
status by geographic location for patients with Reye
syndrome in Ohio. Generally, attack rates were higher
for higher socioeconomic classes within SMSA's and for
low socioeconomic classes outside SMSA's.

TABLE 5

*Reye Syndrome, Rates by Socioeconomic Status
and Geographic Classification, Persons of All Races,
0-17 Years Old, Ohio, 1973-1977*

Location	Low No.	Low Rate*	Middle No.	Middle Rate*	High No.	High Rate*
Total Urban SMSA	21	0.84	80	1.32	43	1.49
Central City SMSA	17	0.86	23	0.78	9	1.41
Urban, Non-Central City SMSA	4	0.75	57	1.84	34	1.51
Rural SMSA	3	0.29	7	0.68	2	0.30
Rural Non-SMSA	8	2.25	10	1.40	2	0.56
Urban Non-SMSA	3	0.39	8	0.51	1	0.13

*Cases per year per 100,000 persons aged 0-17 years,
   Ohio, 1970 Census

Mortality. National surveillance has shown a decreasing trend in the case-fatality ratio for Reye syndrome, from a high of 41% in 1973-1974 to 23% for the
period December 1977 through April 1978. There has also
been a trend toward admitting children to hospitals in
earlier stages of illness. In 1974, 16% of cases of
Reye syndrome were admitted in stage 4-5 (7). In 1978,
only 4% of cases of Reye syndrome were admitted in stage
4-5. This is statistically significant (p<.05). The
case-fatality ratio is also decreasing within stages

(Table 6); thus, the overall decrease in the case-fatality ratio is not fully explained by the children being admitted at earlier stages. Similar trends are seen in Ohio.

TABLE 6

Case-Fatality Ratio by Stage at Admission
Reye Syndrome Patients, United States,
1974, 1977-1978

| | Case-Fatality Ratio | | | | | |
| | 1974 | | 1977 | | 1978 | |
Stage	No.	%	No.	%	No.	%
0	5	0	12	15	1	100
1	53	22	72	19	27	15
2	112	42	106	32	40	18
3	52	50	37	46	21	33
4	28	69	16	69	2	0
5	12	83	8	100	2	100
Total	262	41%	251	34%	93	23%

DISCUSSION

Reye syndrome has been characterized as a winter illness of white, upper-middle-class persons who live in suburban and rural areas (2,3,5). This profile is not entirely supported by the data discussed in this paper.

Although Reye syndrome usually occurs during epidemics of respiratory illness in the winter (9,10), it can and does occur at all times of the year and is reported every month. Reye syndrome occurs in epidemic fashion in periods of influenza B activity; however, 50% or more of the cases occur when there is no influenza B in the community. In periods of no influenza B activity, the "season" for Reye syndrome appears to be more protracted (Figure 3), lasting from early fall to late spring. This long season possibly indicates that

a variety of viruses are responsible for the antecedent
illness.

Previously published observations (4,5) that Reye
syndrome occurs primarily in suburban-rural areas, and
rarely occurs in the inner city, are not supported by
the data in this study. The highest attack rate did
occur in "suburban" areas, however, the combined SMSA
and non-SMSA rural areas had a lower attack rate than
the inner city. The marked difference between rural
SMSA and rural non-SMSA is unexplained.

The attack rate for blacks was not statistically
different from whites. The high attack rate in blacks
under 1 year has been previously unreported and is col-
laborated by the national surveillance data showing 40%
of blacks with Reye syndrome to be less than 1 year of
age. This may be an important relationship and requires
further study.

It is clear that further epidemiologic investigations of defined populations where legitimate attack
rates can be obtained will be necessary to determine
the true epidemiology of Reye syndrome. These populations should be chosen to reflect various demographic
patterns that exist in the United States and that may
lead to a clearer understanding of the etiologic agents
responsible for this illness.

SUMMARY

A 16-month national surveillance period and a 5-
year population-based study of Reye syndrome were analyzed. Data presented show a very high attack rate for
black children less than 1 year of age, a wide distribution of Reye syndrome in all geographic areas, a slight
but significant rise in attack rate for females, a decrease in admissions in stage 4-5, and a decreasing case-
fatality ratio. Further population-based studies are
needed to determine if the relationships found in Ohio
are typical of the United States.

ACKNOWLEDGMENT

     We are indebted to the state and territorial
epidemiologists, hospitals and private physicians who
have reported cases of Reye syndrome to the CDC. Without their cooperation, the national surveillance for
Reye syndrome would not be possible.
     We also wish to thank the physicians and institu-
tions in Ohio for their cooperation and participation
in this population-based study.

REFERENCES

1. Reye,R.D.K,Morgan, G., Baral, J., 1963. Encephalo-
    pathy and fatty degeneration of the viscera, a
    disease entity in childhood. *Lancet 2:* 249-252.
2. Johnson, G.M., Sculetis, T.D., Carrol, N.D., 1963.
    A study of sixteen fatal cases of encephalitis-like
    disease in North Carolina children. *North Carolina
    Med. J. 24:* 464-473.
3. Corey, L., Rubin, R.J., Hattwick, M.A.W., Noble, G.
    R., Cassidy, E., 1976. A nationwide outbreak of
    Reye's syndrome. *Am J Med 61:* 615-625.
4. Corey, L., Rubin, R.J., Thompson, T.R., Noble, G. R.
    Cassidy, E., Hattwick, M.A.W., Gregg, M.B.,Eddins,
    D. 1977. Influenza B - associated Reye's syndrome
    incidence in Michigan and potential for prevention.
    J. Infect. Dis. 155: 1096-1098.
5. Ruben, F.L., Streiff, E.J., Neal, M., Michaels,
    R., 1976. Epidemiologic studies of Reye's syndrome:
    cases seen in Pittsburgh October 1973 - April 1975.
    Am. J. Public Health 66: 11.
6. Walker, S.H., Schleupner, C.J., 1973. Reye's
    syndrome in Baltimore: a review of 16 cases. *MD
    State Med J. 22:* 48-53.
7. Corey, L., Rubin, R.J., Hattwick, M.A.W. 1977.
    Reye's syndrome: clinical progression and cvalu
    ation of therapy. *Pediatrics 60:* 708-714.
8. Weller, T.H. Varicella - herpes zoster virus.
    Viral infections of Humans, 463-466, 1976 (ed.
    Evans, A.S.)
9. Glick, T.H., Likowsky, Jazen W., 1970. Reye's
    syndrome: an epidemiologic approach. *Pediatrics
    46:* 371-377.

10.   Center for Disease Control: Morbidity and Mortal-
      ity Weekly Report 20:101-102, 1971.
11.   U.S. Bureau of the Census: Census of population
      1970: characteristics. Final Report PC(1)-B37
      Ohio, Appendix A, 1971.
12.   Center for Disease Control (unpublished data)
13.   Center for Disease Control: Influenza surveil-
      lance reports 89-91, 1974-1976.
14.   Center for Disease Control: National influenza
      immunization program weekly surveillance reports,
      January-April 1977

DISCUSSION

M.A.W. Hattwick - What was the actual isolate information for the year in which we had an epidemic
   that didn't correlate with the timing of the Influenza A epidemic? When did the influenza B
   isolates occur and, also,how hard were people looking for Influenza isolates during that time period?

      The second thing I find interesting is you
found differences in your urban,rural and racial
findings from the earlier studies in 1974. This may
reflect changes in the study designs but it may,in
fact,be related to real changes in the environment.
I find that particularly interesting because there
have been some changes in our use of toxins in environmental use. Doctor Crocker mentioned once
things become identified as possible problems, they
quickly get eliminated from the environment. I wonder if you have any observations about whether some
of the changes that were seen between 1974 and,say,
1977-78 may be related to changes in the presence
of environmental toxins.

D.B. Nelson -   If we go to the first question, actually the particular curve for 1978 did correspond
   to Influenza A isolates,but it was spread out a bit
   more and there was a significant number of cases
   occurring when Influenza A was not around. There
   were 15 isolates of Influenza B reported to CDC and

they were spread over many states in the winter
months. We looked hard for influenza in the southeast. We had a couple of studies going using ser-
ology and virus isolation,and we did not pick up
any Influenza B. As far as whether environment factors are changing, it is very possible. We have to
be cautious in classifying Reye's as an urban,rural
or suburban disease,because things that may be affecting it are changing.

M.D. Hilty -   I was wondering if you had any different
information on the incidence of chicken pox associated Reye's Syndrome from year to year. There is
some basic information which indicates that there
might be some strain variations in the varicella
Zoster virus and that we may not be dealing with
just one virus.

D.B. Nelson - It is virtually impossible to get any
data on attack rates for varicella but, as far as
per cent of cases due to varicella being reported
annually,it is comparable. In 1977, 13% of the
Reye's Syndrome cases were due to varicella, and in
1978 about 10% were due to varicella. However,that
means that there was more varicella in 1977, since
there was considerably more Reye's Syndrome that
year.

E.L. Arcinue - Doctor Nelson, I probably have misunder-
stood the definition of SMSA. Did you say it is defined as one county with at least one city over
50,000 population?

D.B. Nelson - No. It is usually more than one county.
It is contiguous counties that have within them at
least one city of 50,000 or more population. The
criterion for including counties within an SMSA is
if they are socially and economically related to
that city.

E.L. Arcinue - Detroit proper, would have adjoining
cities where there is more than 50,000 population;
how do you consider these?

D.B. Nelson - Usually,one city is defined as the inner
    city. Generally,centers like Cincinnati, Cleveland
    and Columbus would be the centre for their SMSA;
    with the inner city being defined by the city limits
    and,in the surrounding areas,there may be a very
    heavily populated urbanized fringe. For example;in
    Atlanta,Georgia, the city of Decatur is a highly
    dense,inner city type area that would be considered
    by census statistics as SMSA urban fringe because
    it is outside the city limits of Atlanta.

D.B. Tower - Your data for black versus white, age,
    and suburban versus rural are very reminiscent of
    the situation with polio and with Multiple Sclero-
    sis. In each of those cases, early exposure to ei-
    ther a specific viral agent in the case of polio,
    or a presumed one in the case of Multiple Sclerosis,
    is felt to significantly modify the distribution
    and time of attack. Is it valid to make an assump-
    tion that that may be the case here?

D.B. Nelson - I think that is one possibility. Addi-
    tionally,toxin exposure may be different in young
    black children and those that are going to develop
    Reye's Syndrome may get exposed earlier than white
    children. I feel that one issue that requires fur-
    ther study is the nature of the viral agents in-
    volved in this age group.

M.Thaler   - I noticed that you have clustering of
    varicella at approximately the same time as Influ-
    enza B seems to cluster. Do you have a sufficient
    number of cases of children with both varicella and
    Influenza B to determine whether in those patients
    you have a higher incidence of Reye's Syndrome?

D.B. Nelson - I disagree with that somewhat. The at-
    tack rate or the cluster for varicella is later
    than for Influenza B, so that you actually have
    distinct time differences. Usually varicella is
    what people report;they do not report the respira-
    tory illness.

R.L. Ozere - Are the attack rates for the known Influenza B associated Reye's cases similar between
the state of Ohio and the New England area in recent years?

D.B. Nelson - I am a little reluctant to give attack
rates on the national surveillance because I just
don't know how good our case ascertainment is. I do
know the case ascertainment in Ohio was good, on a
retrospective basis. I think you have to do the
kind of study that was done in Ohio,in other areas,
to get legitimate attack rates.

J.S. Haller - It is a good thing this question was
raised,because I would like to point out at this
point that all your statistics on a national basis
are derived from voluntary reporting. I would plead
with the United States federal representatives that
they put pressure on their Public Health Officers
to make it an obligatory reportable disease.

J.V. Baublis - With regard to Influenza A and B and the
coalescence of these diseases with Varicella Zoster
(VZ) it is a rather frequent occurence based on our
own viral isolation studies from patients. It is
possible that a fortuitous co-occurence of viral
agents could be implicated. Part of the overlap of
Varicella Zoster associated cases late in the
spring may very well be that the patients are also
smitten by flu.

D.B. Nelson - That is very possible. We also have to
be careful about making too many conclusions from
viral isolations. It is not known, if you take a
random selection of children under 18, how many
are going to have isolates of Influenza A, Influenza B or varicella.

REYE'S SYNDROME IN JAPAN: EPIDEMIOLOGY,
CLINICAL FEATURES AND INDICATORS FOR
MORTALITY AND THE SEQUELAE

Fumio Yamashita,M.D.,Masashi Yamamoto,M.D.,
Shojiro Okada,M.D., Ichiro Yoshida,M.D. and
Makoto Yoshino, M.D.

OBJECTIVES

A nationwide survey on Reye's syndrome in Japan
was performed by a research committee on Reye's Syndrome, Ministry of Health and Welfare, to ascertain the
epidemiology,clinical features,prognosis and the indicators for mortality and the sequelae.

METHODS

The nationwide survey, using a questionnaire, was
performed in January 1976 and February 1978. The first
survey was sent to 942 facilities with a pediatric ward
with a reply rate of 39%. Fifty-four percent of the 372
hospitals replied that they had cases with Reye's syndrome* or "Acute Encephalopathy of Obscure Origin"*.
The second survey was sent to 422 hospitals,with a reply rate of 52%. They had had experience with Reye's
syndrome (53 cases) and Acute Encephalopathy (124 cases)
in 142 of 222 hospitals that answered.(N*=144 and 338,
respectively).

The cases reported were rechecked by the following case definition and classified into three groups:
Group A (confirmed by biopsy of the liver or autopsy);
Group B (confirmed by autopsy; however,there was no detailed description of the centrinucleated fatty liver
characteristic of Reye's syndrome); Group C (clinically
diagnosed without liver biopsy).

The case definition was (1) acute onset of encephalopathy demonstrated by normal cells in the CSF (less
than 10 per cubic millimeter) or by cerebral histology
of non-inflammatory edema confirmed by autopsy combined
with (2) centrinucleated fatty liver, demonstrated either by biopsy or autopsy,(3) serum glutamic oxalic
transaminase (SGOT) level greater than 2 times the normal,(4)without clinically recognizable jaundice,(5)no
other explanation for the neurologic or hepatic abnor-
malities.When item (2) was absent,the cases were classified into Group C:Clinical Reye's Syndrome. The cases were classified into five stages as per Corey et al
(1): Stage O, normal consciousness; Stage 1, lethargy,
sleepiness,indifference,amnesia; Stage 2, delirium,com-
bativeness,disorientation; Stage 3,obtundation,decor-
tication; Stage 4,decerebration,loss of oculocephalic
reflexes; Stage 5,seizures,flaccidity,respiratory arrest.

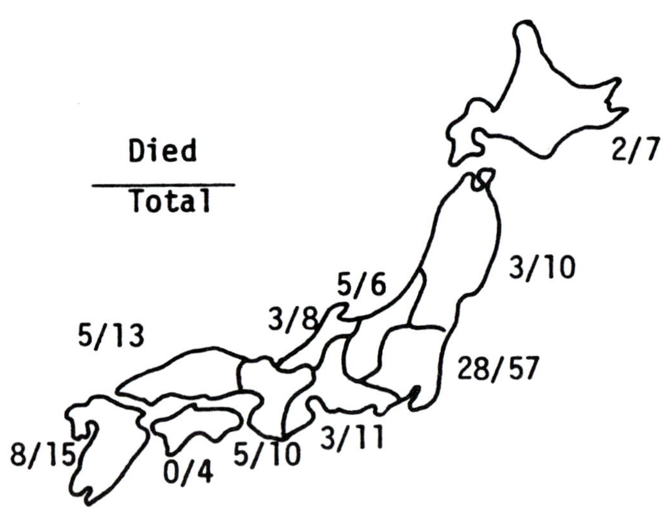

Fig.1. Geographic distribution

RESULTS

Epidemiology:

The total number reported was 141 cases, composed of 32 cases of Group A, 13 Cases of Group B, and 96 of Group C .

The geographical distribution was nationwide.However,the differences in the incidence or the mortality rate by area cannot be discerned,because the number of cases was not large enough for comparative analysis. (Figure 1).

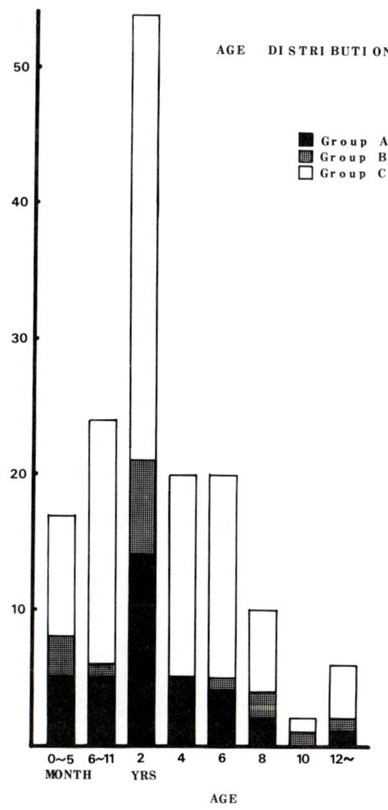

Fig.2

The age distribution revealed the highest peak at
1 - 2 years and the age ranged between 20 days (confirmed case) and 13 years. (Fig.2).

The months of presentation had two peaks in the winter season (December-March) and in the summer season
(July and August). (Fig.3).

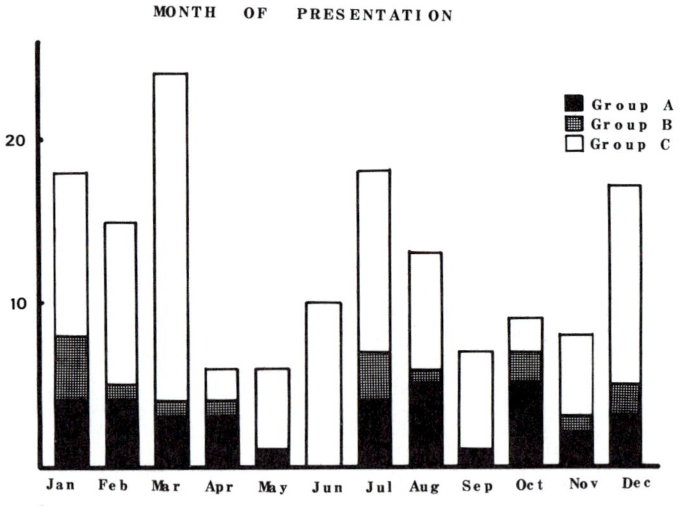

Fig.3

The outbreak of Reye's syndrome could not be correlated with an influenza epidemic, although an epidemic of influenza type A and type B had been experienced
in Japan.One case of Reye's syndrome followed by influenza B has been reported by Hirose et al in 1977
(3).

CLINICAL FEATURES

Antecedent Infection: Seventy-five percent of 112 cases
had a description of an antecedent infection with 67
(59.8%) upper respiratory, 11 (9.8%) febrile illness,
3(2.7%) measles, 2 (1.8%) chicken pox, and 1 (0.9%)
herpes.

Clinical Manifestation:Among the clinical manifestations (Table 1), fever,convulsion and vomiting were
the most common signs, followed by abnormal posture,de-
hydration,hepatomegaly and diarrhea.

Laboratory Findings: Serum glutamic oxalic transaminase (SGOT) and serum glutamic pyruvic transaminase
(SGPT) showed marked elevation of more than 1000 Kar-
men units in 20% and 14.6% respectively.(Table 2). A
small number of cases with lower SGOT levels (less than
100 units) were probably caused by inadequate sampling
of the serum in cases confirmed by liver biopsy or autopsy.

Table 1

CLINICAL MANIFESTATIONS IN REYE SYNDROME

FEVER	92.7 %	(N=137)
CONVULSION	89.1	(138)
VOMITING	62.9	(140)
ABNORMAL POSTURE	55.9	(127)
DEHYDRATION	49.6	(131)
HEPATOMEGALY	42.0	(138)
DIARRHEA	33.6	(131)

DISTRIBUTION OF LABORATORY DATA

Transaminase	GOT (%)	GPT (%)
- 99	7.4	36.2
100-499	63.0	40.0
500-999	9.6	9.2
1000-	20.0	14.6
Karmen U.	N=135	N=130

Table 2

Table 3

DISTRIBUTION OF LABORATORY DATA

LDH	N=108	Ammonia	N=53
- 499	15.7 (%)	$\geqq$ 300	7.5 (%)
500- 999	21.3	< 300	92.5
1000-2999	42.6	ug/dl	
3000-	20.4		
Wroblewski U.			

LDH isozyme

Group N =	A 6	C 18	normal
1.	16.8 ± 15.1 (%)	28.5 ± 12.6 (%)	30-40
2.	16.2 ± 8.3	34.2 ± 10.8	34-48
3.	13.2 ± 3.6	17.5 ± 5.8	15-22
4.	17.1 ± 8.4	8.2 ± 7.3	1- 6
5.	33.9 ± 16.1	11.4 ± 11.7	4- 5
serum level	6425.8 ± 4317.8	5576.6 ± 8916.0 (U)	

Table 4

Table 5

DISTRIBUTION OF LABORATORY DATA

CPK	N=43 (%)	Blood sugar	N=84 (%)		
- 49	23.3	- 9	6.7	-14.6 (- 9 to 30-39)	-18.0 (- 9 to 40-49)
50- 99	11.6	10-19	1.1		
100-149	4.7	20-29	3.4		
150-199	9.3	30-39	3.4		
200-299	14.3	40-49	3.4		
300-	37.2	50-	82.0		
I.U.		mg/dl			

Serum lactic dehydrogenase (LDH) was also markedly elevated ($>$ 3000 Wroblewski units in 20.4%) and the serum ammonium level was more than 300μg/dl (upper limit of the normal level - 100μg/dl) was found in 7.5% of 53 cases (Table 3).

Hypoglycemia (<40 mg/dl) was confirmed in 14.6% of 84 cases (Table 5) and serum creatine phosphokinase (CPK) greater than 300 I.U.(normal upper limit 30 I.U) was found in 37.2% of 43 cases examined. No significant difference in the incidence of hypoglycemia was seen by age.

LDH isozyme pattern showed significant differences between Group A and C:hepatic component (fraction 5) was more dominant in the former than the latter (p $<$ 0.05 in fraction 2,4,5 between two groups). (Table 4).

The acid-base status was checked at the most severe stage in 46 cases, and showed metabolic acidosis in 47.8%; mixed acidosis in 23.9%; respiratory alkalosis in 10.9%, and 13% normal.

Table 6

DISTRIBUTION OF LABORATORY DATA
LUMBAR PUNCTURE: CSF

1. PRESSURE	$\geqq$200(MMH$_2$0)	41.0
(N=78)	NORMAL	59.0
2. PROTEIN	$\geqq$ 50(MG/DL)	12.1
(N=116)	NORMAL	87.9
3. SUGAR	$<$ 40(MG/DL)	9.6
(N=115)	NORMAL	90.4

In 45 cases, serum bilirubin was performed; Group A 0.94± 0.92 (M + 1SD), 12 cases; Group B 1.26 ± 0.62 in 5 cases, and Group C, 0.73 ± 0.63 in 2 cases and 0.84 ± 0.24 was the overall result.

MORTALITY AND INCIDENCE OF SEQUELA

Sixty-two of 141 cases (44%) died and the mortality in Group A plus B and C was 86.7% (39/45) and 24% (23/96),respectively. The surviving 79 cases showed the sequela in 58.2% (46 cases). (Table 7).

No significant difference in the mortality and the incidence of sequela by the mode of therapy was found. Steroids were used in 107 of 141 cases and exchange transfusions were used in 7 of 141 cases with the mortality and the incidence of sequela in both 'used' and 'unused' cases being 46.7% vs 35.5% (mortality) and 64.9% (sequela) vs 45.5% in the former and 42.9% vs. 44.8% (mortality) and 50% vs 60% (sequela) in the latter,respectively.

REYE SYNDROME   NATIONAL SURVEY 1978

TOTAL (A+B+C)	141	
MORTALITY	62/141	(44.0)
SEQUELAE	46/ 79	(58.2)

SEVERELY HANDICAPPED	17/93	(18.3 %)
MENTAL RETARDATION	17/93	(18.3 %)
PALSY	15/93	(16.1 %)
HEMIPLEGIA	4/93	(4.4 %)
M.B.D.S.	3/93	(3.2 %)
EPILEPSIA	3/93	(3.2 %)
ABNORMAL EEG	27/93	(29.0 %)
OTHERS	7/93	(7.5 %)

Table 7. Mortality and sequela.

The mortality and the incidence of sequela were analyzed by the age, staging of the syndrome, the presence or absence of abnormal posture, antecedent infection, clinical features and laboratory findings. (See Tables 8,9,10 and 11).

AGE AND MORTALITY, SEQUELAE

AGE	N	MORTALITY (%)	SEQUELAE (%)
- 5M	14	57.1	5/ 6 83.3
6-11M	20	35.0	10/13 76.9
1- 4Y	71	43.7	25/40 62.5
5- Y	34	47.1	6/18 33.3*

*P=0.01

Table 8
Table 9

DEEPEST STAGE AND MORTALITY, SEQUELAE (%)

STAGE	N	MORTALITY		SEQUELAE	
		N	(%)	N	(%)
0	1	1	100.0	0	0
1	10	5	50.0	5	100.0
2-3	27	7	25.9*	10	50.0
4	93	46	49.5	28	59.6

*P=0.05

Table 10

ABNORMAL POSTURE AND MORTALITY, SEQUELAE

| | | MORTALITY | SEQUELAE |
POSTURE	N	N (%)	N (%)
DECEREBRATE STAGE=4	32	15 (46.9)	12 (70.6)
DECORTICATE STAGE=3	13	3 (23.1)	8 (80.0)
STAGE 2-3	26	13 (50.0)	9 (69.2)
NONE	56	23 (41.1)	15 (45.5)*

*p=0.02

TABLE 11

INDICATORS OF MORTALITY AND THE INCIDENCE OF SEQUELA:
LABORATORY FINDINGS

Prognosticator		Mortality(%)	Sequela(%)
CSF glucose*	< 40	72.7	NSD
(N=115, mg/dl)	≥ 40	33.7	NSD
GOT**	<100	90.0	NSD
(N=135, U.)	>100	35.2	NSD
GPT***	<100	42.6	NSD
(N=130, U.)	>100	24.2	
LDH***	> 3000	59.1	NSD
(N=108, U.)	< 3000	31.4	NSD
Acid Base*,Met.Acidosis		59.1	NSD

Blood Glucose,NH_3,cpk:NSD,*p=0.05,**p=0.01,***p=0.02
NSD:No significant difference.

In summary, the mortality was higher in the patients with vomiting,abnormal posture,(stage 4),lower SGOT and SGPT, very high LDH (more than 3000 Wroblewski units), low glucose concentration (less than 40 mg/dl) in CSF, (Table 6),metabolic acidosis, belonging to Group A(confirmed case). The incidence of sequela was higher in patients less than 4 years old than the cases 5 years of age or older, and was higher in the cases with abnormal posture than the patients without it. (Table 12).

DISCUSSION

The results of our nationwide survey on Reye's syndrome up until February 1978 are described. It is now clear that cases of Reye's syndrome exist in Japan and are increasing yearly, probably by the better understanding and the recognition by physicians of this syndrome. We believe that there are many unrecognized cases of Reye's syndrome and cases treated as acute encephalopathy (or unconsciousness of obscure origin) in primary care practice in our country.

The question of the incidence of convulsions in the above reported cases was proposed by a co-worker who attended the meeting of the research committee on Reye syndrome, February 1978, in Tokyo. He questioned the higher incidence of convulsions in our cases compared to the Reye's syndrome in Cincinnati Children's Hospital. The low incidence of convulsion, at least at the initial stage, in the cases in Cincinnati was confirmed by personal contact with Dr. W.K.Schubert of the Cincinnati Children's Hospital. It is very interesting that the convulsions are very common in the initial stage in the cases in Thailand (4).

We could not draw conclusions on the prognosis by relating the stage at the onset on admission because this was not solicited in the survey. We completely agree with the recommendations by Corey et al (5), which emphasize the importance of uniform staging at admission, during hospitalization, and at discharge,to

TABLE 12

INDICATORS OF MORTALITY AND THE INCIDENCE OF SEQUELA:SUMMARY

ITEM	PROGNOSTICATOR			
	MORTALITY	(P)	SEQUELA	(P)
1. Groups	A, B, (86.7%) C, (26%)	0.001		
2. Age			< 4 yrs.(62.5%) > 5 yrs.(33.3%)	0.01
3. Stage	1 (50%) 4 (49%) 2-3 (25.9%)	0.05		
4. Vomiting	Yes (52.2%)			
5. Posture	No (32.7%)	0.05	Yes (72.5) No (44.5%)	0.02
6. CSF Glucose	<40mg/dl (72.7%) >40mg/dl (33.7%)	0.05		
7. Serum LDH	>3000 (59.1%) <3000 (31.4%)	0.02		
8. Acid-base	Metabolic Acidosis (59.4%) Respiratory Alkallosis (0%) Normal (0%)	0.05		

effectively monitor the results of therapy and the
necessity of multicenter collection of data. Corey et
al (5) reported a higher incidence of sequela in the
younger patients (less than 4 years); however, this
incidence is lower than ours.

The indicators of mortality,we conclude,are in
the deepest stage (stage 4), the presence of vomiting,
low CSF glucose, extremely high LDH (more than 3000
Wroblewski units), lower SGOT, SGPT (less than 100 Kar-
men units), metabolic acidosis,whereas Corey et al (5)
showed the stage of coma on admission, evidence of intracranial pressure (abnormal posture) and blood ammonia levels greater than 300 μg/dl to indicate a poor
prognosis.

REYE'S SYNDROME SIMULATED DISEASES
IN JAPAN - "EKIRI AND EKIRI-LIKE SYNDROME".

In Japan, there was a Reye's syndrome simulated
disorder called "Ekiri", which has been diagnosed often
in the past 50 years. It is called "Ekiri" when trig-
gered by a dysentery infection, and "Ekiri-like" syndrome when the etiology is unknown. ("Eki" means "epidemic"; "ri" means "diarrhea".) It was common between
2 to 5 years of age. In both situations, the clinical
features are characterized by sudden onset of lethargy,
unconsciousness, convulsions, hyperirritability,vomi-
ting of coffee grounds, circulatory failure with elevated diastolic pressure and increased pulse pressure
at the acute stage, and marked hypoglycemia, often
without signs of colitis at the onset; with or without
high fever. It was one of the most common causes of
death for the 2 to 5 year-old in the past, and was
feared by parents because of its high mortality.

The pathological findings are similar to Reye's
syndrome: the brain showed ischemic changes and edema
without any evidence of inflammation. The liver and
kidneys showed fatty degeneration (6,7,8,9). The fatty
metamorphosis in liver cells has the same pattern as

in Reye's syndrome. Unfortunately, no data on the ultrastructure is available since no cases have been reported in the last fifteen years when electromicrosco-
pic techniques have been available. (Figure 4).

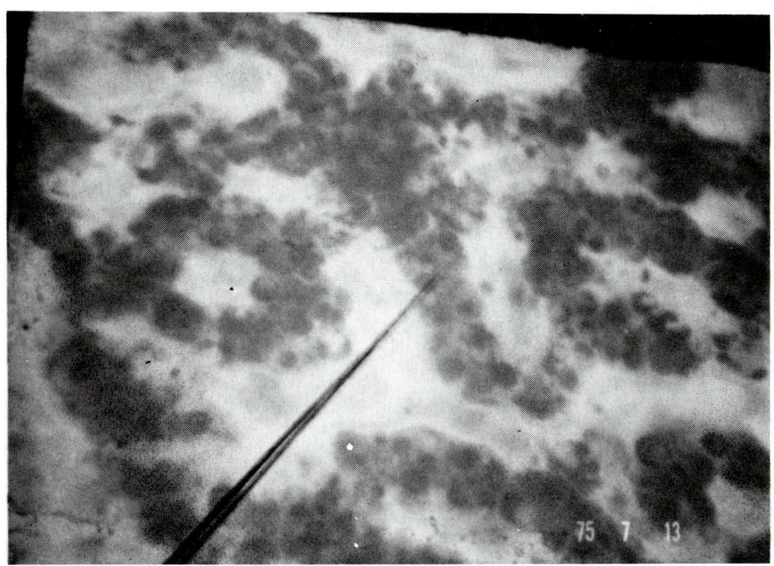

Figure 4. Centrinucleated fatty metamorphosis in the
liver of Ekiri patients. Nucleus is surrounded by
fatty droplets and the dilatated Disse's space is
observed. (Courtesy of Dr. I. Funatsu).

Funatsu (7) has noted that circulatory failure
was more prominent in "Ekiri-like syndrome) than in
Reye's syndrome and also hypoglycemia was more profound. We have succeeded in producing an experimental
model of Reye's syndrome using Shigella flexneri endotoxin in rabbits (11).

"TOXISCHE GRIPPE"

Another Reye's syndrome simulated condition is
"Toxische Grippe" seen by the pediatricians of Kyushu
University. In this situation, infants or younger children usually showed a fulminant course. There are signs
of upper respiratory infection without any sign of cen-

tral nervous system inflammation (normal CSF). All of
the five autopsied cases showed cerebral edema, and 3
of 5 cases had fatty liver similar to Reye's syndrome
(12).

The above Reye's-syndrome-simulated diseases may
suggest to us a clue to the pathogenesis of Reye's
syndrome.

SUMMARY

A nationwide survey on Reye's syndrome in Japan
performed in 1978 by a research committee on Reye's
syndrome, sponsored by the Ministry of Health and Welfare, is reported. Some of the data is compared with
that of the results of a survey by the Bureau of Epidemiology, Center for Disease Control, Atlanta, 1977. The
possible links between Reye's syndrome and other such
diseases such as "Ekiri" syndrome and "Toxische Grippe"
should be considered.

ACKNOWLEDGEMENT

This survey was supported by a research grant for
Reye's syndrome from the Japanese Ministry of Health
and Welfare.

We would like to express our cordial thanks to
pediatricians who offered their information and experience, and the members of the research committee on
Reye's syndrome, Dr. I. Funatsu, for his advice, comments and the courtesy for the permission to print the
liver histology of "Ekiri" patients, and Dr. S. Anraku
of the Brain Institute for histological study and for
his advice.

REFERENCES

1. Corey, L., Rubin, R.J., Bergman, D., Gregg, M.B.
    1977. Diagnostic criteria for influenza B-assoc-
    iated Reye's syndrome; clinical vs pathological
    criteria. *Pediatrics 60:762.*

2.   Ogawa,T.,Shigematsu,S.,and Deguchi,M. 1967. Acute encephalopathy with marked fatty infiltration in viscera (Reye). *Acta Ped.Japonica,70:*894.

3.   Hirose,M. 1977. Study on Reye's syndrome, Annual Rep. of Research Committee on Reye's syndrome. *Ministry of Health and Welfare (Japan); in press.*

4.   Dhiensiri,K.,Sinavatana,P. and Lertsookprasert,S. Reye's Syndrome in North East Thailand. International Conference on Reye's Syndrome, Halifax, Nova Scotia, 1978.

5.   Corey,L.,Rubin,R.J.,Bergman,D., and Gregg,M.B. 1977. Reye's Syndrome: clinical progression and evaluation of therapy. *Pediatrics 60:*708.

6.   Chin,I. 1955. Clinical studies on the pathogenesis of the so-called Ekiri-like syndrome. Advance of the study of Ekiri in Japan.

7.   Funatsu, I. 1962. The pathogenesis of so-called Ekiri-like syndrome and consideration of treatment of the bacillary dysentry. *J. Formosan Med. Assoc. 61:*913.

8.   Suwa,N. 1955. Pathologische Anatomie der Ekir. Advance in the study of Ekiri in Japan.

9.   Kobayashi,N. 1970. Ekiri, the Ekiri-like syndrome and acute encephalopathy of obscure origin. *Pediatria Universitatis Tokyo, 18:*88.

10.   Ogawa,T.A. 1976. A supplement of the neuropathology of the acute encephalopathies in childhood, especially about the relationship of acute toxic encephalopathy and Ekiri and Ekiri-like syndromes. I. The neuropathology of the acute toxic encephalopathy in infancy and childhood. *Psychiatria et neurologia Japonica,78:*125.

11.   Yoshino,M. and Yamashita,F. 1976. Effect of experimental endotoxemia on ureagenesis and the ultramicrostructure in liver induced by Shigella flexneri endotoxin. Annual Report of the Research Committee on Reye's Syndrome. Ministry of Health and Welfare.

12.   Yamashita, F. and Yamamoto,M. 1975. Annual Report of the Research Committee on Reye's Syndrome. Ministry of Health and Welfare.

VARICELLA HEPATITIS IN CHILDREN

R. Hochberger, D.O., P. Tokarski, M. D.,
K. Koranyi, M. D.,   D. Harper, D. O.,
and M. Hilty, M. D.

INTRODUCTION

Reye's syndrome has been associated with many
different viral infections, but varicella zoster and
influenza B are the most common. Chicken pox presents
a most interesting relationship to Reye's syndrome,
primarily because liver damage is known in both situations. Involvement of the liver in chicken pox was
first described in 1927 (1) and focal liver cell
necrosis has been observed by others (2,3,4). The
incidence of hepatic injury or dysfunction as determined by measured elevation of SGOT and SGPT during the
course of chicken pox is not known. To determine the
frequency of enzyme elevation in this easily recognized
common viral infection of children, we measured SGOT
and SGPT in patients with chicken pox and compared
them with levels in unaffected controls.

PATIENTS AND METHODS

A prospective study was conducted during the
winter of 1977-78. Eighty-six patients with chicken
pox were evaluated and compared with 50 controls. All
patients and controls were 3 months to 12 years of age.
Patients with chicken pox were examined by a physician
1-11 days after onset of rash. Forty-five were seen
1-3 days after onset of rash, 38 on day 4-7, and 3 on
days 8-11 after onset of rash. The physician confirmed
the clinical diagnosis of chicken pox, obtained informed consent, and completed a data sheet which recorded
information on past medical history, recent medications
description of the rash, fever, vomiting, and other
constitutional symptoms. Venipuncture blood samples

for SGOT and SGPT were obtained and the enzymes assays
were performed in the clinical laboratories at Columbus
Children's Hospital.

Twelve patients with chicken pox were excluded
from the study because of hemolyzed blood specimens,
incomplete data reporting, and/or inadequate documentation of clinical chicken pox. In 2 patients with
elevated SGOT and SGPT, serum amino acids were quanti-
tated. The 50 control patients were 37 healthy children admitted to the hospital on the otolaryngology
service for surgical procedures and 13 children with
cellulitis whose SGOT and SGPT levels were determined
prior to the administration of antibiotics.

RESULTS

Seventy-four patients with chicken pox were 3
months to 12 years of age and most of the children were
4-8 years of age. Enzyme elevation was most prevalent
in the 4-8 year age group and corresponds to the pre-
dominant age group evaluated.

Forty-eight of the patients had temperatures of
< 101°F, 12 had temperatures 101-102°F, and 14 had
temperatures of > 102°F.

Forty-eight of the patients had a rash considered to be 3+ defined as 4 or more crops of vesicles, 16
patients had 2+ rash consisting of 3 crops, and 10 had
1+ rash with 1-2 crops.

Vomiting occurred in 4 of the 74 children.
Thirty-one took aspirin and 41 used other medications
which included acetaminophen, benadryl, periactin, and
calamine lotion.

The clinical characteristics of 10 children
with SGOT $\geq$ 40 units/ml and SGPT $\geq$ 30 units/ml are
seen in Table 1. The first and fourth patients had
two specimens collected for transaminase activity, and
in both cases the first transaminase obtained on the
third day of illness was higher than the value obtained on the sixth or seventh day. In both of these patients, the rash was more extensive and considered to
be 3+ on the initial examination.

Patients 8 and 9 had the highest SGOT and SGPT
values on the first samples taken on days 1 and 4 of

Table 1

CLINICAL AND LABORATORY STUDIES

Patient	Age	Day of Illness	SGOT	SGPT	Fever	Vomiting	Rash	ASA
1.	4 yrs.	3,7	67,20	34,13	$\leq$101	–	3+	+
2.	7 yrs.	4	44	30	>102	+	3+	+
3.	5 yrs.	3	58	30	>102	+	3+	+
4.	5 yrs.	3,6	54,26	33,14	$\leq$101	–	3+	+
5.	3 mos.	5	40	34	$\leq$101	–	2+	–
6.	10 yrs.	4	40	43	$\leq$101	–	3+	–
7.	5 yrs.	5	38	110	$\leq$101	–	3+	–
8.	8 yrs.	4,10	69,43	43,50	none	–	3+	–
9.	8 yrs.	1,8	58,26	45,25	none	–	3+	–
10.	2 yrs.	2,5	20,66	13,40	101-102	–	2+	+

their illness. Patient 7 had the highest SGPT of the group on day 5. Quantitative serum amino acids were obtained on two children. Patient 8 had elevated serine, alanine, glutamine acid, glycine and ornithine levels, and patient 7 exhibited elevations of threonine, valine, leucine, and lysine in addition to those noted in patient 8. The presence of vomiting did not correlate with elevated serum transaminase levels, however, the clinical severity of the illness as measured with fever and severity of the rash was associated with the higher enzyme levels.

Table 2 illustrates the mean transaminase activity of patients with chicken pox and controls. Children with severe chicken pox (defined in our study as fever > 102°F and 3+ rash) had elevated transaminase levels when compared to control patients. The mean SGOT and SGPT for patients with severe disease was 42.16 ± 14.86 and 22.7 ± 7.1 respectively as compared to SGOT of 19.98 ± 7.51 and SGPT 12.92 ± 5.51 for control patients. The differences are statistically significant (P=<.001 for both enzymes). All patients with chicken pox had slightly higher transaminase activity than control patients.

Table 2

TRANSAMINASE ACTIVITY OF CASES AND CONTROLS

	Severe Illness	Mild Illness	All Patients With Varicella	Controls
Mean SGOT	42.16±14.86	22.25±6.1	28.42±13.03	19.98±7.51
Mean SGPT	22.7±7.1	13.5±3.4	18.04±13.63	12.92±5.51

One of the 50 control patients had an SGOT of 42 units/ml and one had an SGPT value of 38 units/ml with all SGOT and SGPT values being < 32 units/ml. None of the patients with chicken pox or controls developed Reye's syndrome.

DISCUSSION

Reye's syndrome is a disease of childhood characterized by an acute hepatic encephalopathy following a viral illness, most commonly influenza B or chicken pox. Most children have clinical evidence of Reye's syndrome 4-5 days following the onset of chicken pox. These early clinical manifestations usually include vomiting and alteration in sensorium. SGOT and SGPT determinations allow the clinician to assess the degree of hepatic dysfunction and serve as indirect evidence of developing Reye's syndrome. Our results indicate that some patients with chicken pox develop increases in serum transaminase activity which does not result in clinical Reye's syndrome, and may represent varicella hepatitis.

It has been suggested that the varicella virus might be hepatotropic and hepatotoxic (5) causing hepatic liver cell necrosis and/or fatty infiltration of the liver. In 1957, Krugman (4) reported several cases of hepatitis in adults secondary to severe varicella infection and varicella pneumonia. Liver biopsy in one of his patients revealed focal necrosis in the liver. Modest elevations of serum transaminase activity appear to be relatively common in childhood chicken pox. In our series, this occurred in 13.5% of children with chicken pox.

The implications of these elevations in SGOT and SGPT in chicken pox and the relationship to Reye's syndrome is not clear and needs to be examined further. Our preliminary investigation showed that the serum amino acid pattern in chicken pox was abnormal in 2 samples with some differences as well as similarities of the amino acid pattern to that of Reye's syndrome. Further research is needed regarding serum transaminase levels utilizing isoenzyme fractionation of SGOT in varicella and other systemic viral infections. As reported by Dr. Thaler at this meeting, mitochondrial SGOT is released from hepatocytes in patients with Reye's syndrome, and cystosol SGOT is released from hepatocytes during the course of hepatitis. Measurement and identification of the intracellular source of

serum SGOT in patients with chicken pox should assist
in defining the role of a varicella zoster virus in the
development of Reye's syndrome.

REFERENCES

1.   Schleussing, H. 1927. Nekrosen in Leber, Milz und
     Nebennieren bei nicht vereiterten Varizellen. Ver-
     handl. d. deutsch. path. *Œssellsch.,22*:288.

2.   Eschar, J., Reif, L., Waron, M., and Alkan,W.J.,
     1973. Hepatic lesions in chicken pox. *Œstroenter-
     ology, 64*:462.

3.   Landay, S.E.,1977: Varicella Hepatitis and Reye's
     Syndrome:An Inter-relationship. *Pediatrics, 60:*
     746.

4.   Krugman, S., Goodrich, C.H., Ward, R. 1957. Pri-
     mary varicella pneumonis. *N.Engl.J.Med. 257:* 843-
     848.

5.   Griffith, J.F.,Salon, M.B., and Adams, R.D. 1970.
     The nervous system diseases associated with vari-
     cella. *Acta Neurol Scandinav, 46*:279-300.

ACKNOWLEDGEMENT

This research was supported by the Children's
Hospital Research Foundation, Children's Hospital,
Columbus, Ohio.

DISCUSSION

D.B. Tower - Did you do ammonia levels on any of
     these patients,and would this be a significant
     factor in differentiating those that might be
     potential Reye's candidates?

R. Hochberger - We did not do blood ammonias.

E. S. Kang   - I wonder what the significance of the
    difference is between your control and Reye's
    group?

R. Hochberger - I'm sorry; at this point, I can't
    answer. None of the patients or controls devel-
    oped Reye's syndrome.

REYE'S SYNDROME IN NORTHEASTERN THAILAND

Kamnual Dhiensiri, M.D., Poonsiri Sinavatana, M.D.,
Suwat Lertsookprasert, M.D.

INTRODUCTION

Since Reye, Morgan and Baral (1) in 1963 described
the clinical and pathological features of a disease
which was later widely recognized as Reye's syndrome,
numerous publications on this syndrome have been appear-
ing in the literature. Most of the reports have been
from Western countries. Reports from Asian countries
were scanty (2,3,4). In 1968 it was first recognized
that a disease which has been found to be an endemic
disease in northeastern Thailand was similar to Reye's
syndrome (5). Autopsy findings have established its existence since at least 1963 (5). In Khon Kaen, a province in N.E. Thailand, the disease was thought to occur
in striking numbers in 1965. According to an observation
of one of the authors (Dhiensiri) a disease similar to
Reye's syndrome had never been recognized before 1959.
In Bangkok (central region) and Chiengmai (northern region) the disease was first recognized in 1968. It has
never been reported from the southern part of Thailand.

The disease in N.E. Thailand is definitely rural,
occurring with regularity. The distribution of disease
is partly correlated with rainfall. A more definite correlation is observed between the disease and agricultural patterns and the use of pesticides.

CASE MATERIALS

Cases of Reye's syndrome from two periods, eight

years apart, are compared to demonstrate the regularity
and pattern of the disease.

1.   Cases that occurred in 1968-1969 were chosen.
The diagnosis was based on the clinical pictures and the
biochemical changes (Table II).   Only a small proportion
were examined at autopsy.   However, these cases were
considered to be sufficiently reliable because most of
the cases were seen by one of the authors (Dhiensiri).

2.   Cases in 1976 were selected because of their
diagnostic reliability (Table I).   Shown in Table II
and Table III are criteria for the diagnosis, both clinical and tissue diagnosis.   Not included in the series
were ten deaths diagnosed as Reye's syndrome but the records were not available.   Among these were eight females
and two males.

TABLE I

Reye's syndrome cases admission at
Khon Kaen Hospital 1976

	Total	Male	Female
Number	63	27	36
Mortality	35 (55.5%)	13 (37%)	22 (63%)
Autopsy	5		
Liver biopsy or necropsy	37		
Cases that died but records not available for analysis	10	2	8

RESULTS

A comparison of Reye's syndrome occurring during
the two periods demonstrates that the pattern of the
disease has not changed.

Number of patients: The number of cases admitted
to Khon Kaen Hospital each year varies only slightly.

TABLE II

Reye's syndrome - Clinical diagnosis

1. Acute onset of encephalopathy

    - convulsion and coma
    - absence of laterizing signs

2. Hepatic involvement

    - hypoglycemia
    - elevation of transaminases
    - absence of jaundice

3. C.S.F. normal except low sugar

TABLE III

Reye's syndrome - Tissue diagnosis

1. Biopsy of the liver

    - fine vacuolization of hepatocytes
    - necrosis absent or minimal
    - portal infiltration of lymphocytes
      mild

2. Autopsy

    - liver fatty degeneration
    - brain edema
    - kidney fatty degeneration

The average admission has been 80 cases per year.

Race: All were native Thai children.

Sex: During 1968-1969 no definite documentation
on exact numbers in each sex was made. However, it was

thought that the incidence was slightly higher among
females. A limited study in 1970 (6) showed no sex
difference. In 1976 the number of females was definitely higher. Moreover, the mortality was also higher
among females (Table I).

Age. The ages of the patients during the two
periods are shown in Figure 1 and Figure 2. A similarity between those periods was noted. The majority of
cases were from one to seven years old. This was also
noted in the study at Udorn in 1969 (7). The youngest
patients during those periods were six months old.

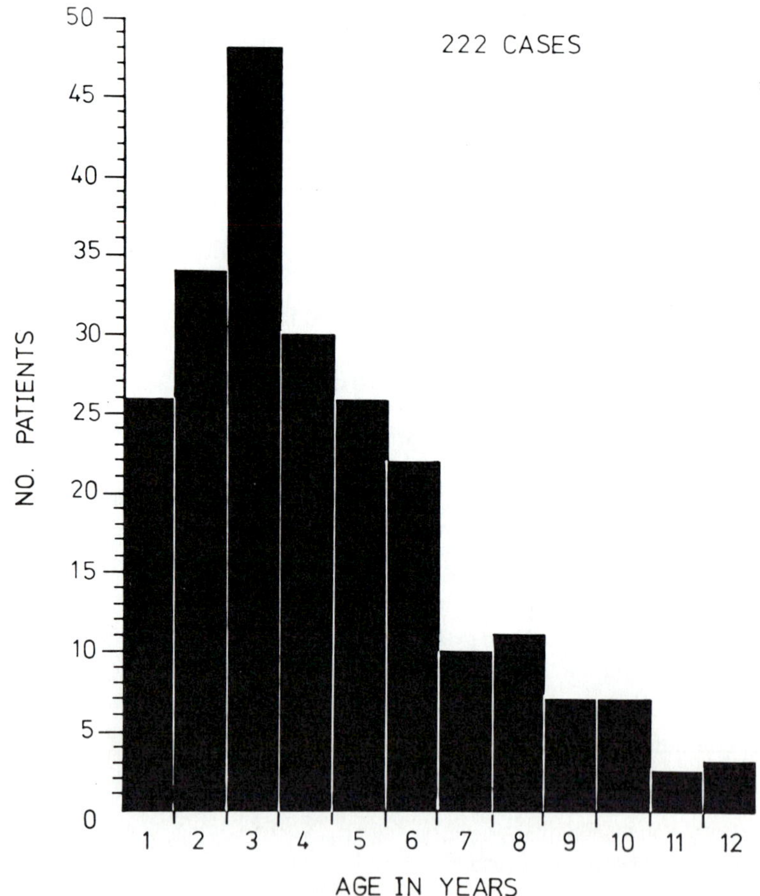

Figure 1. Reye's syndrome 1967 - 1969
            Age incidence

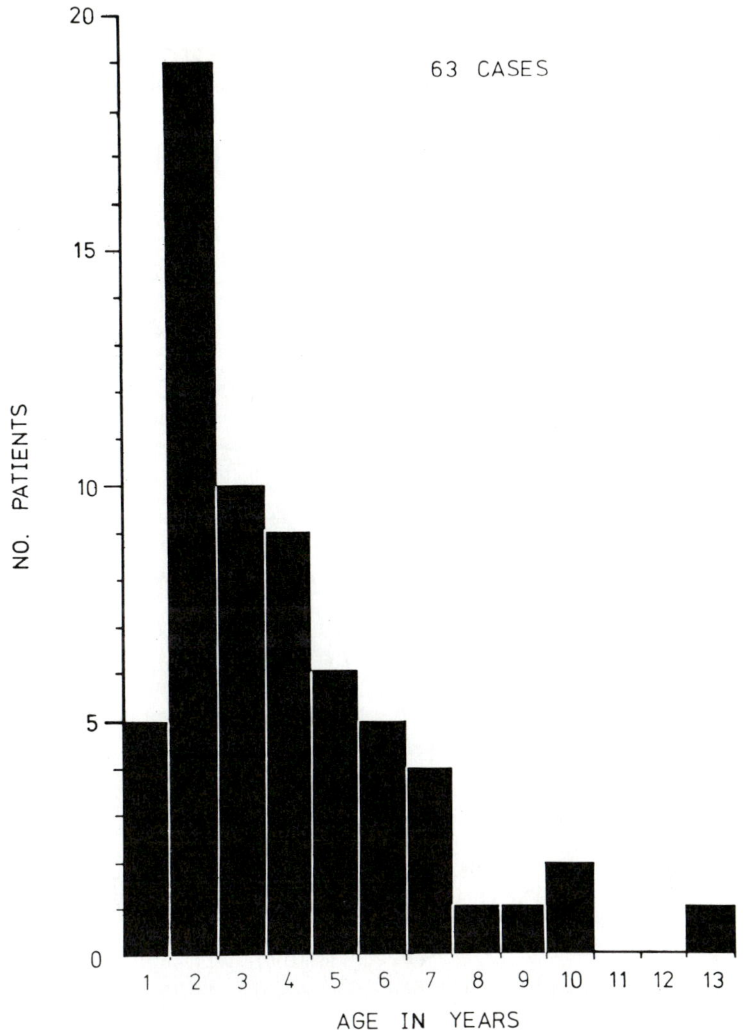

Figure 2.   Reye's syndrome 1976   63 cases
                 Age   Incidence

     Geographic distribution;   Records were available
for analysis only in 1976 (Figure 3).   All patients
were from rural villages, none from city areas. The
pattern was thought to be the same during the past
years.   The majority of cases were from the villages
located close to the hospital.   In four nearby districts

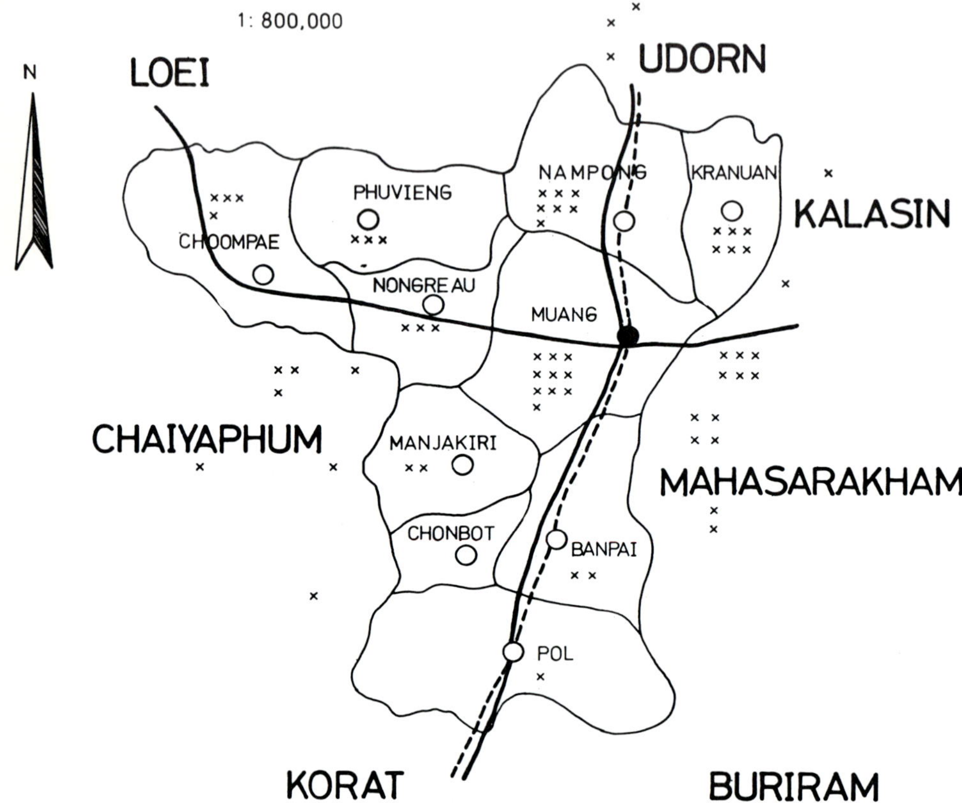

Figure 3.   Geographic distribution of Reye's
            syndrome in 1976.

(Manjakiri, Chonbot, Banpai and Pol) where transport-
ation is considered convenient, only five cases were
admitted to the hospital. It might be possible that
some cases from those districts did not come to the
hospital but instead were seen at local health centers.
It was also possible that the incidence was actually
low because there were more patients from far away
districts admitted to the hospital during the same
period. An interesting observation on the four
districts mentioned earlier is that rice cultivation

is much less in these districts due to the lack of an
adequate irrigation system (8).

   <u>Seasonal distribution.</u> The majority of cases occurred during May to November with a cluster of cases
between July and October (51 - 58%) (Fig.4). Upon a
closer look it was apparent that the incidence of cases
was more closely related to the amount of rainfall except during the later part of the rainy season in which
case the number of patients remained high despite the
decline in the amount of rain water (Fig.5).

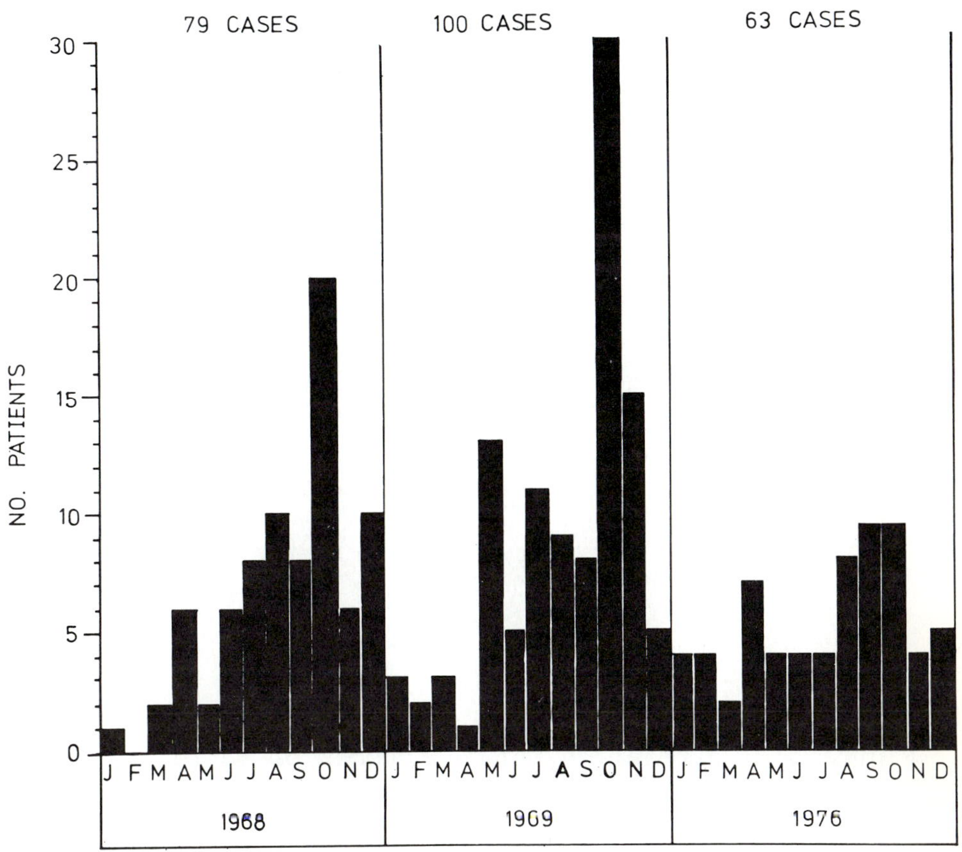

Figure 4. Number of children with Reye's
           syndrome admitted per month to
           Khon Kaen Hospital

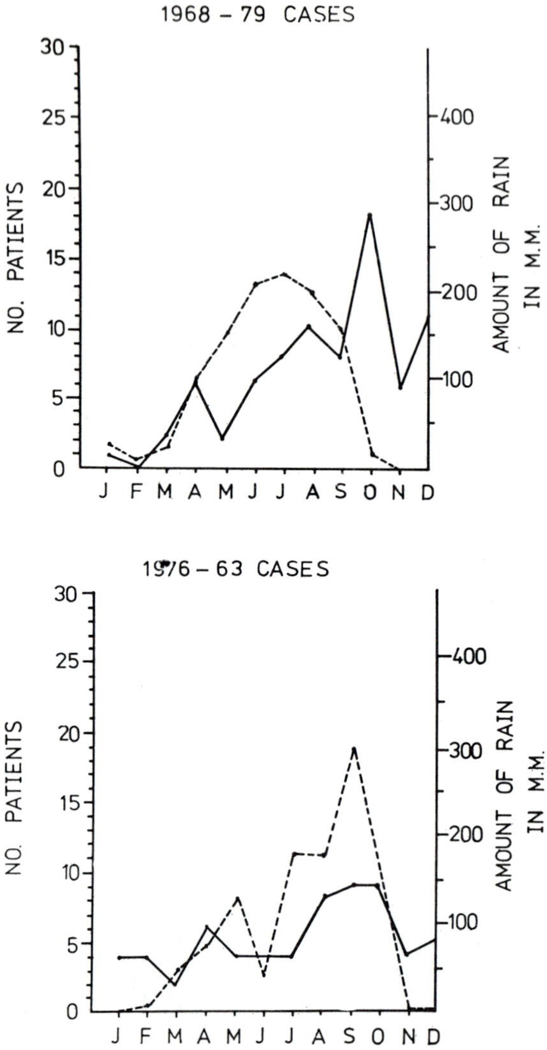

Figure 5.   Correlation between number of patients
and the amount of rainfall
----- rainfall
______ number of patients

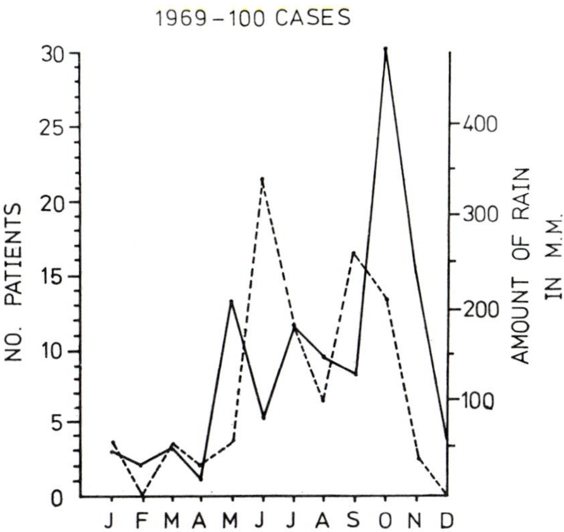

Figure 5. (continued)

    <u>Exposure to pesticides.</u> In N.E. Thailand agri-
culture depends mainly on the rainfall. A year of
good rainfall means a year of good agriculture. Rice
cultivation accounts for the major agriculture. Cultivation of vegetables (cucumbers and string beans) is
also widely practiced among villagers though to a much
lesser extent. Figure 6 displays the pattern of cult -
ivation of rice and vegetables and the use of pesticides
and a single herbicide. Pesticides were used all
year round but the use was heavy during July to October.
Greater exposure to pesticides was certain to occur
during this period. Folidon E 605 (Parathion) is the
most common pesticide used among the villagers. Other
pesticides used to a lesser extent were Sevin (carba-
mate) and Endrin (organochlorine).

    <u>Treatment and mortality.</u> Our standard treatment as
of 1976 consists of an immediate administration of
50% glucose solution. Insulin is used in conjunction
with glucose at the proportion of one unit of insulin
per five grams of glucose. Maintenance fluid is 10%
dextrose in 1/2 or 1/3 N.S.S. The amount of fluid used

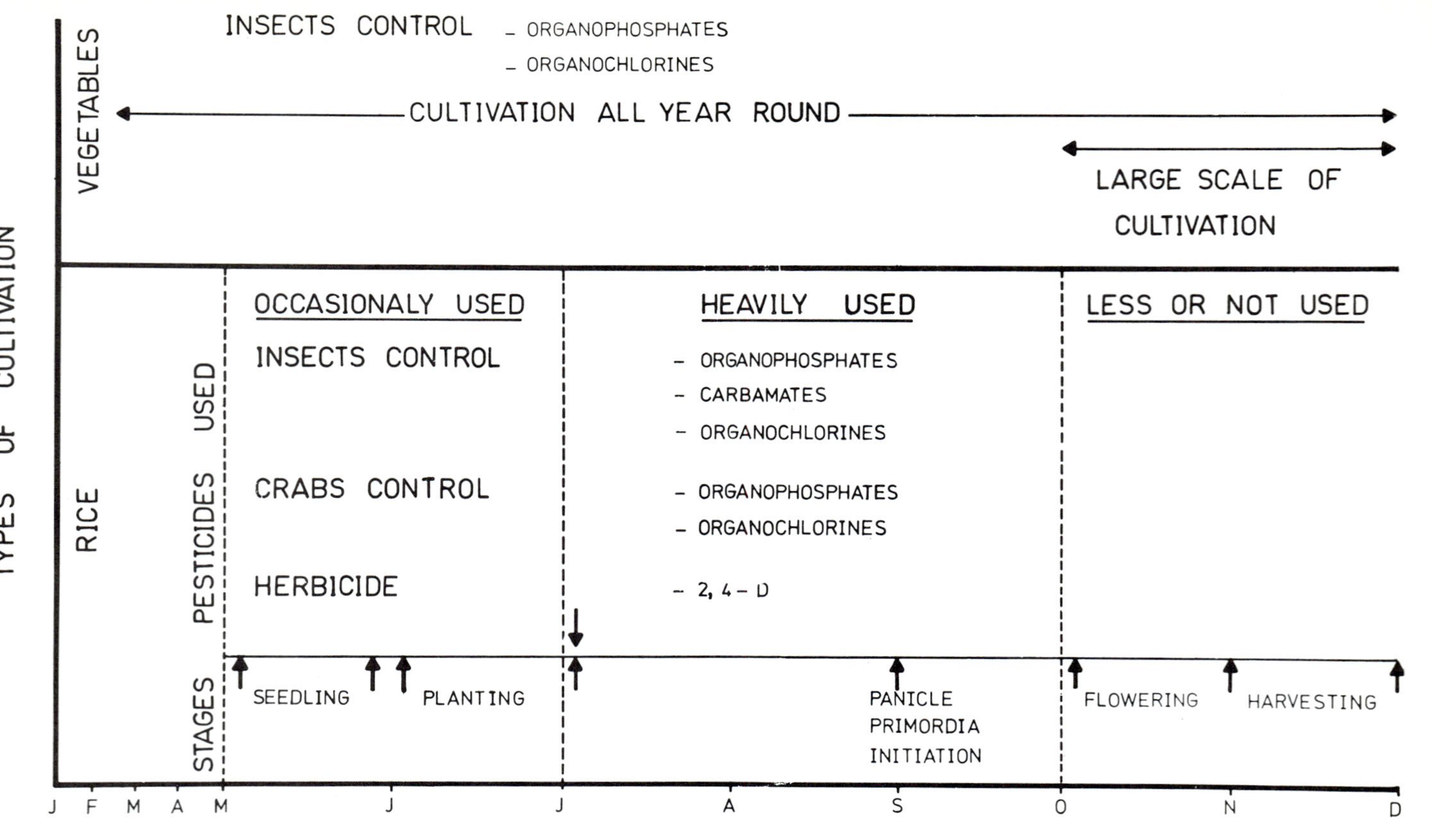

Figure 6. The use of pesticides and herbicide in agriculture in N.E. Thailand.

is two-thirds of the calculated maintenance need. Sodium bicarbonate is not usually given. Mannitol is given in a dose of one gram per kilogram body weight every four to six hours. Steroid usually in the form of dexamethasone is also used. Vitamin K is given intravenously as a single dose. Nasogastric intubation and gastric lavage are used at the time of admission. Neomycin is given by a nasogastric tube. Exchange blood transfusion has never been used because of the scarcity of blood. The overall mortality is still high at 60%.

In 1968-69 the treatment was less uniform. All of the patients received 50% glucose solution. Used from time to time were mannitol, steroids and insulin, neomycin by nasogastric tube,and enemas. The mortality was 80%.

DISCUSSION

In N.E. Thailand, the characteristic features of the disease enable an early presumptive diagnosis. Immediate treatment can be given in most cases. Non-histologic diagnosis is possible when the criteria for diagnosis are met (6). Since 1970, prothrombin time has not been performed routinely due to limitation of the laboratory facilities. We have used the criteria for clinical diagnosis of Reye's syndrome as in Table II.

In general, the clinical features of the syndrome have not changed from earlier case reports from N.E. Thailand (6,7,9). We wish to bring up some observations which are still unique and very consistent. An overall observation indicates a higher incidence and mortality rate in females. Hypoglycemia is still a consistent laboratory finding (71% in 1976). Most of the patients were admitted to the hospital because of convulsion and coma. The onset of convulsion and coma is usually abrupt and occurs in the morning in about two-thirds of the cases.

Typically, the parents will give the following history:
"The child was well in the evening. She ate her supper
and went to sleep in the usual manner. She woke up during the night asking for water, and went back to sleep
again. In the morning she appeared to be lethargic and
did not eat her breakfast. Suddenly, convulsion occurred, followed by a deep and sustained coma."

We observed some degree of immediate improvement
in the majority of cases after an intravenous administration of 50% glucose solution. For example, an improvement of respiration or a decrease in decorticate
or decerebrate posture were usually observed. However, the patients usually remained unconscious. Only
ı few regained consciousness shortly after I.V.glucose.

Hyperkalemia has been reported in a significant
number of patients with this syndrome in N.E. Thailand,
and indicated a poor outcome (6,7). In 1976 we found
44% of the patients had serum potassium higher than 5.6
mEq/liter.

Hepatomegaly, which is a consistent finding in
most series, is less striking in our series. In most
cases, liver was not enlarged on admission, although
later in the course of the disease it became enlarged.

Vomiting which is very consistent in most series
and being pernicious, is less so in our series. A history of vomiting prior to the onset of convulsion and
coma was obtained in two-thirds of the cases.

ETIOLOGIC CONSIDERATION

Viruses. Most of the cases reported in the literature had preceding illnesses similar to viral infections. Viruses commonly implicated in the etiology of
Reye's syndrome include influenza B virus and varicella
virus. In N.E. Thailand, no particular viruses were
found to be related to the disease (9). In Bangkok,
influenza A virus was thought to be the cause (10).
However, the number of patients studied was small. In
Thailand, where thousands of cases of varicella occur
annually, no report of Reye's syndrome has ever been

associated with this infection.

Mycotoxin. Aflatoxin B1 was proposed as a possible etiologic agent (11). Argument against this possibility was made by Glasgow (12). We would like to
point out some further observations about aflatoxin. In
N.E.Thailand, infants are usually fed with a pre-
chewed form of a sticky rice as early as 2 - 3 days of
age. In this connection, young animals are known to be
more susceptible to this toxin. Hence, we might expect
to see more cases of Reye's syndrome in the N.E. in
young infants. But the youngest patients recorded were
aged six months and, even then, the number of cases were
very few. Another point is that the native children who
live in town actually have the same foods as the children in the villages,thus exposing them similarly to
aflatoxin. We have not seen a single patient from the
city area.

Drugs. Salicylates and phenothiazine were mentioned to be associated with Reye's syndrome (13,14,15).
In Thailand serum salicylate level was measured in only
few cases, and the level was usually below the toxic level (10,16). In N.E. Thailand measurement of salicylate
is not considered necessary, since the drugs are usually
not given or else given in a small amount for a short
duration, due to rapidity of onset of convulsion and coma. Phenothiazine is not commonly used for vomiting.

Viral-toxin interaction. A synergistic interaction between an acute viral infection and a subclinical chronic exposure to an exogeneous toxin has
been suggested by Colon et al (17). Crocker et al (18)
demonstrated a synergistic interaction between insecticides and viral infection. A maximum effect was noted
when insecticides were used in combination.

Evidence of viral-like infection was obtained in 80% of our cases. Prodromal symptoms were fever, URI, diarrhea,vomiting and lethargy. The duration of pro-drome was from one to three days. Prodrome was negative in 20% of the cases. However,the lack of prodrome does not necessarily deny the existence of mild preceding illness. In N.E.Thailand the presence of a mild URI or diarrhea may not be noticed or considered by the parents to be an illness. Among the cases reported from Bangkok prodrome was present in 100% of the cases (10,16,19).

Reye's syndrome in Thailand is thought to be a new disease. Its occurrence has coincided with the wide use of pesticides. Shown in Figure 7 is the amount of pes-ticides imported into Thailand. The amount was signifi-cantly increased after 1965, the year in which we be-lieved the syndrome was first observed in striking num-bers. A definite decrease in the amount of imported pes-ticides was noted during 1971-1976. DDT and toxaphene which were used in malarial control and cotton farming accounted for this drop. The amount of other pesticides used in another agriculture productivity was thought to be unchanged.

Evidence of a prolonged exposure to pesticides was obtained in 100% of the cases of Reye's syndrome in N.E. Thailand. In rural villages the use of pesticides is extensive,prolonged and with inadequate precaution taken. In city areas, on the other hand,pesticides are used less and probably with better precaution. More convin-cing evidence is shown in Figure 6. Agriculture is the main occupation in N.E.Thailand. Rice cultivation,par-ticularly a glutinous variety,accounts for the major agriculture. Cultivation of rice is usually started in May or June depending on the rainfall. Pesticides and sometimes a herbicide are used during the seedling,up to the heading stages. The use is heavy during tilling and booting stages which are usually between July to October. This period coincides with the peak incidence of the disease. Vegetable (cucumbers and string beans) cultivation is also widely practiced by farmers.The cultivation of vegetables is much more common during the early winter season because of the good weather. When

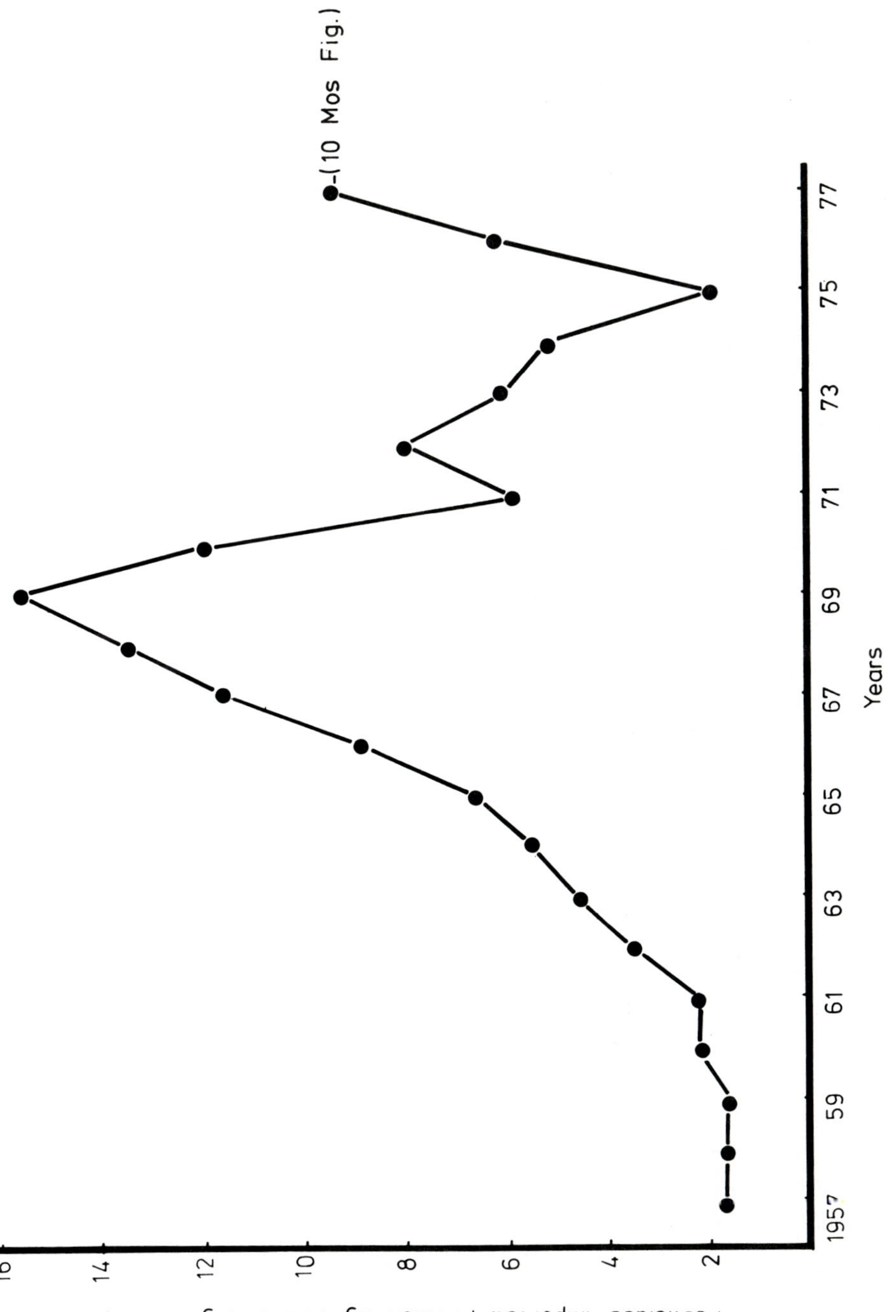

Figure 7. Pesticide Importation in Thailand (1957-77) (Analysed from data of pesticide regulation division, Ministry of Agriculture and Cooperatives)

compared to rice, the cultivation of vegetables is
done to a much less extent.Pesticides are also used
with inadequate precautions. Children,therefore, continue to be exposed to pesticides after the rice farming season,but to a lesser degree. This may account
for the sporadic occurrence of the syndromê outside
the rice farming season. We have also observed that
sporadic cases usually come from the villages which
have natural water reservoirs,or a canal,that provides them with water for cultivation.

Villagers frequently use pesticides improperly.
There is a tendency to use a solution with a higher
concentration than recommended by the manufacturing
companies,in order to achieve a maximum effect. A
combination of pesticides is not uncommon. Folidon
(organophosphate) and Endrin (organochlorine) are the
most common combinations.

During the rice farming season, whole families go
to the paddy where there is a small resting shelter.
The mother or an older sibling stays at the resting
area to take care of small children and prepare food.
Water for drinking is normally obtained from a small,
shallow, dug pond containing rainwater. For washing
or cleaning themselves, the family uses water from the
pond but, in some instances, water from the rice field
is used. Older children are allowed to play around the
shelter and in the rice field, which usually is flood-
ed with water. If pesticides have been used, the water
is certainly contaminated, allowing skin contact or un-
intentional swallowing to occur while playing in the
water. It is obvious that older children are at risk.
The spraying of pesticides is done by a simple hand-
spraying instrument. The disposition of pesticide con-
tainers, in some cases, is by leaving them carelessly
scattered around the shelter area. Again,children from
two to six years old are at a higher contact risk,be-
cause of their curiosity.

Children in rural areas in N.E.Thailand are required by law to go to school at seven years of age.

Schools open at the beginning of the rice farming season, and continue up to harvesting time. This will make the children stay out of the paddy and, consequently, school children get less exposure to pesticides. The occurrence of disease is markedly reduced after seven years of age. In the case of infants,the exposure to pesticides by the above-mentioned means is unlikely. Infants over the age of six months (after teething) are usually allowed to nibble unpeeled cucumbers fresh from the farm. These vegetables are usually sprayed with pesticides. We would like to emphasize that our cases of Reye's syndrome do not occur in infants younger than six months.

There are some differences in methods of rice cultivation in the central,northern and southern regions. Pesticides are usually used with better precaution,and children are usually not brought to the rice fields. Only children in rural villages in N.E.Thailand go with the parents to the paddy during the rice farming season, usually every day. Taking more precautions and not taking children into the paddy probably account for the less frequent occurrence of the syndrome in these other regions.

In Bangkok, with a population of 4.8 million, the incidence averaged 50 cases or less per year. The incidence of the disease,when compared to the province of Khon Kaen with a population of 1.2 million, is much lower. With far better medical services and a greater awareness of this disease among pediatricians in Bangkok itself, the possibility that the cases may pass unrecognized is less likely. The urban incidence is thought to be declining in the past few years. The age incidence in Bangkok cases (10,16,19) was mostly under two years. The majority of cases have occurred during the rainy season (16,19). The children affected were from families of low socio-economic status. The mosquito population is high during the rainy season, particularly in the area where the standard of living is low. The use of DDT for mosquito control is higher during that period. Infants are expected to get highest

exposure then, since they stay inside a room most of
the time. Another route of entry of DDT in infants is
breast milk. The milk of lactating women who are exposed to DDT usually contains a significant amount of
insecticide (20). In Thailand, breast feeding is common sometimes up to two years, especially among the
low-income group.

CONCLUSION

The existence of Reye's syndrome in N.E.Thailand
has been established. The disease may have existed previously, however, the incidence increased after 1960.
A comparison between two periods, eight years apart,
demonstrates a regularity and a repeating pattern of
the disease. The disease is rural. Distribution of the
disease relates closely to the types of agriculture
practiced by villagers. A correlation between the geographic use of pesticides and the incidence of the disease is emphasized. Our findings would tend to support
the hypothesis of viral-toxin interaction as a possible
etiologic factor of Reye's syndrome. However,many aspects of the syndrome are still left unexplained;e.g.,
the occurrence of only a single case per village, racial predilection, and sex prevalence. It is possible
that genetic, nutritional or other unidentified environmental factors may equally play a role in the etiology of this syndrome.

ACKNOWLEDGEMENT
We wish to express our gratitude to Dr. Allen Glasgow whose initial work and continuing interest in Reye
syndrome in Khon Kaen has encouraged us to pursue the
study. Contributions of Drs. Aroon Veerasethakul, Su-
wali Sripo, Sirichit Vasanavatana, and Miss Sumamarn
Chareonka are gratefully acknowledged.

<u>REFERENCES</u>

1.   Reye,R.K.D.,Morgan,G.,and Baral,J. 1963. Enceph-
     alopathy and fatty degeneration of the viscera:A
     disease entity in childhood. *Lancet 2:*749.

2. Mathewson,I.,1968. Encephalopathy and fatty degeneration of the viscera. *Far East Med.J. 4:7.*

3. John,T.J.,Mammen,K.C.,Date,A.,and Kamath,K.R. 1969. Acute encephalopathy with fatty degeneration of the viscera: A study of three cases in India.*Ind.J. Med. Res. 57:10.*

4. Burns,R.R.,Silverberg,S.G. 1970.Encephalopathy and fatty degeneration of the viscera (Reye's syndrome) A clinico-pathologic entity?*S. Med.J.63:183.*

5. Olson,L.C.,Bourgeois,C.H,Keschamras,N.,Harikul,S, Sanyakorn,C.K.,Grossman,R.A.,Smith,T.J. 1970.Encephalopathy and fatty degeneration of the viscera in Thai children.*Am.J.Dis.Child. 120:1.*

6. Glasgow,A.M.,Cotton,R.B.,Dhiensiri,K. 1972. Reye's syndrome. Blood ammonia and consideration of the non-histologic diagnosis.*Am.J.Dis.Child. 124:827.*

7. Olson,L.C.,Bourgeois,C.H.,Cotton,R.B.,Harikul, S., Grossman,R.A. and Smith,T.J. 1971. Encephalopathy and fatty degeneration of the viscera in northeastern Thailand:Clinical and epidemiology.*Pediatrics 47:707.*

8. Report from the Department of Agriculture, Khon Kaen Division.

9. Bourgeois,C.H.,Olson,L.C.,Comer,D.,Evan,H., Keschamras,N.,Cotton,R.B.,Grossman,R. and Smith, T. 1971. Encephalopathy and fatty degeneration of the viscera A clinicopathologic diagnosis of 40 cases.*Am.J.Clin. Path. 56:588.*

10. Visudhiphan,P.,Chatiyanonda,K. 1975. Isolation of influenza A virus in Reye's syndrome.*Southeast Asian Jrnl.Trop. Med.Pub.Health 6:260.*

11. Bourgeois,C.H.,Shank,R.C.,Grossman,R.A.,John,D.C., Wooding,W.P. and Chandhavimol,P. 1971. Acute aflatoxin Bl toxicity in the macaque and its similarities to Reye's syndrome.*Lab.Invest. 24:206.*

12. Pollack,J.D., Ed., 1975. Reye's syndrome, N.Y., Grune & Stratton, Inc.   p.170.

13. Mortimer,E.A. and Lepow,M.L. 1962. Varicella with hypoglycemia possibly due to salicylates. *Am.J.Dis. Child. 103:91.*

14. Glick,T.H.,Likowski,W.H.,Levit,L.P.,Mellin,H. and Reynolds,D.W. 1970. Reye's syndrome:An epidemiologic approach. *Pediatrics 46:371.*

15.   Giles,H.McC. 1965. Encephalopathy and fatty de-
      generation of the viscera. *Lancet 1:*1075.
16.   Tuchinda,C., 1977. Reye's syndrome. *Med.Practice
      M emo. 1:*350.
17.   Colon,A.R.,Ledesma,F.,Pardo,V. and Sandberg,D.H.
      1974.Viral potentiation of chemical toxins in ex-
      perimental syndrome of hypoglycemia, encephalo-
      pathy, and visceral fatty degeneration. *Am.J.Dig.
      Dis. 19:*1091.
18.   Crocker,J.F.S.,Rozee,K.R.,Ozere,R.L.,Digout,S.C.
      and Hutzinger,O. 1974. Insecticides and viral in-
      teraction as a cause of fatty visceral changes and
      encephalopathy in the mouse. *Lancet 2:*22.
19.   Sunakorn,P.,Rajadanurak,K. 1975. Reye's syndrome.
      *J. Med.Ass.Thailand 58:*393.
20.   Casarett & Doull. Toxicology: The basic science of
      poisons. New York: Macmillan Publishing Co.Inc.,
      1975. p 433.

<u>DISCUSSION</u>

F.L. Ruben -   A few years ago, work or researchers in
      Thailand were commenting on Aflatoxins as being
      the etiologic agents, and set the picture of rur-
      al distribution as opposed to urban. Why has your
      region of Thailand chosen to use pesticides and
      herbicides, whereas the other regions of Thailand,
      I take it, are not using these chemicals?

K.Dhiensiri - Actually, we use them in every part of
      the country. The difference is the method of how
      we carry it out. In Northeastern Thailand,usually
      the whole family goes to the paddy every day,but
      in the other parts usually they don't take the
      children to the paddy; I think that explains why
      the children in the other parts of the country
      are not exposed to pesticides like in the north-
      east.

J.D. Pollack - I can't bring myself right now to sub-
        scribe to the aflatoxin theory .. at least, in
        our own studies. I do know that the toxogenic
        strains of Aspergillus flavus and other Aspergil-
        lus species will only produce aflatoxin in situ-
        ations of high humidity; that,when it is dry,they
        don't produce any toxin, even those that are ca-
        pable of it. When it is wet at a 20 - 40% rela-
        tive humidity, either in the lab or in the field,
        those strains which can produce aflatoxin do,
        particularly on grain such as rice. That's just
        a comment. My question is; did you find any afla-
        toxin or these pesticides in the children?

K.Dhiensiri - We did not do any measurement of either
        toxin or insecticides in our patients. Our hos-
        pital doesn't have such a facility. As for afla-
        toxin, Dr.Glasgow in the last meeting in Columbus
        made an observation against aflatoxin as the
        cause of Reye's Syndrome in Northeast Thailand.
        I would like to add further evidence that seems
        to indicate that aflatoxin may not relate to the
        syndrome. First, in N.E. Thailand infants as
        young as two or three days are fed with sticky
        rice. If aflatoxin in sticky rice is the cause
        of the syndrome, we would expect to see the syn-
        drome in young infants. Still, we have not seen
        Reye's syndrome in infants younger than six
        months. Secondly, if children move from the rice
        farming area to the city, they don't get the dis-
        ease. It seems to me that children get the dis-
        ease only when they live in the rice farming area
        or when they ingest cucumber freshly taken from
        the farm.

F.Yamashita - This morning, I mentioned that in Ja-
        pan we have had Akee syndrome which has the same
        symptoms as in Reye's syndrome,so I would like to
        ask you; have you dysentery infection in these
        cases?

K.Dhiensiri - We have quite a number of patients who
        have a prodrome of vomiting and diarrhoea, and
        some of them pass stools containing mucous, but we

are not able to culture or to isolate any
other pathology or bacteria. So we conclude
that it is probably non-specific.

F. Yamashita   -   I am impressed with the high in-
stance of convulsion in your study.

K. Dhiensiri   -   Yes; most of our cases come in with
convulsions and coma, and that is the symptom
that brings the patient to the hospital. We
rarely see patients like you see in Western
countries with chicken pox, improving and then
getting progressively lethargic with pernicious vomiting.

Unidentified   -   Has anyone measured the concentration of insecticide in the breast milk of Thai
women?

K. Dhiensiri   -   No; I don't think so.

Unidentified   -   The same argument that you used a-
gainst aflatoxin can be used against insecticides, in that the babies could be getting
tremendous amounts of insecticides in the
breast milk.

K. Dhiensiri   -   I don't think anyone in Thailand
has done this.

SECTION II

CLINICAL EXPERIENCE

REYE'S SYNDROME IN INFANCY.
STUDIES ON AMMONIA METABOLISM.

Claude L. Morin, M.D., M. Sc.,
Michel Weber, M.D., Ijaz Qureshi,
Ph D., and Jacques LeTarte,M.D.

Between January 1970 and May 1978, 39 children
(23 boys and 16 girls) were treated at Sainte-Justine
Hospital in Montreal for Reye's syndrome. For all
these patients,with the exception of two who were symp-
tomatic siblings of referred patients, a liver biopsy
was done during the acute phase of the syndrome and
frozen sections, stained with oil-red-o, showed massive
micro-vesicular fatty infiltration. The diagnosis
rested also on clinical and biological data; i.e., an
acute onset in a previously healthy child of central
nervous system dysfunction and hepatic involvement as
evidenced by an increase in transaminase activities.We
have dealt with a very young population with a mean age
of 2.6 years, going from three weeks to eleven years.
Of these 39 patients, 19 were under one year with a mean
age of 0.36 years. The older group comprised 20 children with a mean age of 4.8 years.
The purposes of this work were to, 1) review some
biological and clinical features of this very young
population with the syndrome, especially emphasizing
the high incidence of neurological sequellae in the
patients under one year of age, 2)draw special attention to the occurrence of relapses in some patients,
3)present results of studies on ammonia metabolism in
families with children recovered from Reye's syndrome.
Table 1 and Figure 1 show some clinical and laboratory data obtained from patients under one year of age
as compared with those of the older group. As previously reported, vomiting was a cardinal clinical feature of the children over one year of age. 95% of them

presented this symptom as they enter the second phase
of the illness. However, only 52.6% of the children
under one year presented this symptom. Seizures occurred in 52.6% of the children under one year and in
35% of the older group. For all these patients but one,
an E.E.G. was recorded as soon after admission as possible and scored according to criteria published by
Aoki and Lombroso (1). No difference was observed between the two groups. Coma staging was done according
to criteria set by Schubert and co-workers (2). Even
though the encephalopathy with a mean score of 3.6 was
more severe in the younger population as compared with
2.6 of the older group, no statistical difference was
observed between the two groups.

TABLE 1—*Clinical and Laboratory Data*

	< 1 year	> 1 year
Vomiting	10/19 (52.6%)	19/20 (95%)
Seizures	10/19 (52.6%)	7/20 (35%)
E.E.G. grading ($\bar{X} \pm$ SD)	2.4 ($\pm$ 1.3)	2.1 ($\pm$ 1.6)
Coma stage ($\bar{X} \pm$ SD)	3.6 ($\pm$ 1.3)	2.6 ($\pm$ 1.9)

The S.G.P.T. activity, blood sugar and prothrombin
time as determined during the initial work-up of both
groups of patients are shown in Figure 1. The numbers
in parentheses represent the numbers of patients in
whom the determination was done. The small number of
blood sugar determinations is due to the exclusion of
patients already receiving glucose infusion at the time
of determination. S.G.P.T. activity in the younger
group was twice as high as in the older group while
mean blood sugar was 51.9 mg/dl as compared to 74.6
mg/dl in the older group. There was, however, no statistical difference between the two groups. The
prothrombin time was identical and abnormal in both
groups of patients, being respectively 53% and 56% of
normal.

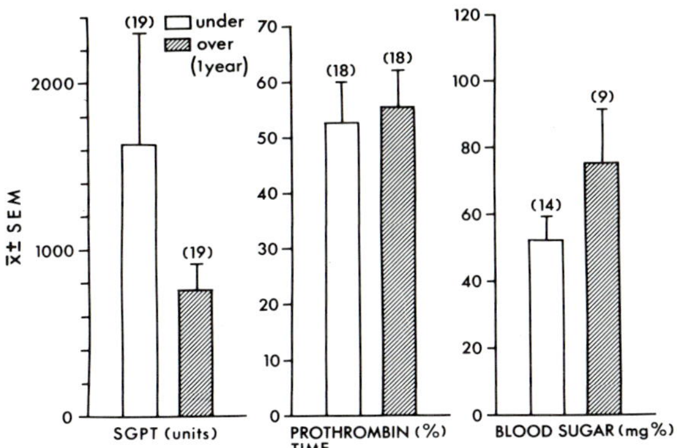

FIG. 1-*Biological Data*

Table 2 shows the outcome in the 39 children with this syndrome. 21 of these children, for 53.4%, recovered completely from their illness. 25.6% had neurologic sequelae while 20% died during the acute phase of the illness. In comparing the children grouped according to age, a very high incidence of neurologic sequelae in the children under one year of age stands out. Of 19 children below one year, 8, that is 42.1%, as compared to 10% for the older group, recovered with severe residual neurologic dysfunction. As a whole the prognosis was very bad in the patients under one year since only 42.1% recovered completely from their syndrome as compared to 65% for the older group. The course of the disease was identical for the 10 patients with neurologic sequelae. They remained comatose for a period of two to three weeks with multiple seizures poorly controlled by medication. Thereafter they showed marked spasticity with a lack of interest and communication or a loss of all cognitive brain function.

TABLE 2-*Outcome in the 39 Children*

	< 1 year (19)	> 1 year (20)	Total (39)
Alive and well	8 (42.1%)	13 (65%)	21 (53.4%)
Neurologic sequelae	8 (42.1%)	2 (10%)	10 (25.6%)
Died	3 (15.8%)	5 (25%)	8 (20%)

An electroencephalogram was performed in all children within a few hours after admission to hospital and
the results are shown in Table 3. If the initial
E.E.G. was considered abnormal, five grades of abnormality were considered as described previously by Aoki
and Lombroso (1). The interpretation of the E.E.G. was
done by a neurologist who was not aware of the clinical
condition of the patient. In our hands, the E.E.G.
grading was a better tool than the initial clinical
staging as a predictor of the final outcome. As shown
in Table 3, no child with an E.E.G. beyond grade II recovered completely from the syndrome. Of 13 patients
with an initial grade II E.E.G., four had neurologic
sequelae while the others recovered completely. One
patient with grade I who died was admitted in shock
with dehydration following a severe diarrhea.

TABLE 3—*Outcome and E.E.G.*

	Alive	Sequelae	Died
Normal	5	–	–
Grade I	7	–	1*
Grade II	9	4**	–
Grade III	–	5	–
Grade IV	–	–	3
Grade V	–	1	4

  *   dehydration, shock
  ** one patient with subdural hematoma

Table 4 shows the outcome in the patients of this
study in relation to treatment. The patients have been
classified according to both treatment and initial
E.E.G. Supportive therapy consists of correction of
coagulation defects with plasma, neomycin administration and 10% dextrose infusion. In the early period of
this study, peritoneal dialysis and supportive therapy
was used while exchange transfusion and supportive
therapy was the treatment used lately. It appears that
beyond an initial E.E.G. of grade II, the outcome of
the children was not influenced by the mode of therapy.

Of seven grade II children with supportive therapy, three had neurological sequelae while of the six treated either by peritoneal dialysis or exchange transfusion, five recovered completely and one had residual neurological damage. However, the number of patients is too small to draw any conclusion.

TABLE 4—*Outcome and Treatment*

	Supportive Therapy	Peritoneal Dialysis	Exchange Transfusion
Normal	o(5)		
Grade I	o(6), +(1)*		o(1)
Grade II	o(4), ●(3)	o(4), ●(1)	o(1)
Grade III	●(2)	●(2)	●(1)
Grade IV	–	+(1)	+(2)
Grade V	+(1)	+(1)	+(2)

    o Alive and well,   ● Sequelae,   + Died
    * Dehydration, shock,   ( ) Number of patients

During this study, four of the 39 children were rehospitalized for a relapse of the syndrome between one to twenty-one months after their initial episode. At discharge following the first episode, all had normal liver function tests and had, with the exception of one patient who suffered from neurologic sequelae, resumed a normal E.E.G. pattern. At relapse, all four presented with a clinical picture similar to the initial, but of lesser severity. Of these four patients, one presented with multiple relapses as shown in Figure 2. The initial episode as well as the five relapses were preceded by an upper respiratory tract infection followed within a week by vomiting. Echovirus 11 and a parainfluenza type 3 were isolated at the time of two of the six episodes of Reye's syndrome. Four of the six episodes were documented by liver biopsy. E.E.G. stage II and stage I along with seizures and coma were documented for the first two episodes while irritability and periods of drowsiness were observed during the last four relapses. For each bout of Reye's syndrome, a rise in S.G.P.T. activity and an abnormal prothrombin

time were observed. Hypoglycemia was observed for the
first four episodes. This child is now six years old
and had his last bout of Reye's syndrome at 20 months.
Since then, he went through many infections, apparently
of viral origin, without any clinical problem and without any rise of S.G.P.T. activity. His liver and
spleen remain slightly enlarged but a recent investigation including liver function tests and a liver biopsy
showed normal results.

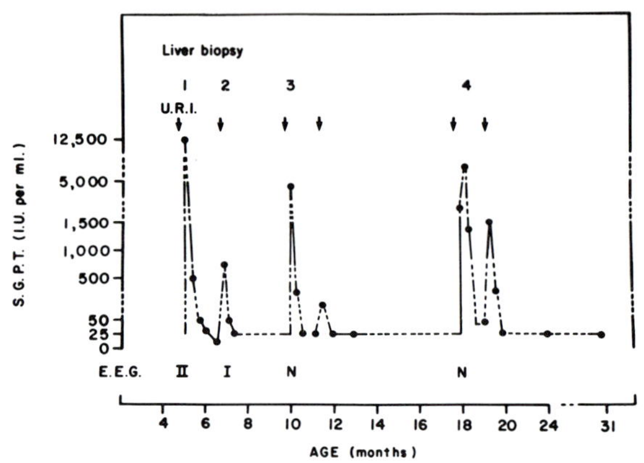

FIG. 2-*A Patient Presenting with Six Episodes of
Reye's Syndrome Following Upper Respiratory Infections
(URI) Indicated by Arrows.

* Reprinted from Pediatrics 59:244-249, 1977 (3)
by kind permission of the American Academy of
Pediatrics.

A study was done on ammonia metabolism in families
with children recovered from Reye's syndrome. This
work was undertaken following the suggestion of Thaler
(4), that patients with Reye's syndrome may suffer from
an inherited defect in ammonia metabolism located in
mitochondria.

Ten of the 39 children just presented were available
for the following study along with 16 male and female
siblings and 19 parents. Control families comprising
20 children and 20 adults were selected from among the
hospital staff and laboratory personnel. As shown in
Table 5, an effort was made to match the ages and com-

position of control families with that of the affected
ones. Among the 10 propositi, 8 had a single bout of
Reye's syndrome while PB (Figure 2) had 6 episodes of
the syndrome. MD had two episodes and one brother who
died from the illness.

A protein-loading protocol was devised for home conditions and consisted of a test menu of mixed protein
providing around 1.5 to 3.0 grams of protein per kilogram of body weight. After the test meal, all urines
were collected for a period of 12 hours. Urinary urea,
ammonia and α-amino nitrogen along with orotic acid
were measured in these specimens and were expressed as
mg or µg of metabolite per mg of urinary creatinine.
Creatinine coefficient was calculated in each case to
verify if the samples were valid. There were no significant differences in values of the creatinine coefficient and protein intake between the affected groups
and respective controls. A protein tolerance test for
hyperammonemia and a measurement of the activity of
liver ornithine transcarbamylase were also performed in
some children.

TABLE 5-*Subjects of Studies on Ammonia Metabolism in
Families with Children Recovered from Reye's Syndrome*

a)	Children		
	Propositi	(8)	: 7.6 ± 1.1 years
	PB		: 3.8
	MD		: 6.4
	Siblings	(16)	: 9.5 ± 0.9
	Controls	(20)	: 7.8 ± 0.7
b)	Adults		
	Parents	(19)	: 34.7 ± 1.1
	Controls	(20)	: 36.2 ± 0.9

PB had 6 episodes of Reye's syndrome as shown in
Figure 2; MD had two episodes and one brother who
died from the illness. ( ) shows the number of
subjects.

Excretion of various urinary nitrogenous metabolites
in children surviving from Reye's syndrome, along with

that of their siblings and controls are shown in Fig -
ures 3 and 4. The results, expressed as per mg of urinary urea and α-amino N (Figure 3) of the eight propositi, were significantly lower as compared to the values of the controls. The siblings in affected families also showed a similar pattern of excretion. The
two children with relapses, PB and MD, showed values
within the range of the other propositi and normal children. Ammonia nitrogen and orotic acid (Figure 4) were
similar in all the groups and PB and MD. The lower urea
excretion in the eight propositi and their siblings
could be interpreted as a residual defect in urea synthesis mechanisms. However, this would be inconsistent
with lack of evidence for concomitant increase in the
excretion of urinary ammonia, α-amino nitrogen and orotic acid. The results obtained in the parents were
similar to those of the adult controls and are not
shown here.

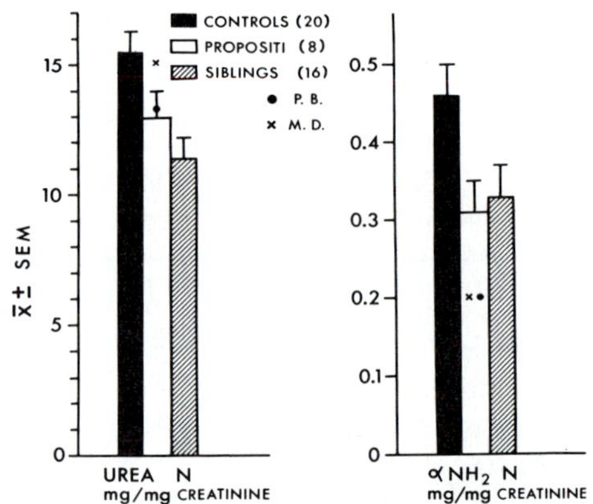

FIG. 3 - *Excretion of Urinary Urea*
        Nitrogen and α-Amino Nitrogen

PB had 6 episodes of Reye's syndrome
as shown in Figure 2; MD had two
episodes and one brother who died from
the illness. ( ) shows the number of
subjects.

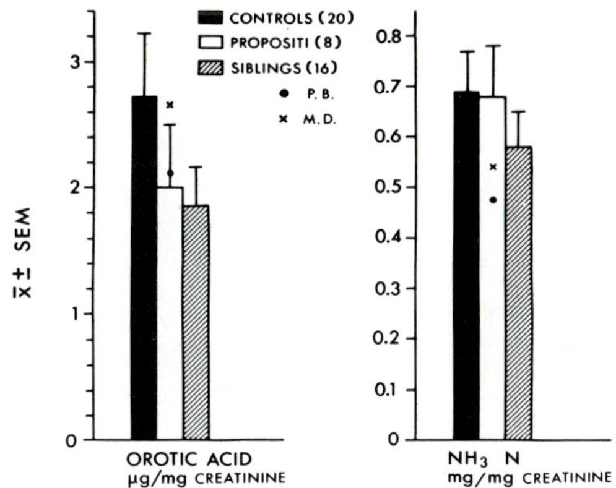

FIG. 4-*Excretion of Urinary Ammonia Nitrogen
and Orotic Acid*

PB had 6 episodes of Reye's syndrome as
shown in Figure 2; MD had two episodes
and one brother who died from the illness.
( ) shows the number of subjects.

The results of the protein loading test for hyperammonemia using a commercial solution of casein-
hydrolysate are shown in Figure 5. A load of 1.5 grams
of protein per kg of body weight was given after a 12-
hour overnight fast. Plasma ammonia and urea nitrogen
were measured before and two hours after the protein
load. The results for the children with relapses, PB
and MD, were within the range of those of 13 normal
children represented by the shaded area. The results
obtained in a confirmed heterozygote of ornithine
transcarbamylase (OTC) deficiency are also shown for
comparison. In this case, the post-loading plasma ammonia nitrogen was higher than the normal range,where-
as urea nitrogen was lower. The heterozygote child with
OTC deficiency had a liver OTC activity of 5.3 μmol/mg
protein/h (5) as compared with normal values of 39.5±
7.1 (X̄ ±SEM) in five controls. PB, who had six episodes of Reye's syndrome, had a normal value of 47.5
from liver tissue obtained while he was in remission.

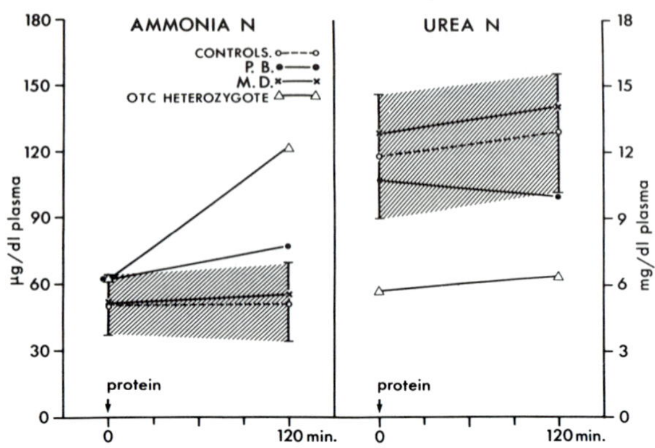

FIG.5 – *Fasting and Post-load Levels of Plasma
Ammonia and Urea Nitrogen*

Shaded areas represent Mean ± SD from
13 control children.

The results of the present study do not indicate
any underlying or residual defect of enzymes related
to ammonia metabolism in affected families.

ACKNOWLEDGEMENT

This work was supported in part by the Fondation
Justine Lacoste-Beaubien.
Doctor Qureshi is the recipient of a research
fellowship from Le Conseil de la Recherche en Sante
du Quebec, Montreal, Quebec.

REFERENCES

1.   Aoki,Y., Lombroso, C.T. 1973. Prognostic value of
     electroencephalography in Reye's syndrome.*Neurology
     23:333.*
2.   Schubert, W.K., Bobo, R.C., Partin, J.C., Partin,
     J.S. 1975. Reye's Syndrome.*Disease-a-Month (Dec.)*

3. Van Caillie, M., Morin, C.L., Roy, C.C., Geoffroy,
    G., McLaughlin, B. 1977. Relapses and Neurologic
    Sequelae in Reye's Syndrome.*Pediatrics 59*:244.
4. Thaler, M.M., Hoogenraad, N.J., Boswell, M. 1974.
    Reye's syndrome due to a novel protein tolerant
    variant of ornithine transcarbamylase deficiency.
    Lancet 2:438.
5. Qureshi, I.A., Letarte, J., Ouellet, R.   1978.
    Study of enzyme defect in a case of ornithine
    transcarbamylase deficiency. *Diabete et Metabol.*
    (In Press).

DISCUSSION

Unidentified Speaker-   In making these studies, one
    should remember that one of the side products of
    the urea cycle is, in fact,creatinine which comes
    from arginine and, if the cycle isn't working very
    well, the creatinine production can go down. As a
    result, many of the indices that you're using can
    be altered; not because one of your metabolites is
    high, but because creatinine is low.

C.L. Morin -   Well, we express the results not
    only by creatinine but also by the amount of pro-
    tein intake.

S.Mayo   -   I wondered if you had any informa-
    tion on the number of cases and relapses of
    Reye's syndrome reported in the Gaspé Peninsula
    area of Quebec. There has been large scale aerial
    insecticide spraying of the forests in that area
    for about the past 10 years.

C.L. Morin -   All of our patients with relapses
    were from the City of Montreal. We had two pa-
    tients from Gaspé, but you have to remember that
    Reye's syndrome is a very acute disease and Gaspé

to Montreal is rather distant. I don't know if
they had time to reach our city.

A.M. Glasgow   -   Have you measured carnitine levels
in your recurrent patients?

C.L. Morin   -   No, we didn't.

A.M. Glasgow   -   We had one patient who seemed to
have recurrent episodes similar to Reye's syndrome,
who had systemic carnitine deficiency, and there
has been one other patient reported. I think this
is a possibility that should be looked at in
these recurrent cases.

C.L. Morin   -   That's very interesting, but I don't
know if that would be likely in 4 patients out of
39.

A.M. Glasgow   -   I think it's another disease in the
differential diagnosis, especially in recurrent
cases. I don't know how common it is; there have
been only three cases reported, and two of those
cases had two episodes similar to Reye's syndrome.

Unidentified Speaker - Did you find abnormal lipid accumulation in the liver, between attacks?

C.L. Morin   -   Between attacks, the liver was normal in the one patient that we studied. One biopsy during one of the acute episodes, at least on
light microscopy, looked like Reye's syndrome with
some subtle differences. Our patient with recur-
rences was not quite as sick, and her transaminases were not as high. In addition, these patients
also manifest muscle weakness that usually began
at about 10 years of age. One little girl, however,
is five now and has a very subtle muscle weakness.

Unidentified Speaker - Looking at Reye's syndrome incidence from the standpoint of urban vs. rural,
is Montreal homogenous, or is it a mixture of suburbs and central core areas like our standard met-

ropolitan areas in the U.S.A.?

C.L. Morin   -   When I say "metropolitan", that includes suburbs, also.

CLINICAL AND ENZYMATIC INDICES OF

HEPATIC DYSFUNCTION IN REYE'S SYNDROME

M.Michael Thaler, M.D.

I dedicate this paper to Ralph Douglas Kenneth
Reye, an Australian pathologist whose legacy has
brought us all together almost exactly one year after
his death. In attempting an assessment of progress a-
chieved in the 15 years since Reye published his observations on the syndrome which bears his name, the fact
emerges that the original report continues to provide
a surprisingly thorough and accurate guide to the established findings. His last published words contain
a clear challenge to us: "We hope that the experience
of others may help to suggest an answer to the problems
of etiology, prevention and treatment." (1) Let us begin to measure the distance travelled by looking over
Reye's shoulder at the moment the "distinctive" histopathological picture captured his expert microscopist's
eye:

"In the liver it is the uniformity and com-
pleteness of the fatty change that is such a
striking feature; every cell in every lobule
is packed with fatty droplets...Despite this
extensive fatty change,there was no necrosis
either of zonal distribution or of individual

115

cells, nor were mitotic figures or binucleate
liver cells present as indirect evidence of
prior cell dissolution." (1)

Most striking in this account is his emphasis on the
contrast between the totality of fatty changes in the
liver in the presence of an otherwise remarkably normal
parenchyma. This perceptive observation clearly points
toward a storage phenomenon, an impression reinforced

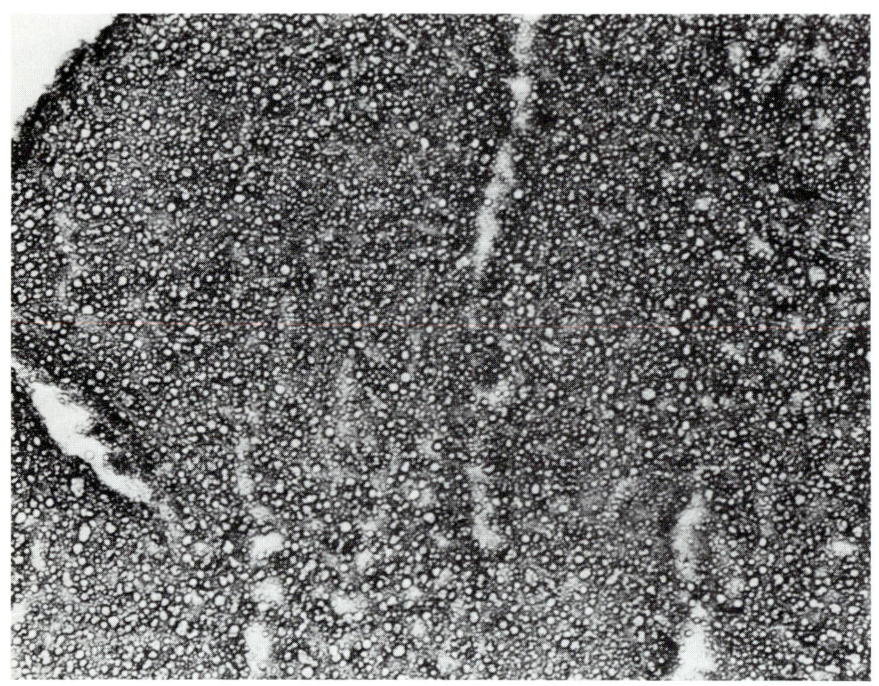

Fig.1. Liver in Reye's syndrome not stained for
       fat, in order to demonstrate "packed" effect
       described by Reye. The lipid deposits, visua-
       lized as globules, are uniform in shape,nearly
       uniform in size, and evenly distributed through-
       out this biopsy specimen obtained approximately
       12 hours after onset of coma.The alternating
       portal and central structures are typical
       "palisades" observed in subcapsular regions
       (capsule at upper left).Fresh frozen section.
       (Giemsa, x80).

by uniformity both in amount and in lobular distribution of the fat. (Fig.1), and by the "owl's eye" appearance of hepatocytes in sections unobscured by fat stains. Reye suggested on the basis of a tissue specimen obtained after recovery from the acute illness,that the fatty changes may disappear after a relatively brief period,revealing an histologically unimpaired parenchyma.(1).

These observations received confirmation when the first ultrastructural studies of the liver in Reye's syndrome (Figs. 2B,2C,3B) became available to us in 1970.(2). In addition, the findings suggested that the outcome of the disorder was not correlated with the degree of fatty deposition in the liver parenchyma during the illness: identical changes were observed in the liver of twins who developed Reye's syndrome within 8 hours of each other,although one twin had just died and the other had been rapidly improving at the time the tissue was obtained. However,light and electron microscopic examination of a follow-up liver biopsy performed after a 3-week interval in the surviving twin indicated clearly that the fatty deposits had nearly disappeared, with only a few microdroplets remaining in the hepatocytes located exclusively in the perisinusoidal cytoplasmic regions.(Figs.3A, 3B). In contrast, the Kupffer cells were now "packed" with lipid microdroplets.

Besides these course-related changes in the cellular distribution of fat, the most striking acute ultrastructural feature was an abundance of peroxisomes, which also disappeared with time.(Compare Figs.2B and 3B). Alterations in other organelles,including the mitochondria, were relatively unimpressive in these initial specimens (Fig.2C) and were seen by us as consistent with the severe metabolic, respiratory and circulatory disturbances associated with the acute illness. Deposits of young collagen within sinusoidal spaces were also interpreted in this light. Since Norman et al (3) and Bourgeois et al (4) had shown that the stored fat in Reye's syndrome consisted of triglycerides, our ultrastructural findings suggested an acute

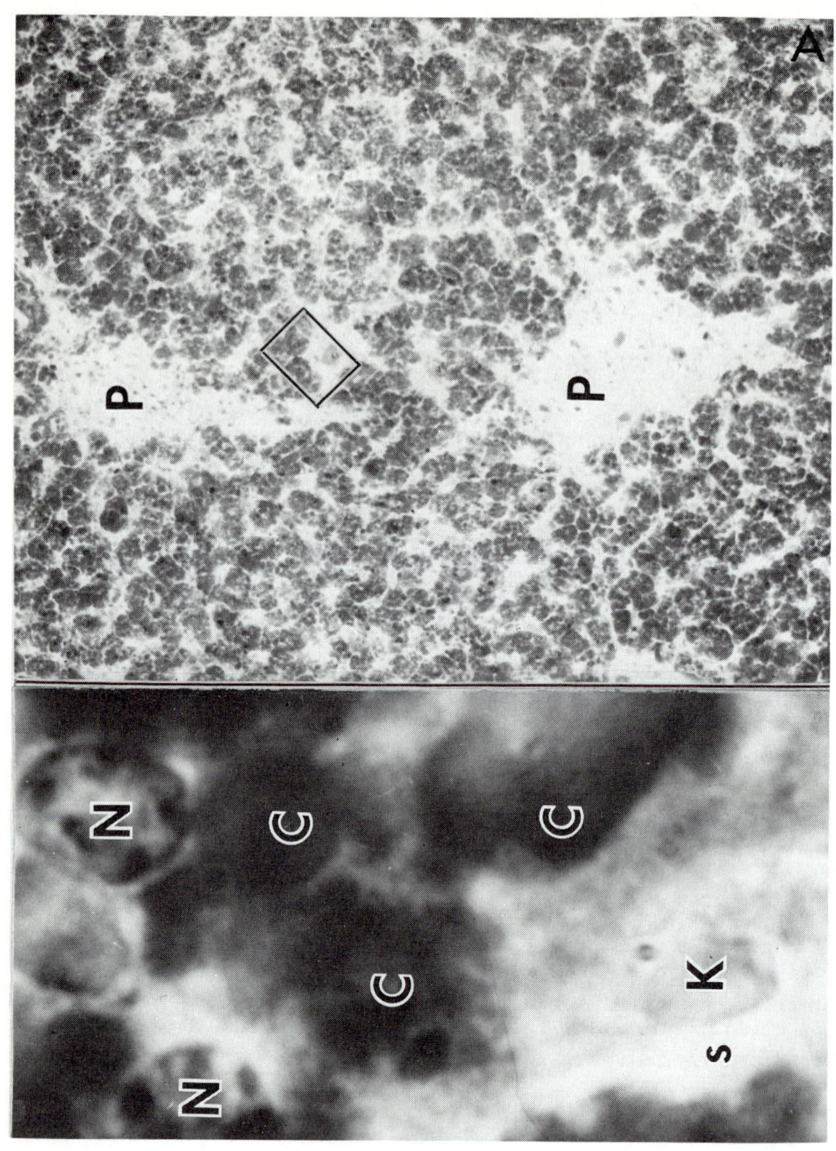

Fig.2A. Liver from one of twins with Reye's syndrome
(details in Reference 2). <u>Right</u> low power view
of parenchyma stained for fat,showing confinement
of lipid to hepatocytes. Structures in portal
triads (P) are uninvolved.(Oil red O,x150). <u>Left</u>
10-fold greater magnification of sinusoidal area
in midzone between two portal areas (enclosed in

black border).Lipid-laden liver cells
contrast sharply with lipid-free Kupffer
cell. C,hepatic cytoplasm; N, hepatic nuclei;
K,Kupffer cell lining sinusoid (s).

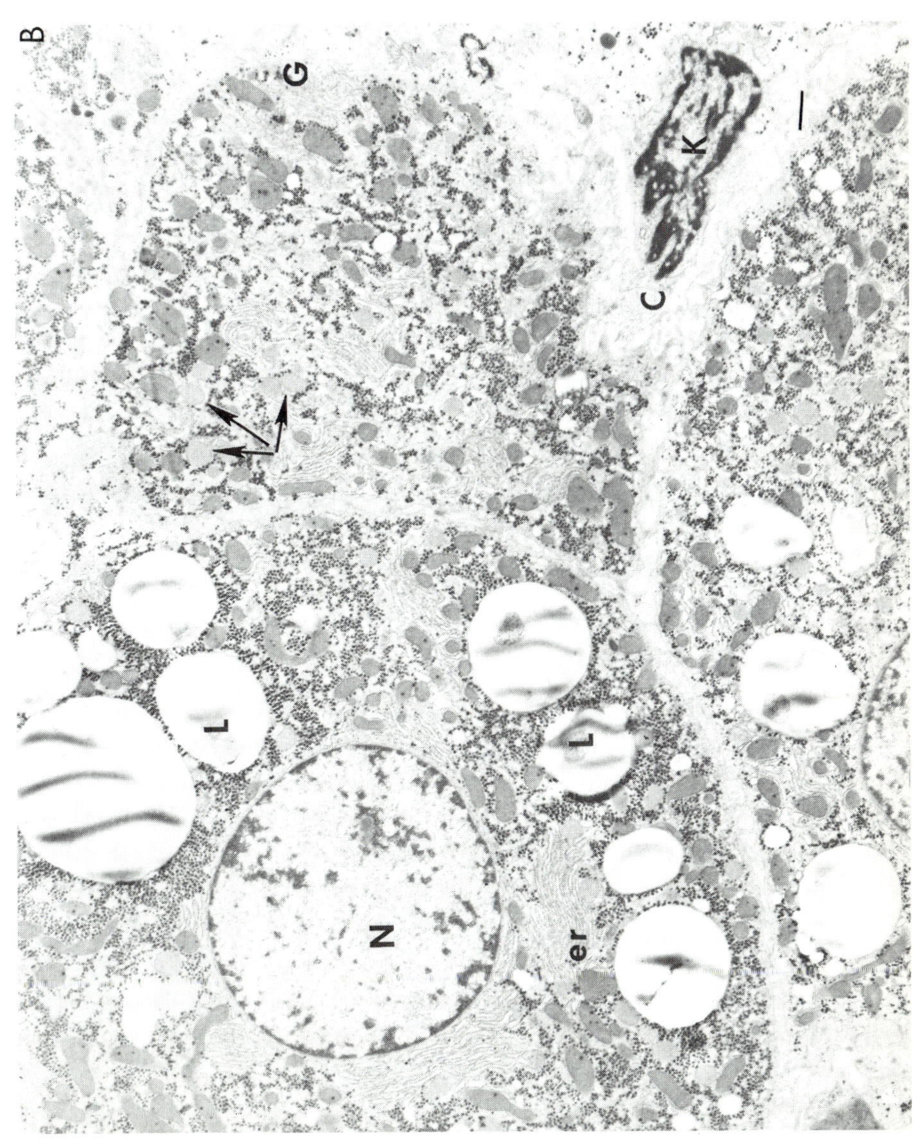

Fig. 2B. Ultrastructural appearance of liver
          shown in Fig.2A. Discrete lipid droplets
          are stored in the cytoplasm without dis-
          placement of other structures. Features
          notable at this magnification include
          abundant glycogen and rough endoplasmic
          reticulum,and numerous relatively translu-
          cent peroxisomes (arrows) which contrast
          with relatively dense mitochondria. Collagen
          deposits are located in the space of Disse.
          Marker represents 1 micron (x9,000).
          L, lipid droplets; N,hepatocyte nucleus;
          K,Kupffer cell nucleus; G,Golgi apparatus;
          C,collagen; er,rough endoplasmic reticulum.

and transitory insult causing severe inhibition of hepatic triglyceride export, with gradual clearance of
the accumulated fat by direct or indirect transfer to
Kupffer cells,and lipid peroxidation within peroxisomes.

The focus of attention shifted to mitochondria in
1972,with the publication by Partin et al (5) of ultrastructural material from a substantial number of patients. On the basis of striking alterations in mitochondrial morphology (swelling, pleomorphism) which
seemed to be correlated with survival or death,these
authors concluded that generalized damage to mitochondria was intimately related to the pathogenesis of
Reye's syndrome. The correlation between the appearance of mitochondria and prognosis turned out to be
relatively uncertain, since morphological changes in
mitochondria often disappear even in non-survivors (6).
Nonetheless, the involvement of mitochondria in the
disease process was clearly established by these and
other studies. In this connection, the same group recently reported morphological changes in brain and muscle mitochondria (J.C.Partin and J.S. Partin, elsewhere

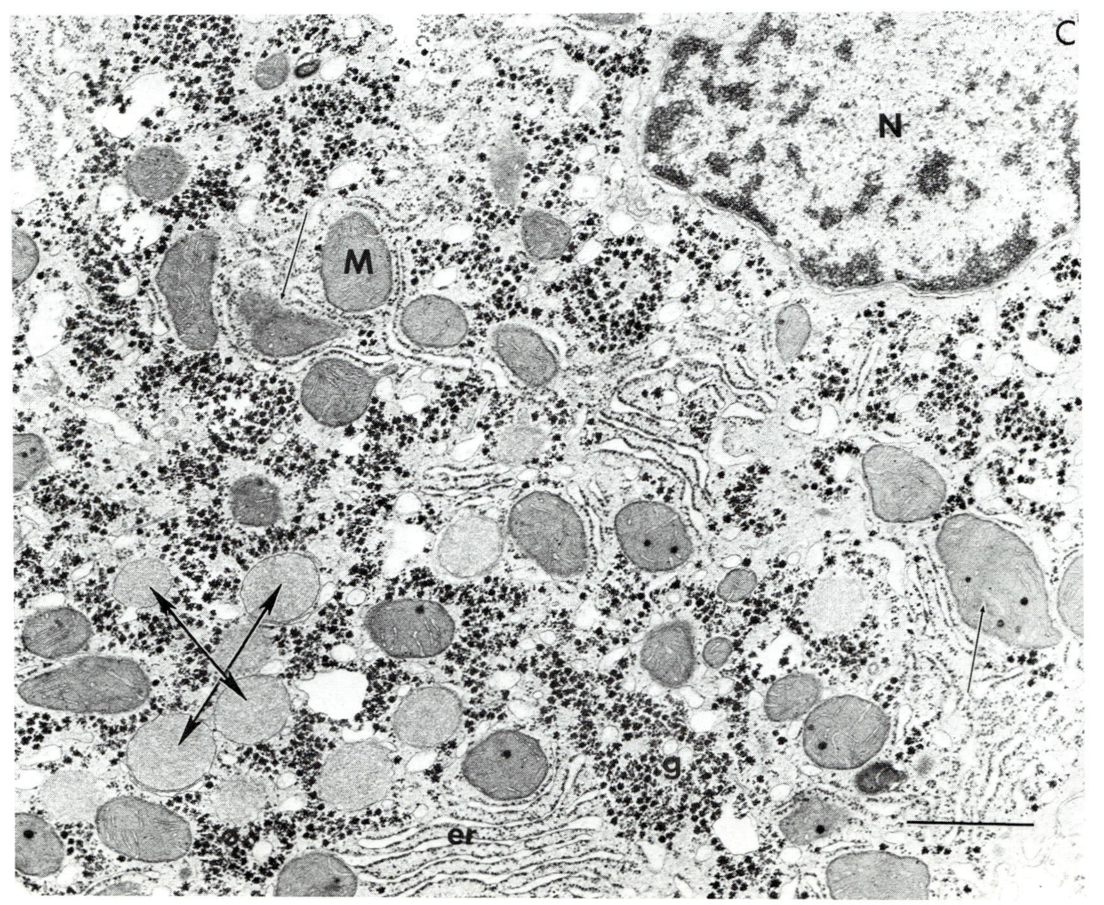
C
N
M
g
er

Fig.2C. Higher power view of the liver shown in
         Fig.2B. Note numerous peroxisomes associated
         with smooth endoplasmic reticulum (crossed
         arrows). Mitochondria appear relatively well
         preserved (M), with occasional evidence of
         mild enlargement,pleomorphism or loss of mem-
         brane (single small arrows). N, nucleus;
         g, glycogen; er, rough endoplasmic reticulum.
         Marker represents 1 micron (x30,000).

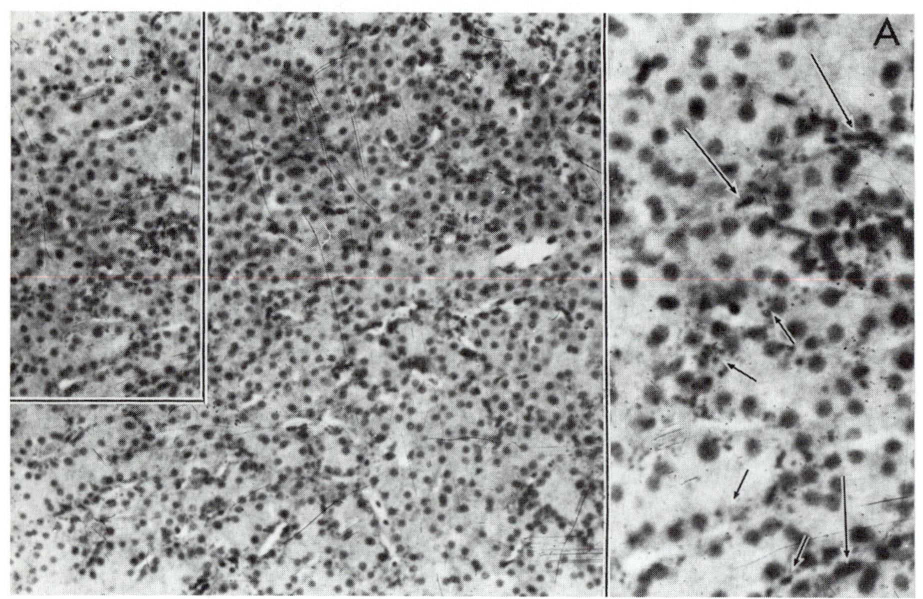

Fig.3A. Liver from patient shown in Fig.2A after 9
        weeks of convalescence. Left, low power view
        of parenchyma stained for fat reveals a strik-
        ing reduction in hepatocellular lipid in com-
        parison with Fig.2A. The fat appears to have
        been relocated in Kupffer cells and perisinu-
        soidal regions of hepatocytes.(Oil red O,x150).
        Right, 3fold greater magnification of the area
        in the upper left corner (enclosed in black
        border) shows residual microdroplets arranged

along sinusoidal aspects of liver cells
(short arrows) and within Kupffer cells
(long arrows).

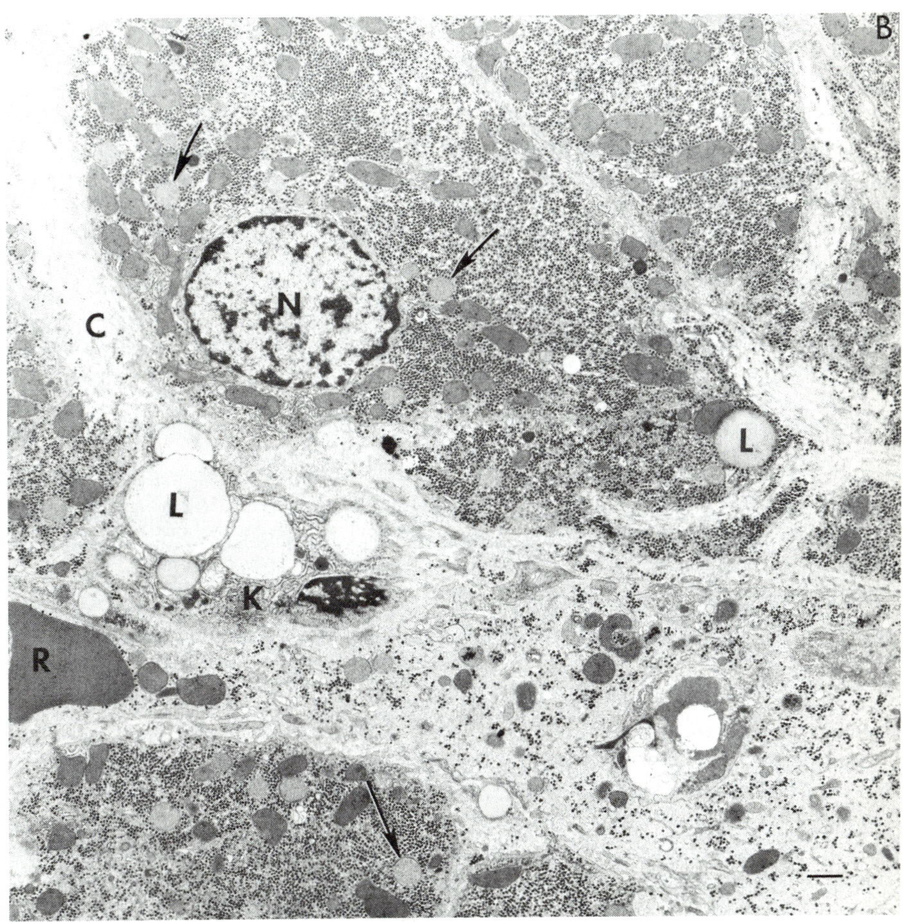

Fig.3B. Ultrastructural appearance of liver shown
in Fig.3A. Lipid is concentrated in Kupffer
cells. One small lipid droplet is observed
in the perisinusoidal cytoplasm of a liver
cell. Peroxisomes are present in reduced
numbers (arrows). N,hepatocyte nucleus; L,
lipid droplets;K,Kupffer cell; R,red cell in

>   sinusoidal space; C, collagen in the
>   Space of Disse. Marker represents
>   1 micron.

in this book), which raises the possibility of a generalized rather than of a primarily hepatic disease process. The evolution of Reye's syndrome in one of our
patients, in whom elevation of serum transaminase and
blood ammonia first occurred on the fourth day of coma,
is consistent with this possibility (7).

At this point, I believe it is worthwhile to recall Reye's careful reservation that the "clinico-
pathological entity" he had discovered may not represent the manifestations of a single etiological factor.
As he warned, "We are not, of necessity, entirely convinced that the etiology is identical in every case."
(1). The sheer variety of the information presently a-
vailable suggests that this relatively uniform and distinctive syndrome may be precipitated by several unrelated factors such as viruses,toxins, abnormal metabolites,chemical agents, and drugs, acting separately
or in concert,apparently modulated in their pathological expression by an age-related constitutional susceptibility which we do not as yet understand. After
considerable efforts have failed to establish a unique
etiology, we may be compelled to follow the thorny alternative possibility raised by Reye.

The information derived from morphological observations during the 15 years since Reye's article appeared may, therefore, be summarized in a single sen-
tence: in its acute phase, the disorder involves a
transient sequestration of neutral fat in the liver,
kidneys and myocardium, associated with greatly increased numbers of hepatic peroxisomes and mitochondrial changes in liver, brain and muscle. The relationship
between steatosis and the changes in mitochondria remains obscure. Thus, it seems that the unique histopathological features of Reye's syndrome have thus far

guarded their secrets jealously, yielding few concrete indications which may resolve the triple challenge bequeathed by their discoverer. Since structure reflects function, an explanation for these morphological changes may become evident after clarification of the functional disorder in Reye's syndrome.

On the clinical level, three functional indices are generally recognized as being consistently disturbed during the acute phase: prothrombin time, the serum transaminases, and blood ammonia. Since all three involve the liver, the assumption remains that this organ is the primary locus of the disease. Prolongation of the prothrombin time is usually associated with severe hepatocellular damage. Therefore, this finding may have been unexpected in Reye's syndrome, with its well-preserved hepatic parenchyma, and may reflect selective inhibition of clotting factor synthesis or release. Similarly, plasma lipoprotein levels are markedly reduced during the acute illness, suggesting interference with formation or export of these proteins. Thus, the possibility of an inhibitory effect involving certain short-lived classes of hepatic proteins should be kept in mind, and additional examples searched for among hepatic export proteins with relatively rapid turnover rates.

The serum transaminases in Reye's syndrome are elevated across a wide range of values, which often change with remarkable rapidity. Not infrequently, transaminase activities in Reye's syndrome reach extremely high levels usually found only with extensive necrotic or inflammatory processes involving the liver. Therefore,the sources of these striking and rapid elevations in circulating transaminase in Reye's syndrome are difficult to explain. Glutamic-oxaloacetic transaminase (SGOT) consists of two distinct cytoplasmic and mitochondrial isozymes, which normally coexist in the circulation in proportions ranging from 5:1 to 20:1. This ratio between cytoplasmic and mitochondrial SGOT remains relatively constant in liver diseases associated with hepatocellular damage, such as acute viral he-

patitis, chronic aggressive hepatitis, fulminant hepatitis and cirrhosis.(8,9). Analyses of the isozymic
activities of SGOT in normal children, and in children
with Reye's syndrome, acute fulminant hepatitis, and
chronic aggressive hepatitis, revealed a reversal in
the cytoplasmic-to-mitochondrial SGOT ratio in Reye's
syndrome only, whereas the usual predominance of the
cytoplasmic enzyme was maintained or augmented in children with fulminant or aggressive hepatitis.(Fig.4).
The cytoplasmic-to-mitochondrial SGOT ratio was gradually restored to normal in the course of recovery from
Reye's syndrome.

These preliminary findings suggest an extensive
increase in permeability of mitochondrial membranes
during the acute phase of Reye's syndrome, with dislo-
cation of proteins such as SGOT from the mitochondrial
matrix to the cytoplasm. Thus,losses of other, osmoti-
cally more active molecules from mitochondria may explain the swelling of these organelles early in the
course of the disease.

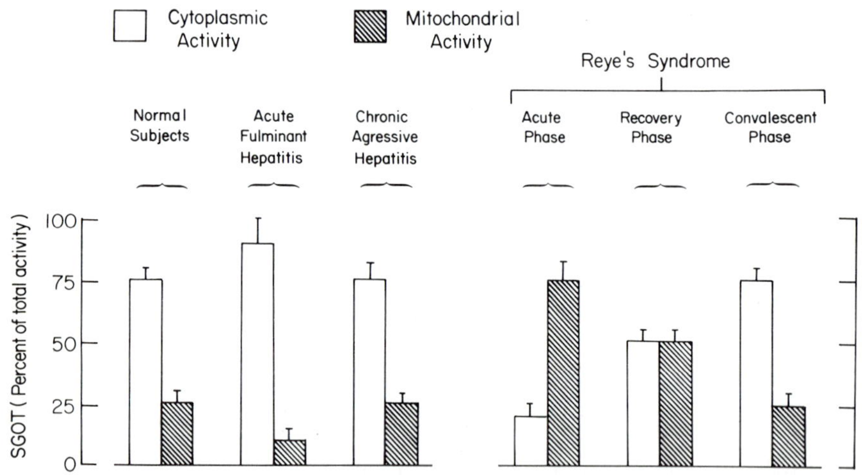

Fig.4. Relationship between cytoplasmic and mito-
     chondrial activities of SGOT in normal subjects,
     and in children with necrotic and non-necrotic
     liver disease associated with coma.The normal
     ratio between the 2 isozymic activities is re-
     versed in Reye's syndrome during the acute ill-
     ness,with gradual return to the normal pattern

during recovery and convalescence. In
contrast, cytoplasmic/mitochondrial SGOT
ratios remain unaltered in chronic aggressive hepatitis, and appear to be increased
in acute fulminant hepatitis.

Less likely is the alternative possibility that the increase in mitochondrial SGOT reflects prolongation of
the relatively brief turnover rate of this isoenzyme
compared with its cytoplasmic analog.(10). The tendency of SGOT to change with unusual rapidity in Reye's
syndrome may be due to this property of the mitochondrial enzyme. It will be important to determine which of
these possibilities is correct, and whether reversals
of the SGOT isozyme ratio occur in other disorders
which may be related to Reye's, including infections
with varicella, influenza B and other common viral a-
gents, as well as in genetically transmitted enzyme deficiencies associated with hyperammonemia.

Huttenlocher's (11) observation in 1969 that blood
ammonia is elevated in Reye's syndrome may yield valuable clues for resolution of "aetiology, prevention, and
treatment". While the brain disorder may occur independently of liver dysfunction, the consistent and early
hyperammonemia in Reye's syndrome suggests a possible
link between hepatic metabolism and the CNS manifestations in this disorder. To explore this possibility,we
began assaying the enzymes constituting the urea cycle
in liver from patients with Reye's syndrome in 1973. Of
special interest were findings obtained in a 9.5 year
old girl with post varicella Reye's syndrome, reported
in 1974 (12): in addition to an 80% reduction in ornithine transcarbamylase (OTC) activity, kinetic analyses
performed to rule out X-linked OTC deficiency demonstrated a complex defect,consisting of reduced affinity of
the enzyme for one of its 2 substrates (ornithine),and
substrate inhibition by ornithine and carbamyl phosphate
the other substrate. In addition to this unique patient,

we have subsequently examined 2 unrelated boys with
Reye's syndrome who had severe OTC deficiency (20%
of control values) which persisted upon reassay 4 months
after recovery from the acute illness. In one of these
children, to be discussed later, kinetic analysis revealed a defect qualitatively similar to that discovered in the girl described above. Clinically, such
variants of OTC deficiency differ from classical X-
linked OTC deficiency by their tolerance for, or even
dependence on, dietary protein.

While these kinetic defects in OTC demonstrate
that multiple etiologies may underlie the clinical and
pathological manifestations of Reye's syndrome, they
appear to be extremely rare. All other patients with
the syndrome have displayed transient reductions in activity of the mitochondrial urea cycle enzymes, with
normal kinetics. (13,14,15). Two major patterns of enzymatic involvement have emerged, which may provide a
basis for categorization of Reye's syndrome along functional lines.

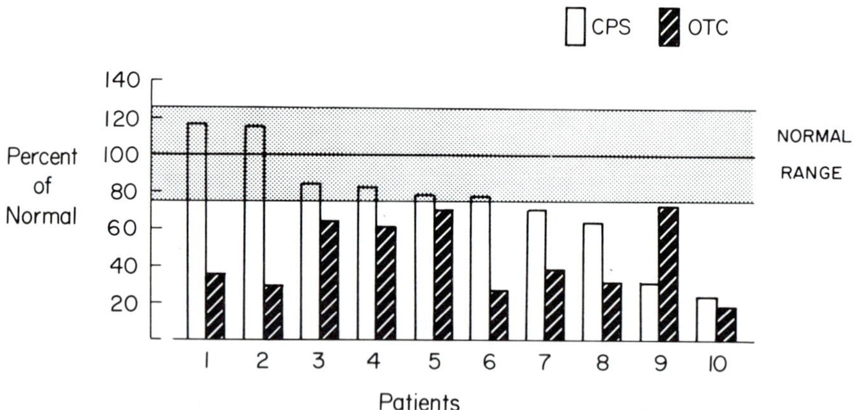

Fig.5. Relative activities of carbamyl phosphate
        synthetase (CPS) and ornithine transcarbamylase
        (OTC) in liver from 10 patients with Reye's
        syndrome.

As the results obtained in 10 of our patients demonstrate (Fig.5), cases with clearcut isolated OTC deficiency may be grouped as belonging to type A (Nos.1,2 and 6), and cases with deficiency of both mitochondrial enzymes of the urea cycle,i.e.,OTC and CPS (carbamyl phosphate synthetase) may be classified as type B (No. 10). Patients with relatively modest reductions in both enzymes (Nos.3,4,5) or those in whom deficiency of one enzyme predominates over the other (Nos.7,8,9) can be denoted as types C and D, respectively.

Splitting of cases into operational subgroups according to enzyme deficiency patterns offers the opportunity to analyze the metabolic processes which may participate in the pathophysiology (as distinct from etiology) of Reye's syndrome. The two mitochondrial ureagenic enzymes (CPS & OTC) found to be consistently deficient in patients with this disorder, participate in formation and removal of carbamyl phosphate (CP),a precursor for citrulline within mitochondria, and for orotic acid (OA) within the cytoplasm:

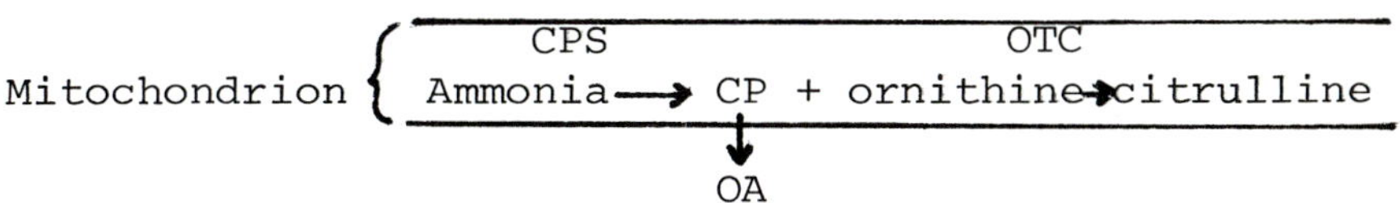

In either homeostasis or in the presence of CPS deficiency, urinary OA concentrations are practically undetectable. A block at the OTC step shifts more CP toward production of excess OA which is then excreted in the urine. It may be postulated that such a block could be due to either a deficiency of the enzyme or an insufficient supply of ornithine, an amino acid derived from arginine in the cytoplasm,and then transported into mitochondria,where ornithine concentrations may exert an important regulatory effect on the urea cycle _in vivo_ (16,17).

These considerations suggest that patients with Reye's syndrome type A (isolated OTC deficiency) may be clinically distinguishable from type B patients (combined CPS and OTC deficiency) by the presence of orotic

aciduria in Type A and its absence in Type B. Treatment
with arginine may ameliorate the hyperammonemia and reverse the orotic acidemia in Type A, and may also influence the clearance of ammonia in other types of Reye
syndrome. Correlations between urinary OA levels,and
hepatic activities of CPS and OTC, may reveal potential
rate-limiting factors,such as ornithine, in patients
with intermediate (Type C) or uneven (Type D) deficiencies of both enzymes. Ornithine may participate in inhibition of the urea cycle in all types of Reye's syndrome,since this amino acid may be present in rate-
limiting concentrations within mitochondria even under
normal circumstances (16,17,18) and may facilitate conversion of CPS to citrulline in hyperammonemic states
(19). Moreover,changes in mitochondrial permeability,
suggested by swelling and leakage of mitochondrial SGOT,
may interfere with the transport of ornithine into mitochondria during the prodromal phase of Reye's syndrome.
Thus,a partial block at the OTC step due to insufficien-
cy of ornithine may be uniformly present, and may be responsible for increased intrahepatic OA concentrations
even without striking elevations in urinary OA. Since
OA is an inhibitor of lipoprotein synthesis, its accumulation in the liver prior to the overt clinical manifestations of the acute illness may be responsible for hy-
polipoproteinemia, failure of triglyceride export, and
formation of the storage-type fatty deposits which are
the diagnostic hallmark of Reye's syndrome. If this hypothesis (20) is correct, the primary insult in this
disorder must occur several days prior to the onset of
clinically detectable symptoms.

Current clinical studies by our group are designed
along the lines indicated by these postulates, and are
intended to evaluate the physiologic significance of enzyme activities measured in vitro, to determine limiting
factors or steps in the disposal of ammonia in Type B,C
and D patients, and to correlate these findings with responses to arginine therapy. While the numbers of patients investigated thus far are too small for definitive answers, data obtained from a boy with OTC deficiency due to a protein-tolerant kinetic variant described
previously in a girl (12) and from a representative patient with Type B deficiency may illustrate various im-

portant aspects of these studies. Patient A is the OTC-deficient boy representing the Type A enzyme pattern, and patient B is a boy of approximately similar age representing combined enzyme deficiency, Type B.

Patient A (6 years old) and patient B (7.5 years old) were both hospitalized in stage 3 coma which had developed on the day of admission following a mild,febrile illness associated with vomiting in both, and acute diarrhea in patient B. The pertinent laboratory values during the acute illness are shown in Tables I and II.

Laboratory Values in Patient A

Day	Blood Ammonia	SGOT	Alkaline Phosphatase	Bilirubin	Prothrombin Time
1	220	400	140	1·0	15
2	240	450		1·1	16
2·2	140	400	120	1·0	14
3	100	250	130	0·8	12
Normal range	50-80 (µg/100ml)	5-40 (I.U./L)	50-150 (I.U./L)	0·3-1·0 (mg/100ml)	12·0 (sec)

Table I. Pertinent liver function tests in a patient with Reye's syndrome associated with selective OTC deficiency.

Laboratory Values in Patient B

Day	Blood Ammonia	SGOT	Alkaline Phosphatase	Bilirubin	Prothrombin Time
1	130	850			12·7
2	117	355	106	0·7	14·9
3	150	250	110		12·2
4	80	200			12·0
5	64	120			11·5
Normal range	50-80 (µg/100ml)	5-40 (I.U./L)	50-150 (I.U./L)	0·3-1·0 (mg/100ml)	12·0 (sec)

Table II. Pertinent liver function tests in a patient with Reye's syndrome associated with combined CPS and OTC deficiency.

Assay of liver obtained by needle biopsy on the first
day in both patients revealed 107% CPS and 6.2% OTC activity in patient A, and 44% CPS and 18% OTC activity
in patient B (normal activity = 100%). In patient A,
moderately elevated prothrombin time, SGOT and blood ammonia values were associated with striking elevations
in urinary OA excretion (Fig.6). Oral arginine therapy

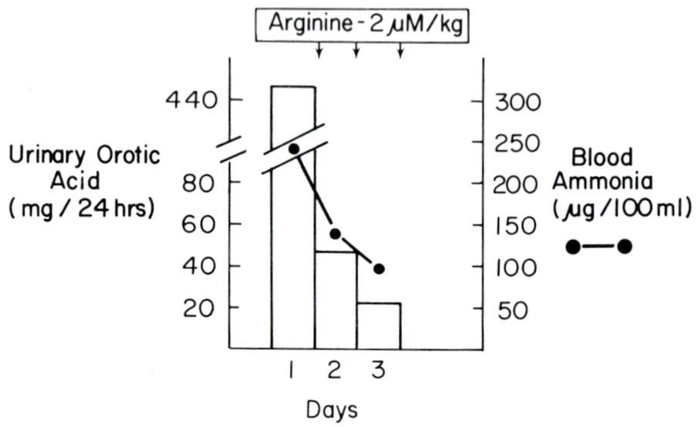

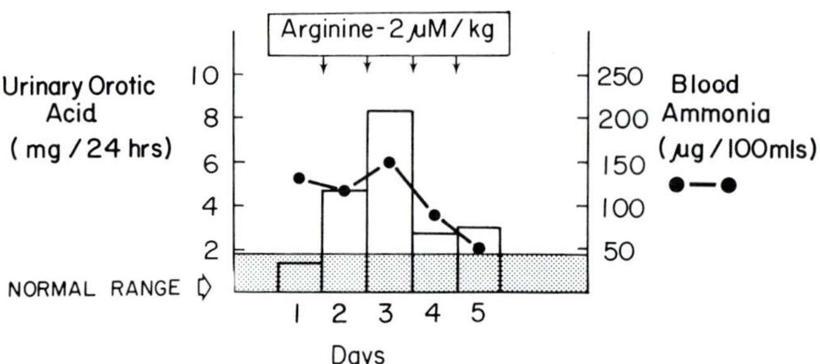

Fig.6. Urinary orotic acid excretion and blood
ammonia concentrations in a patient with
selective OTC deficiency (patient A) and in
a patient with combined CPS and OTC deficiency
(patient B).Arginine treatment was administered
orally at the indicated dose at the intervals
denoted by arrows.

was instituted on the morning of the second day. A precipitous decline in urinary OA, and a more graduated decrease in blood ammonia, occurred during the next two days while receiving arginine. In contrast, urinary OA was only marginally elevated in patient B. (Fig.6). Arginine therapy had no effect on urinary OA excretion nor blood ammonia, which persisted at nearly constant levels for 3 days. Patients A and B recovered from coma on days 3 and 5, respectively.

Several months after recovery from the acute illness,a protein-rich (1g protein/kg) breakfast was administered to each patient. Urinary OA concentrations in patient A increased 5 and 10-fold during the next two 6-hour periods,respectively. (Fig.7). In contrast,the urinary OA concentration in patient B increased approximately 3-fold in the first six postprandial hours,returning to normal thereafter. Blood ammonia and SGOT levels remained within normal limits in both patients.

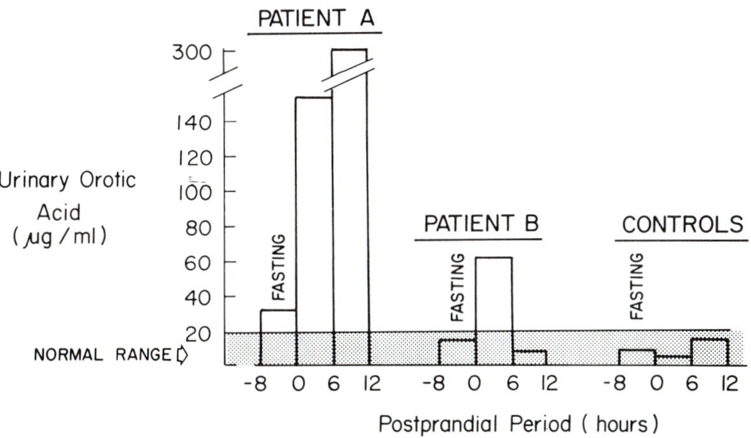

Fig. 7. Urinary orotic acid excretion in patients
A and B,before and after ingestion of a protein-
rich meal,administered 4 and 6 months,respec-
tively,after recovery of each patient from
Reye's syndrome.Controls are normal related and
unrelated age-matched subjects.

Summarizing these findings, OA excretion appeared to correlate with enzyme patterns, being markedly elevated in isolated, severe OTC deficiency, and only modestly increased in the presence of combined OTC and moderate CPS deficiency. The decline in urinary OA and blood ammonia at the time of arginine administration in patient A was consistent with a kinetic defect which produces an increased requirement for ornithine (12). Finally, a protein load following recovery from the acute illness produced increased OA excretion in patient A, reflecting persistence of the block at the OTC step, whereas a similar load in patient B induced a brief, marginal OA response suggesting nearly complete recovery from the acute disorder. Thus, the observed parallels between OTC and CPS activity patterns and urinary OA appear to validate the use of _in vitro_ enzyme assays as indices of conditions _in vivo_, and provide evidence for the rate-limiting role of enzyme or substrate in the conversion of ammonia to urea in the acute phase of Reye's syndrome. Conversely, urinary OA determinations may be useful in indicating an isolated defect in OTC (type A) or its absence (type B and possibly types C and D), thereby supplementing or replacing tissue assays. Such data may aid in the identification of arginine-responsive patients, and in monitoring functional status of such patients during convalescence from Reye's syndrome.

In closing, it must again be acknowledged that current advances in Reye's syndrome are producing more questions than answers. Apart from the etiological unknowns, these questions include the role of liver in the pathogenesis of the brain lesions, the biochemical events which precede and precipitate the main illness, and the relationship between these prodromal insults and eventual prognosis. The evidence for involvement of mitochondria in Reye's syndrome seems convincing. Whether the morphological and functional abnormalities of these essential organelles reflect causes or consequences remains the crucial part of Reye's challenge to the future.

REFERENCES

1. Reye,R.D.K.Morgan,G,and Baral,T. 1963. Encephalopathy and fatty degeneration of the viscera..a
   disease entity in childhood.*Lancet II:*749.

2. Thaler,M.M.,Bruhn,F.W.,Applebaum,M.N. and Goodman,
   J. 1970. Reye's syndrome in twins.*J.Pediat.77:*638.

3. Norman,M.G.,Lowden,T.A.,Hill,D.E. and Bannatyne,R.
   1968. Encephalopathy and fatty degeneration of the
   viscera in childhood.II. Report of a case with isolation of influenza B virus.*Can.Med.Assoc.J.99:*549.

4. Bourgeois,C.,Olson,L.,Comer,D.,Evans,H.,Keschamras,
   N.,Cotton,R.,Grossman,R. and Smith,T. 1971. Encephalopathy and fatty degeneration of the viscera: a
   clinicopathologic analysis of 40 cases.*Am.J.Clin.
   Pathol. 56:*558.

5. Partin,J.C.,Schubert,W.K. and Partin,J.S. 1971.
   Mitochondrial ultrastructure in Reye's syndrome
   (encephalopathy and fatty degeneration of the viscera). *New Eng.J. Med. 285:*1339.

6. Partin,J.C. 1974. Liver ultrastructure in Reye's
   syndrome.p. 117 <u>In</u> J.D.Pollack (ed.), Reye's Syndrome, Grune & Stratton, New York.

7. Applebaum,N.M. and Thaler,M.M. 1977. Reye's syndrome without initial hepatic involvement. *Am. J.
   Dis.Child. 131:*295.

8. Gabrieli,E.R. and Orfanos,A. 1968. A clinical study
   of serum glutamic oxalacetic transaminase isoenzymes in liver diseases.*Proc.Soc.Exp.Biol.Med.128:*
   803.

9. Idio,G.,Franchis,R.D.,Bellobuono,A. and Tormaghi,G.
   1971. Asparate aminotransferase isoenzymes in human
   serum in various liver diseases. *Enzyme 12:*529.

10.   Schmidt,E.,Schmidt,W., and Otto,P. 1967.Isoenzymes of malic dehydrogenase, glutamic oxaloacetic transaminase and lactic dehydrogenase in serum in diseases of the liver. *Clin. Chim. Acta. 15:*283.

11.   Huttenlocher,P.R.,Schwartz,A.D., and Klatskin,G. 1969. Reye's syndrome: ammonia intoxication as a possible factor in the encephalopathy. *Ped.43:*443.

12.   Thaler,M.M.,Hoogenraad,N.J.,Boswell,M. 1974.Reye's syndrome due to a novel protein-tolerant variant of ornithine-transcarbamylase deficiency.*Lancet II:* 438.

13.   Sinatra,F.,Yoshida,T.,Applebaum,M.N.,Hoogenraad, N.J. and Sunshine,P. 1975. Abnormalities of carbamyl phosphate synthetase and ornithine transcarbamylase in liver of patients with Reye's syndrome. *Pediatr.Res.9:*829.

14.   Snodgrass,P.J. and DeLong,G.R. 1976. Urea-cycle enzyme deficiencies and an increased nitrogen load producing hyperammonemia in Reye's syndrome. *New Eng.J. Med. 294:*255.

15.   Brown,T.,Hug,G.,Lansky,L.,Bove,K.,Scheve,A.,Ryan, M.,Brown,H.,Schubert,W.K.,Partin,J.C. and Lloyd-Still, J. 1976. Transiently reduced activity of carbamyl phosphate synthetase and ornithine transcarbamylase in liver of children with Reye's syndrome.*N.Eng.J.Med. 294:*861.

16.   Snodgrass,P.J. 1968. The effects of pH on the kinetics of human liver ornithine-carbamyl phosphate transferase. *Biochemistry 7:*3047.

17.   Raijman,L. 1976. Enzyme and reactant concentrations and the regulation of urea synthesis. p.243.<u>In</u> S. Grisolia,R.Baguena,and F.Mayor (Eds.) The Urea Cycle. J.Wiley & Sons. New York.

18.   Morris,J.G. and Rogers,Q.R. 1978. Ammonia intoxication in the near-adult cat as a result of a dietary deficiency of arginine. *Science 199:* 431.

19.   Tremblay,G.C.,Grandall,D.E.,Knott,C.E. and Alfant,M.
      1977.   Orotic acid biosynthesis in rat liver:
      studies on the source of carbamyl phosphate. *Arch.*
      Biochem. Biophys. 178:264.

20.   Thaler,M.M. 1976. Metabolic mechanisms in Reye's
      syndrome. End of a mystery? *Am.J. Dis.Child. 130:*
      241.

DISCUSSION

J.S. Partin   -   Doctor Thaler, can I ask you about
           the peroxisomes? We,too,have found that perox-
           isomes persist longer than the mitochondrial
           alteration in the liver. Do you think that this
           is just non-specific, or can it be correlated
           with any of these other changes?

M.M. Thaler   -   Obviously this is just an opinion,but
           I feel that the peroxisomes are non-specific
           because they occur in most situations where
           there is severe steatosis. Their presence in
           fatty livers indicates that secondary or resi-
           dual pathways of lipid removed by peroxidation
           have been activated. In the context of Reye's
           syndrome, the persistence of peroxisomes means
           that the liver is capable of catabolizing all
           this fat which should,therefore, disappear.

I.Yoshida   -   I was very much interested in your
           data on GOT isozymes in plasma. We also have
           found quite similar results which have already
           been published. I think the plasma mitochondri-
           al GOT isozyme activity is a good indicator of
           mitochondrial injury,because we had one pa-
           tient with very bizarre mitochondrial config-
           uration with myopathy and we noticed that the
           mitochondrial isozyme of GOT is very much el-
           evated during the attacks.

M.M. Thaler   -   That's right. Because it is indeed
           an index of mitochondrial injury, the mito-

chondrial SGOT might help us sort out whether the mitochondrial injury precedes the disorder or whether it is the disorder that causes the mitochondrial injury. One has to be cautious about one aspect of interpretation, however. As you probably know, the turnover of the mitochondrial isozyme is much more rapid than the cytoplasmic isozyme.

W.K. Schubert -   I may have missed this, but do the patients with recurrent disease that you describe have the mitochondrial isozyme abnormality and, if so, does it persist?

M.M. Thaler   -   It persists only during acute episodes. It is only when their transaminase is elevated that the pattern switches.

W.K. Schubert -   So they have the same isozyme pattern as the "environmental" Reye's syndrome cases?

M.M. Thaler   -   Yes, they do. Of course, take that for what it's worth, because we haven't really had a chance to look at many cases. We've studied only three. Now we are going to look at the other well-known inherited ones.It's just the beginning of our study. But so far, I can say it suggests that whenever these patients have an elevated transaminase, it is elevated because of an increase in the mitochondrial portion.

Unidentified   -   And is their ultra structure similar in both types of Reye's syndrome?

M.M. Thaler   -   Well, the ultra structure during the acute episode is clearly similar considering the broad range that one can see,as described yesterday. They differ in Stage 1 and Stage 2 and 3 and, as we heard today,a similar appearance can be induced by solvents and by endotoxins and,perhaps,by certain viruses.

HEMOCARBOPERFUSION (HCP) IN HEPATIC

DECOMPENSATION AND CEREBRAL EDEMA

A.R. Colon, M.D., M.C. Gelfand, M.D.,
and J.F. Winchester, M.B.

INTRODUCTION

In our institution we have cared for patients
with Reye's syndrome by using conservative measures for
hepatic support (1), containment of cerebral edema (2)
and expectant treatment (3). Since the referring
medical community is attuned to the early manifestations
of Reye's syndrome these children generally arrive in
Lovejoy stages (4) I to II. This allows aggressive
treatment at an early stage in the course of the disease
and a more favorable response, although mortality rates
remain at best 15% and overall 40%.

The pathological axis of Reye's syndrome is
hepatic decompensation coupled with cerebral edema.
Although the biochemical processes appear to be perhaps
unique to Reye's syndrome, the same complex can appear
with other forms of hepatic disease (6). Circulating
toxic moities have long been considered prime factors
contributing to hepatocerebral decompensation and the
safe and prompt removal of these moities from circulation
has long been a major therapeutic goal. Activated
charcoal was used as an experimental extracorporeal
sorbent in the mid-sixties and over the ten years that
followed technical refinements have eliminated the
associated complications of platelet depletion and charcoal embolization. HCP has now been used in a few
major centers for the treatment of hepatic coma in

adults, however, to our knowledge only one child, a 15
year old (7), had been treated with HCP prior to our
studies. We have used hemocarboperfusion in three
children with hepatocerebral decomposition. One was a
13 year old boy with halothane hepatitis, another a 12
year old boy with Reye's syndrome and the last a 10
year old girl with fulminant hepatitis and cerebral
edema. This report is based on the results of treating
these patients.

METHODS

    In all patients HCP was used only if there was
no response to established modalities of treatment.
Informed consent was obtained and all patients had an
arteriovenous shunt created in the leg. Blood was
pumped through a column (Hemacol, Warner-Chilcott,
Morris Plain, N.J.) containing charcoal coated with
2% acrylic hydrogen polymer at flow rates between 100
to 250 ml/min. Whole blood clotting times were kept
between 20 to 30 minutes by the use of heparin, sulfate
and each HCP lasted four hours. Following perfusion,
patients were given fresh frozen plasma and platelets,
both in a dose of 0.1 unit/kg/body weight. HCP was
repeated 24 hours later.

CASES

    Case 1: A 13 year old black male was exposed
to halothane during drainage of a right frontal abscess.
One month later fever, eosinophilia (16-20%), right
upper quadrant tenderness, jaundice, vomiting and
lethargy appeared. Transaminases rose to over 2400
units and coagulation (PT-PTT) became abnormal. Bilirubin was 25.5 mg/dl with a direct fraction of 19.2
mg/dl.

    The patient lapsed into stage IV hepatic coma
and received two exchange transfusions and two hemodi-
alysis treatments without benefit. He was then hemoper-
fused on two consecutive days and awoke from coma. He
is well two years later.

Case II: A 12 year old white male developed a flu-like syndrome five days prior to admission (PTA). Three days PTA he complained of fatigue and nausea, and two days PTA he began vomiting. He was given promethazine by his private doctor. Ten hours PTA he became combative and was admitted to a local hospital where a routine chemistry screen revealed an SGOT of 168 I.U. and serum ammonia of 240 μgm/dl. He was then transferred to our care and arrived in a decerebrate state. A diagnosis of Reye's syndrome was made and confirmed by hepatic needle biopsy.

Treatment with steroids, mannitol, exchange transfusion and other supportive modalities was instituted. After two exchange transfusions there was no change in status. Because of the rapidity through which the patient progressed from stage I to stage IV Reye's syndrome, we decided to employ HCP. After two perfusions there was no change. 24 to 48 hours later both EEG's were isoelectric and all life support systems were stopped.

Case III: A 10 year old white female underwent tonsillectomy two months PTA. She had persistent bleeding for three days requiring whole blood transfusion. Five weeks later she became jaundiced. SGOT was 2300 I.U., SGPT 800 I.U., monospot and HGsAg were negative. Coagulopathy increased and bilirubin total was 20 mg/dl. She lapsed into coma and was transferred to our institution.

On arrival she was febrile, severely icteric, unresponsive and showed posturing and pupillary dilation suggesting an early decerebrate state. There was no papilledema. A Richmond screw was inserted over the right frontal cranial area and intracranial pressure measured at 45 mmHg. Hypothermia, hyperventilation and mannitol failed to control the cerebral edema and increased pressures. EEG showed diffuse slowing and HCP was performed without change in her CNS state. Pupils remained fixed and non-reactive to light. EEG became progressively flatter and the patient expired 24 hours after admission.

RESULTS

Laboratory results are listed in Tables I through III.

TABLE I.   Results pre and post HCP of hemograms and coagulograms.

CASE	I		II		III	
	Pre	Post	Pre	Post	Pre	Post
Hct	29	30	36	37	21	21
WBC x 10^3	12	11	10	7.0	20.5	12.8
Segs	60	54	59	39	71	79
Bands	21	26	30	27	12	6
Lymphs	6	7	4	6	16	11
Plates 10^3	95	65	50	31	450	451
PT	19/12	22.5/12	14/12	22/10	41/10	--
PTT	113/37	120	33/30	180	150	--

Platelet counts remained the same or showed a small but clinically insignificant drop following HCP. PT and PTT increased in part due to heparinization. All patients showed a drop in total proteins. Serum ammonia decreased in cases I and III but appeared to be increased in the child with Reye's syndrome. Serum amino acids were almost all reduced in concentration towards normal levels.

DISCUSSION

The rationale behind the use of HCP is the removal of circulating cerebro and hepatotoxic moieties from circulation. These compounds include ammonia, inert amines, short-chain fatty acids, amino acids and other as yet unidentified moieties interacting or acting independently to produce toxicity. The major compounds considered to be toxic will be reviewed.

TABLE II: Results pre and post HCP of selected chemistry values

CASE	I		II		III	
	Pre	Post	Pre	Post	Pre	Post
Glucose	202	107	130	185	148	--
BUN	74	96	15	17	1	5
CO_2	28.2	27.0	28	30	24.6	19.5
Na	144	150	154	157	136	126
K	3.1	3.3	4.2	3.7	5.2	4.7
Cl	97	99	108	109	91	99
TP	4.6	4.0	5.2	4.3	6.0	3.6
Alb	--	--	3.4	2.4	3.7	1.89
Alpha-1	--	--	--	--	.21	.16
Alpha-2	--	--	--	--	.29	.22
Beta	--	--	--	--	.52	.54
Gamma	--	--	1.7	1.9	1.27	.79
SGOT	79	79	195	123	1590	660
SGPT	84	87	258	202	895	315
Alk phos	22	25	83	77	40	20
NH_3	146	97	405	536	381	174
Bilir.	18.3	18.6	0.6	0.8	38.6	18.0
" D.	10.7	9.3	0.1	0.1	32.2	13.1
Mg	1.4	1.5	2.2	2.2	--	1.9
Ca	6.3	6.4	8.0	8.3	8.7	6.9
P	3.7	5.5	4.7	3.4	3.4	4.8
Creat	2.5	2.1	0.8	0.6	0.7	0.8
Choles	171	182	111	91	212	72
TG	105	180	38	52	--	--
Uric Acid	11.9	11.6	8.1	2.9	--	--

TABLE III. Serum Ammonia and Amino Acids Concentrations Before and After HCP.

	Before first Perfusion	After first Perfusion	After second Perfusion
Coma Grade	IV	III	0
Alanine	*6.85	3.97	0.46
α-amino-n butrate	0.53	0.34	trace
Arginine	1.80	ND	0.50
Aspartic acid	present	present	present
Citruline	present	present	present
Cystine	2.20	1.83	1.92
Ethanolamine	*1.10	ND	trace
Glutamic acid	*9.17	2.55	1.45
Glutamine	3.12	3.15	3.14
Glycine	3.80	2.85	2.79
Histidine	2.00	ND	1.19
Hydroxyproline	*4.51	0.82	1.45
Isoleucine	1.03	0.63	0.81
Leucine	1.29	0.94	1.00
Lysine	6.30	ND	3.98
Methionine	*2.98	2.16	2.04
Ornithine	*2.40	ND	1.07
Phenylalanine	*2.33	1.41	1.25
Proline	*6.88	3.68	2.88
Serine	1.42	1.07	1.02
Taurine	*13.45	0.20	0.46
Threonine	2.47	1.67	1.67
Tyrosine	*2.34	1.25	1.00
Valine	2.34	0.52	0.45
Ammonia	146	120	97

Ammonia: The urea cycle is the major pathway of ammonia detoxification in man.   The cycle begins with ammonia and bicarbonate to form carbamyl phosphate and ends with the formation of urea and ornithine from arginine and water.   (Figure I.)

Evidence has accumulated that at least some patients with Reye's syndrome (8,9) have a single or combined deficiency of ornithine transcarbamylase and carbamyl phosphate synthetase leading to hyperammonemia.   This metabolic defect has been postulated to be one factor in the encephalopathy in these patients. Walker and Schenker (10) have postulated that there are five sites of ammonia cerebrotoxicity.   (Figure II)

Hyperammonemia however is not necessarily associated with cerebral edema and therefore elevated ammonia is not a sine-qua-non for the diagnosis of Reye's syndrome.   Hyperammonemia therefore, appears to be only one of the factors in Reye's encephalopathy.

HCP failed to significantly change the levels of ammonia in our patient with Reye's syndrome, but in the other two patients significant drops in serum ammonia were registered.   These results were similar to those noted by Gazzard et al. (7)   The fact that the patient with Reye's syndrome failed to show a decrease in concentration with HCP lends support to the concept of urea cycle enzyme dysfunction.

Inert amines: Fischer (11) and Williams (12) have proposed that false neurochemical transmitters contribute to hepatic encephalopathy.   Transmitters in the peripheral adrenergic system require a phenolic ring with a short carbon and a hydroxyl at the beta position of the chain (Figure III.)   During hepatic decompensation many amines from the action of bacterial enzymes on gut proteins escape hepatic metabolism and persist in the circulation.   These amines may form octopamine and phenylethanolamine, both of which are false neurochemical transmitters, (13) which replace the active dopaminergic or adrenergic neurotransmitters. (14)   Gazzard (7) demonstrated that with HCP three

Figure I: The Urea Cycle

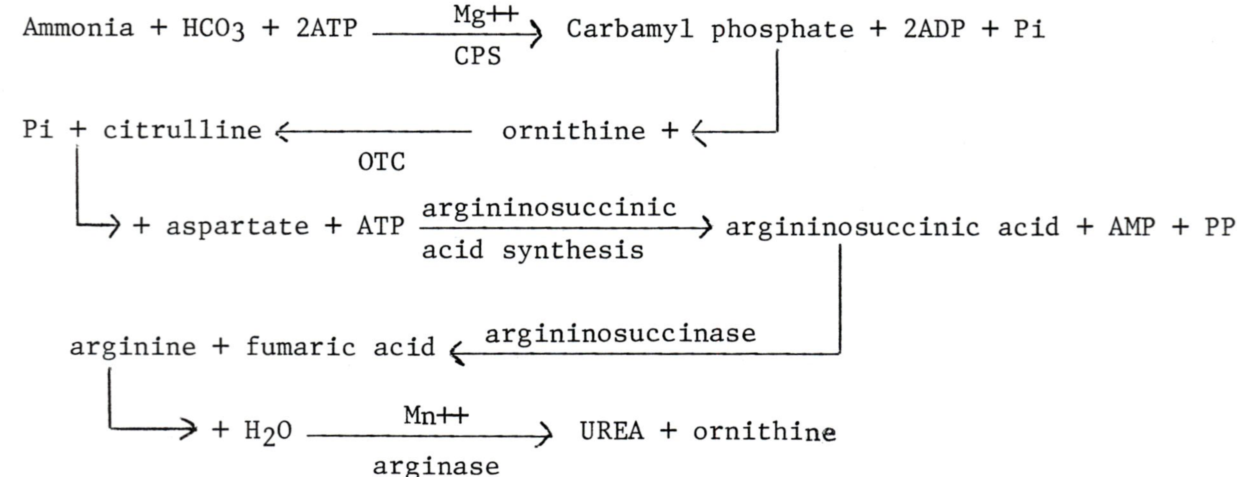

Figure II: Postulated sites of CNS ammonia toxicity

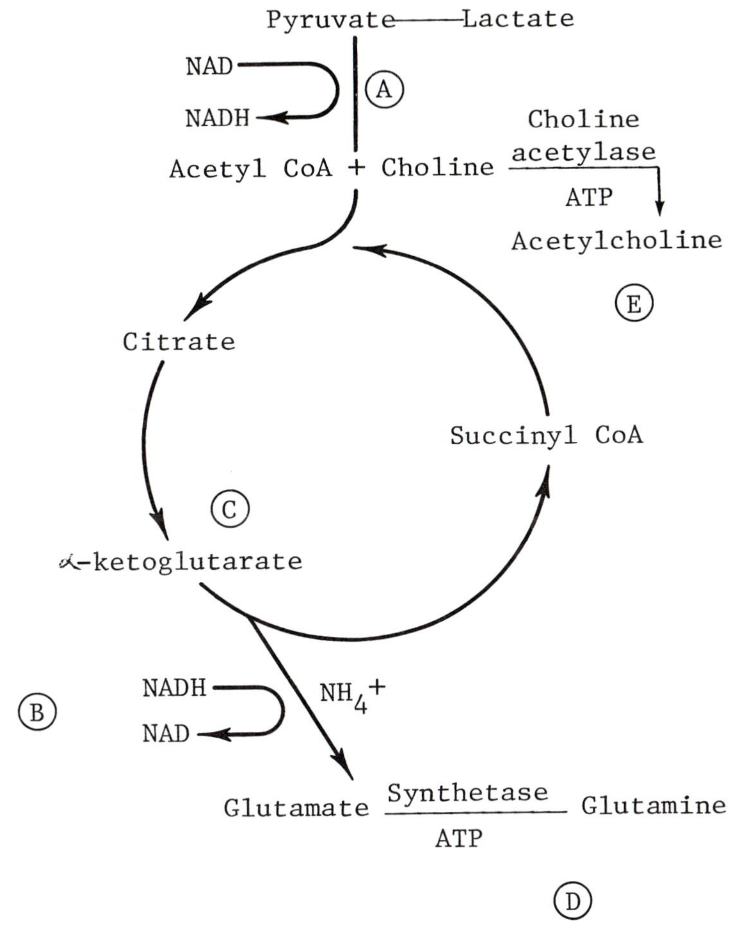

A: Impaired oxidative decarboxylation of pyruvate
B: NADH depletion
C: α-ketoglutarate depletion
D: Greater ATP utilization than at E
E: Decreased acetylcholine formation

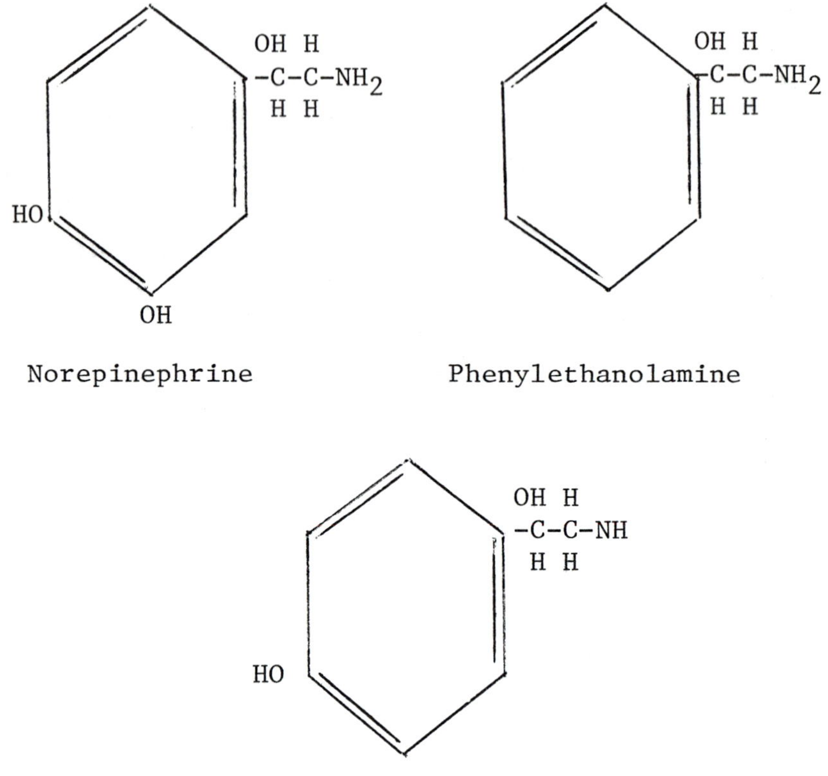

Figure III: Transmitters demonstrating the phenolic ring and hydroxyl group at the position of side chain.

amino acids (tyrosine, phenylalanine and methionine) concerned with dopamine metabolism are all decreased. We noted similar findings in the serum amino acids of one patient. No samples were obtained from the patient with Reye's syndrome.

Shortchain fatty acids (SCFA): Butyrate, valerate, and octonoate may be elevated in the CSF of patients with liver associated encephalopathy. SCFA are also known to be elevated in patients with Reye's syndrome and Trauner et al (15) demonstrated a correlation between a fall in serum SCFA and clinical improvement in a patient with the syndrome. However, experimentally administration of these same SCFA to volunteers does not produce encephalopathy and some investigators feel a conjoined action of SCFA plus ammonia is necessary for encephalopathy (16). No SCFA levels were done on our patients, however, moieties with molecular weights below 125 Dalton are probably poorly removed by HCP (17).

Amino acids: Hyperaminoacidemia for phenylalanine, tyrosine, tryptophan and methionine (aromatic amine precursors) (18) is noted in hepatic coma, while in Reye's syndrome alanine, glutamine, lysine and alpha-amino-n-butyrate are elevated. (19) The amino acid changes noted in Reye's syndrome may be related to a deficiency of OTC.

HCP has a significant effect on hyperaminoacidemia. Serum amino acids measured in one of our patients showed a reduction in almost all amino acids. We have subsequently documented this finding in other patients and, in addition, we have shown both plasma and CSF increases in branched chain: aromatic amino acid ratio in patients undergoing HCP adding further support to the concept of blood brain barrier disruption in hepatocerebral decompensation. (20)

That both patients with cerebral edema expired is consistent with data from other investigators. Silk et al (21) found HCP failed in 81% of patients with cerebral edema.

Earlier HCP was associated with thrombocytopenia and charcoal emobilization, but the use of a biocompatible polymer coating has greatly eliminated these problems. None of our patients had significant thrombocytopenia.

Besides the aforementioned problems other complications of HCP include hypotension and hypothermia. None of our patients suffered these complications.

While both patients with cerebral edema did not recover and would suggest that HCP has no place in the treatment of hepatic decompensation with cerebral edema, the following syllogisms should be examined: A) Several investigators feel that hyperaminoacidemia, hyperammonemia and SCFA are the main biochemical abnormalities producing encephalopathy in Reye's syndrome; B) HCP has been shown to reduce at least two of these classes of moieties and therefore; c) HCP may aid in the treatment of Reye's syndrome encephalopathy.

The question which must be asked is whether or not to treat early Reye's syndrome (or at the very least, those progressing rapidly through stages I-III) with HCP. With the current plethora of treatments, a controlled trial employing HCP would be hard to implement.

REFERENCES

1. Trey, C. 1970. The critically ill child: Acute hepatic failure. *Ped. 45*:93-98.
2. Rogers, M. 1978. The management of increased intracranial pressure. *Johns Hopkins Med.J. 142*: 99-102.
3. Steigmann, F., Clowdus, B.G. Hepatic encephalopathy. Charles Thomas (Springfield, 1971).
4. Lovejoy, F.N., Smith, A. et al 1974. Clinical staging in Reye syndrome. *Am.J.Dis.Child 128*: 36-40.
5. CDC. Reye Syndrome - United States MMWR 27:15-16, 1978.

6. Ware, A.J., et al 1971. Cerebral edema: A major complication of massive hepatic necrosis. *Gastroent 61:*877-884.

7. Gazzard, B.G. et al 1974. Charcoal hemoperfusion in the treatment of fulminant hepatic failure. *Lancet I:*1301-1306.

8. Thaler, M.M. et al 1974. Reye's syndrome due to a novel protein-tolerant variant of ornithine transcarbamylase deficiency. *Lancet II:*434-440.

9. Thaler, M.M. 1976. Metabolic mechanism in Reye syndrome. *Am J Dis Child 130:*241-243.

10. Walker, C.O., Schenker, S. 1970. Pathogenesis of hepatic encephalopathy with special reference to ammonia. *Am J Clin Nut 23:*619-624.

11. Fischer, J.E., Baldessarini, R.J. 1971. False neurotransmitters and hepatic failure. *Lancet II:* 75-79.

12. Parkes, J.D. et al. 1970. Levodopa in hepatic coma. *Lancet II:* 1341-1343.

13. Kopin, I.J. 1968. False adrenergic transmitters. *Ann Rev Pharm 8:*377-394.

14. Conn, H.O. 1973. Current diagnosis and treatment of hepatic coma. *Hosp Prac 8:*65-72.

15. Trauner, D.A. et al 1977. EEG correlations with biochemical abnormalities in Reye syndrome. *Arch Neurol 34:*116-118.

16. Zieve, L.T. et al 1974. Synergism between ammonia and fatty acids in the production of coma. *J Phar Exp Ther 191:*10-16.

17. Leber, N.W. et al. Chronic uremia - haemodialysis or haemoperfusion. Artificial organs (ed: Kenedi, R.M. et al) MacMillan (London, 1977) pp. 220-226.

18. Iber, F.L. 1957. Plasma amino acids in patients with liver failure. *J Lab Clin Med. 50:*417-425.

19. Hilty, M.O. et al 1974. Reye's syndrome and hyper-aminoacidemia. *J Peds 84:*362-365.

20. Gelfand, M.C. et al. Reversal of hepatic coma by charcoal hemoperfusion. Trans Am Soc Artificial Organ. (in Press)

21. Silk, D.B. et al 1977. Treatment of fulminant hepatic failure by polyacrylonitrile membrane haemodialysis. *Lancet II:*1-3.

DISCUSSION

M.R. Hurley   -   I was a little confused; how many
        patients have you perfused now, and how many
        of those had Reye's syndrome?

A.R. Colon   -   We perfused only one patient with
        Reye's syndrome. As I said in the beginning,
        all of our patients are treated with estab-
        lished modalities, but we had this one pa-
        tient for whom, out of desperation, we used
        the perfusion technique.

M.R. Hurley   -   The second point; what column were
        you using?

A.R. Colon   -   The hemocol, made by Warner-Chillcot.
        There are about three different brands avail-
        able.

M.R. Hurley   -   What do you really think you are
        getting out?

A.R. Colon   -   I don't know; that's why we're so
        fascinated with Dr. Aprille's work. I am
        tempted to send her the columns to see what
        she can elute from them.

M.R. Hurley   -   Yes; I don't want to put a damper on
        enthusiasm, but it makes you think of the
        peritoneal dialysis story.

A.R. Colon   -   Oh, absolutely. I'm giving you ne-
        gative data. I appreciate that, and I am in
        no way going to suggest hemocarbonperfusion
        as a primary modality of treatment for Reye's
        syndrome. What I am saying though, is that we
        probably are not in a situation where we can
        test it as a "virginal technique".

M.R. Hurley   -   I wonder if you know if anyone is
        trying to remove just the ammonia and leaving
        all the other things in? Because I think you

could think of doing that by using, for example, a dialysis system.

A.R. Colon   -   Well, we have a specific resin column that we have employed in dogs, but it
hasn't been for ammonia. I'm afraid we've
been working with short chain fatty acids,
but I think you're right. One should be able,
theoretically at least, to use a quaterary
agent to preferentially remove ammonia.

Unidentified   -   I have a comment about the rising
ammonias as a result of your dialysis. You
know, you really shouldn't be surprised that
the ammonias go up as a result of these
things. I think people should recall that the
catabolism of one gram of protein for calories (that's four calories) is equivalent to
60,000 μgms of nitrogen, 65,000 μgms of ammonia. That's a lot when you look at how much
is circulating in the blood.

Unidentified   -   Just a brief question. Did you mention the size and molecular weight cut off in
your perfusion?

A.R. Colon   -   Yes; we think it is 125 daltons but
we're not sure.

Same Speaker   -   The reason I ask is because I'm
sure you're aware of Opolong's work in Paris
with the acrinolectol membrane in patients
with hepatic coma, which removes moities up
to 15,000 molecular weight and the patient
improves,but then dies because of bleeding.

A.R. Colon   -   How does he elute them out? I
thought he was using the nitrite column.

Same Speaker   -   Yes; but he gets the perfusate and
then he uses a fractionation procedure.

A.R. Colon   -   It's difficult to elute things out
of this carbon column. Very difficult; it
holds on tenaciously. Well, it is unfortunate
that this other technique isn't available in

the United States, because it might be an
ideal way of doing this. Silk and his colleagues, working with Roger Williams, have
tried the acrylonitrile column for cerebral
edema. They have not had much luck. The
treatment works for hepatic coma in 75% of
the cases but, since there is no functional
liver tissue left, they don't survive.

MANAGEMENT OF REYE'S SYNDROME:
CINCINNATI EXPERIENCE

William K. Schubert, M.D., John C. Partin, M.D. and
Jacqueline S. Partin, M.S.

Multiple therapeutic regimens have been proposed for the treatment of Reye's Syndrome. None is completely satisfactory and none is likely to be developed that is satisfactory until further research defines the precise etiology of the disease. At the Cincinnati Children's Hospital Medical Center we have diagnosed Reye's Syndrome with increasing frequency since Reye's original paper in 1963 as shown in Table 1 (1) below:

REYE'S SYNDROME: CINCINNATI

YEARLY INCIDENCE

1963	1
1964	-
1965	1
1966	1
1967	1
1968	-
1969	8
1970	10
1971	4
1972	7
1973	9
1974	24
1075	12
1976	9
1977	20
1978 (to June)	16
TOTAL	123

There have been at least two clear cut epidemics in 1974 and 1977 but the increased number of cases diagnosed

yearly is almost certainly a reflection of parent,
emergency room and physician awareness of the disease
with consequent increase in cases diagnosed rather than
an increase in actual number of cases. Many cases presently being diagnosed and treated supportively would
previously have gone undiagnosed or in some instances
with serum transaminase elevations in the absence of
jaundice would have been diagnosed as "anicteric hepatitis". In the six year period from 3/63 to 3/69 nine
patients were diagnosed clinically and three additional
patients not seen by the authors were diagnosed at post-
mortem examination. From 3/69 to 6/78 all patients
diagnosed had equal consideration for exchange transfusion and are presented as a separate group. Diagnosis
was made based on the typical clinical history of a prodromal illness,either influenza or varicella, followed
within three to seven days by severe vomiting, progressive signs of cerebral dysfunction, and serum transaminase elevations,as previously described (6). Liver
biopsy was performed to confirm the diagnosis in 99 of
112 patients seen from 3/69 to 6/78 as discussed by Dr.
John Partin in this book.   The importance of liver
biopsy to confirm the diagnosis of Reye's Syndrome if
we are to fully understand its pathogenesis cannot be
overstated. Even in neurological grade I or so-called mild
Reye's Syndrome, the liver lesion may be severe and the
patient progress to coma despite early institution of
supportive therapy with intravenous glucose and observation. It seems clear to our group that early recognition of Reye's Syndrome with hospitalization and such
supportive therapy can result in definite reduction of
severe cases and thus simplify treatment (2,3).

     Exchange transfusion has been used for the treat-
ment of Reye's Syndrome with more severe central nervous
system signs since March of 1969. Our procedure consists of surgical placement of one or two large bore
(8-10 French) radiopaque plastic catheters into the
right atrium or vena cava (2). When the catheter(s) has
been placed and fresh whole blood is available, the liver biopsy is performed for light and electron microscopy,
histochemistry on frozen sections, and such biochemical
studies as are possible on the remaining tissue. A two
volume exchange is performed,and repeated at 8-12 hour

intervals thereafter until definitive clinical improvement or signs of irreversible brain damage have occurred. The exchange is performed in 20-120 cc aliquots, depending on body weight. The blood is fresh (0-48 hrs), complete and citrated. As this is what is available to us, we have not used heparinized blood. Utilizing a system of three-way stopcocks, venotubes, and pressure cuffs on the plastic blood bags, it is possible for one operator to withdraw blood from the patient while the second withdraws from the blood bag and then to simultaneously inject the fresh blood into the patient and the withdrawn blood into a discard bottle. With this procedure, the exchange transfusion can usually be accomplished within two hours. Calcium as heptagluconate is administered in a dose of 200 mgm per 200 cc of blood exchanged. We have utilized a Scribner anterio-venous shunt in one patient, a 17 year old boy who received a total of 102 units of blood in a 2.5 day period (4). The advantage of the shunt is the increased facility with which the exchange can be performed; the disadvantages are the time involved to place the shunt which delays therapy, the potential loss of the artery, and the difficulty of shunt placement in smaller children.

In our opinion, of great importance is the presence of a senior physician at the bedside during and at intervals after the procedure. The procedure has been relatively uniform since March 1969 (2,3). The decision to treat with exchange transfusion is based on clinical evaluation on admission, and improvement or deterioration in neurologic status during support with intravenous glucose while the diagnostic studies and whole blood crossmatch are being performed. Patients with grade III disease (see below), or grade II disease with progression to grade III during this relatively short time period, are exchanged. We have not used hypothermia but have maintained normal body temperatures in febrile patients with a cooling blanket. Since early 1974 patients with grade III or more severe disease are intubated electively as described by DeVivo, et al (5,6). Mannitol has been used intermittently in a dose of 0.5 to 1.0 grams/Kg in bolus doses to control sudden increases in intracranial pressure. More recently (1976) in patients with neurologic diseases of grade III and

above, intracranial pressure has been monitored (12
patients) with an extradural fiberoptic pressure monitor
inserted in the operating room through a temporal burr
hole. Using this monitor, the dura is not penetrated.
The main advantage to intracranial pressure monitoring
has been to allow use of mannitol electively as pressure rises and to anticipate catastrophic increase in
pressure. The total amount of mannitol used has thus
been decreased with avoidance of the complication of
hyperosmolarity and hypovolemia. Monitoring of intracranial pressure has confirmed our impression that the
encephalopathy is metabolic and that patients may remain comatose with normal intracranial pressure for prolonged periods (Fig. 1) (below) (7).

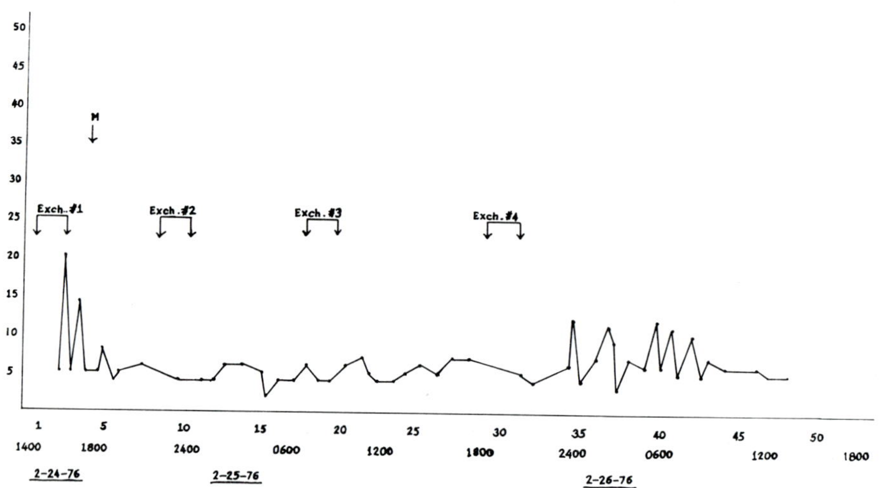

On this and subsequent charts intracranial pressure is
plotted as centimeters of water so that normal is 10 or
less. Except for a brief initial pressure of 20, this
patient remained in stage 4 coma for 48 hours with a
normal intracranial pressure before making a complete
recovery.

Figure 2.

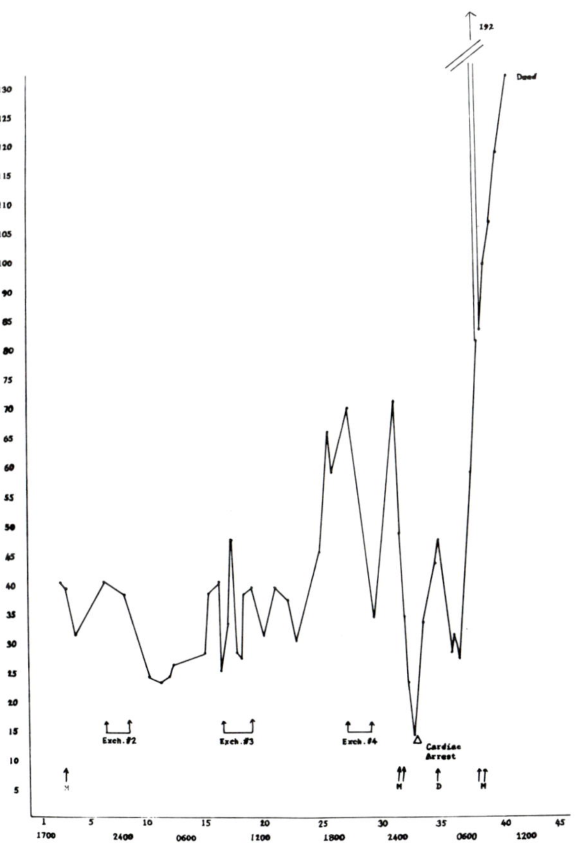

Patient number two (Fig. 2) entered the hospital in stage 4 coma with a high intracranial pressure only partly responsive to mannitol. Despite exchange transfusion, mannitol, barbituate and intensive supportive therapy, the intracranial pressure remained elevated and death occurred 42 hours after admission. We interpret these results to indicate an increased severity of the cerebral mitochondrial injury although in these two patients we do not have histologic confirmation of this by brain biopsy and ultrastructural analysis. Such studies, i.e. brain biopsy with the examination presented by Jacqueline Partin, are vitally needed in those patients in whom intracranial monitors are placed if a more complete understanding of the encephalopathy in Reye's Syndrome is to be achieved. As mentioned,

mannitol was used for measured or clinical increased
signs of increased intracranial pressure. Corticosteroids were used in 13 patients but have not altered
morbidity or mortality and have produced complications
with infection and gastric ulcer and are not used at
present.

Although our data agree with Huttenlocher in that
severity of this disease may be estimated by the initial
blood ammonia concentration (9), the blood ammonia may
come rapidly to normal as the liver mitochondrial injury recovers,although the patient remains comatose and
dies. With this fact and the histologic evidence that
the encephalopathy is not that of blood ammonia elevation (10), we do not attempt to control blood ammonia
elevation. Evaluation of any treatment of Reye's Syndrome requires clinical staging of the degree of neurologic dysfunction as shown in Table II.

REYE'S SYNDROME NEUROLOGICAL STAGING - CINCINNATI

   I Quiet, lethargic, responds to commands.
      Won't eat, will walk.

  II Stuporous, thick speech, difficulty in counting.
      Unwilling to walk, clumsy motor activity.

 III Agitated delirium, unable to count, may have
      seizures.
      Intermittent coma, clonus and Babinski reflex.
      Fundal veins distended.
      Dilated, rapidly responsive pupils, dolls eye
      reflex.

  IV Coma, decerebrate posturing, may have seizures.
      Brain stem type respiration, tachycardia.
      Fundal veins engorged, blurred optic discs.
      Pupils dilated, slowly responsive, dolls eyes
      reflex preserved.

   V Coma, flaccid paralysis, spinal reflexes, later
      decorticate.
      No spontaneous respiration.
      Fixed dilated pupils, dolls eyes reflex lost.
      Fundal veins distended, papilledema possible.

Our staging has been according to the above criteria
at the time of admission to Cincinnati Children's
Hospital Medical Center recognizing that some patients
deteriorate after admission, but that this is one constant in the patient's hospital course not blurred by
therapeutic manipulation. From 1963-1971, such staging
was retrospective from hospital records; from 1971-1978,
the staging was prospective and done by two of the authors in conference at the time of admission.   The
staging is similar to that proposed by Plum and Posner
(12) and used by Lovejoy and colleagues (13).

The distribution of all patients by neurological
stage on admission who were seen at Children's Hospital
Medical Center from March 1963 to June 1978 is shown
in Figure 3.   (below)

DISTRIBUTION BY NEUROLOGICAL STAGE OF

123 CONSECUTIVE REYE'S SYNDROME CASES, CINCINNATI CHILDREN'S HOSPITAL

March 1963 – June 1978

Neurological Stage	I	II	III	IV	V	Totals
Number of Patients	31	13	32	37	10	123
Number Survived	31	13	30	28	0	102
Living and Well	31	13	29	21	0	94
Severe Brain Damage	0	0	1	7	0	8
Number Died	0	0	2	9	10	21
Percent Survival	100%	100%	94%	76%	0%	83%

Of 123 patients, 102 survived and 94 are living and well
without brain damage.   From March 1963 to March 1969,
eleven patients were seen.   Of these, one survived without brain damage, 2 suffered severe brain damage, and 8
died.   The overall survival not dead or brain damaged
was then 10%.   These 11 patients are included in figure
3.   The prognosis in patients with neurological grade I
or II on admission is excellent.   The survival rate is
lessened and the incidence of brain damage increased
progressively in neurological grades III and IV.   No

patient presenting with neurological grade V symptoms
survived in the entire series. From March 1969 until
June 1978, all patients were considered equally for
treatment by exchange transfusion. The distribution of
these cases by neurological stage is shown in Figure 4:

DISTRIBUTION BY NEUROLOGICAL STAGE OF

112 CONSECUTIVE REYE'S SYNDROME CASES, CINCINNATI CHILDREN'S HOSPITAL

March 1969 - June 1978

Neurological Stage	I	II	III	IV	V	Totals
Number of Patients	31	13	32	33	3	112
Liver Biopsy	21	11	31	33	3	99
Exchange Transfusion	1	3	28	33	3	68
Survival of Exchanged	1	3	26	25	0	55
Total Survival - %	100%	100%	94%	76%	0%	88%

One hundred and twelve consecutive patients comprise
this group. Patients with neurologic grade I and II
disease did well whether treated by exchange transfusion
or not. Of 28 grade III patients treated by exchange
transfusion, 26 or 94% survived and of 33 patients with
grade IV disease 25 or 76% survived. No patient with
grade V disease survived. The overall survival rate is
91% but 6 patients were left with significant neurologic damage. Of interest is the change in stage of recognition of the disease in the latter period (1969-
1978) compared to the former (1963-1969). In the earlier period, 7 of 11 patients (64%) seen presented with
neurologic stage V disease while in the latter period
only 3 of 112 patients, or less than 3%, presented with
stage V disease presumably due to the public awareness
of the disease in our area (3).

The age distribution of the total group 1963-1978 is shown in Figure 5. The average age was 6 years. There were 60 males and 63 females. Figure 6 presents the age of onset and treatment results in the 112 consecutive patients equally considered for treatment by exchange transfusion. There is a significant improvement most notable in the infants 0-2 years of age. Figure 7 presents the outcome for infants 0-2 years of age in the total group of 123 patients and Figure 8 compares the results of the infants from 1969-1978 considered equally for exchange transfusion. The diagnosis may be delayed in infants because of difficulty in interpretation of neurologic dysfunction. Hypoglycemia initially emphasized by Reye was present in only 11 of the group of 112 (9.8%) patients equally considered for exchange transfusion but only three of the 11 hypoglycemic patients were over two years of age. Furthermore of these 8 infants presenting with hypoglycemia, 6 died or were left with severe brain damage while only two are living and well. That the disease may occur as early as one month is apparent. From comparison of figures 7 and 8 it can be seen that all 5 infants not considered for exchange transfusion suffered death or brain damage while 7 of 15 infants equally considered for exchange transfusion had brain damage or death. This experience with 112 cases of Reye's Syndrome equally considered for exchange transfusion with an overall survival of 88% and a survival of 94% in stage III and 76% in stage IV, is compared with the experience of DeVivo, Keating and colleagues in St. Louis using an intensive care supportive regime in Figure 9. This illustration is furnished by Dr. Darryl DeVivo of Washington University in St. Louis and St. Louis Children's Hospital. Unfortunately the neurological grading system is different. The neurological stages from several institutions including St. Louis are compared in Table III.

Figure 5

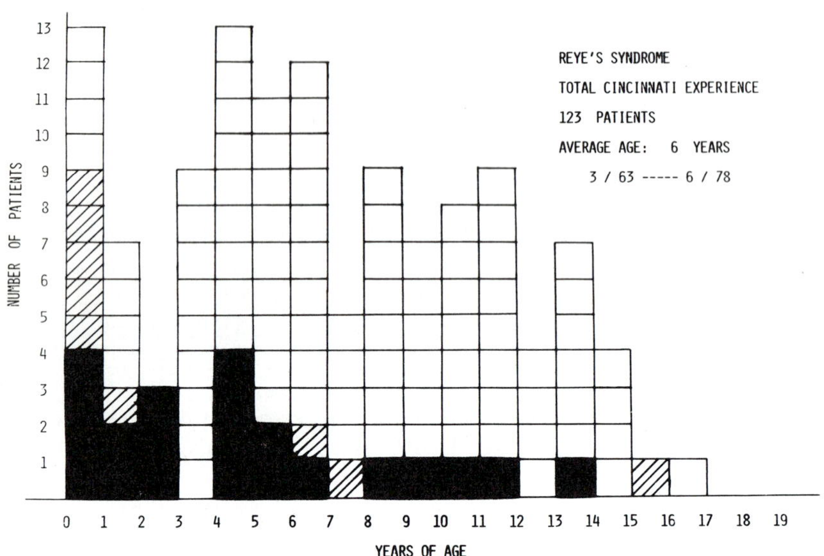

Figure 6

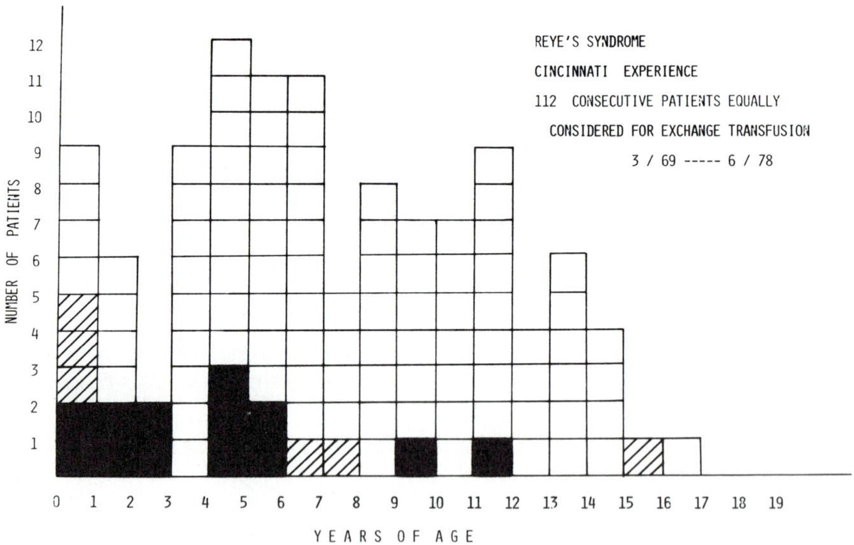

Clear square - one child living and well.
Black square - one child who died from Reye's Syndrome
Hatched square - one child with moderate to severe
brain damage.

Figure 7

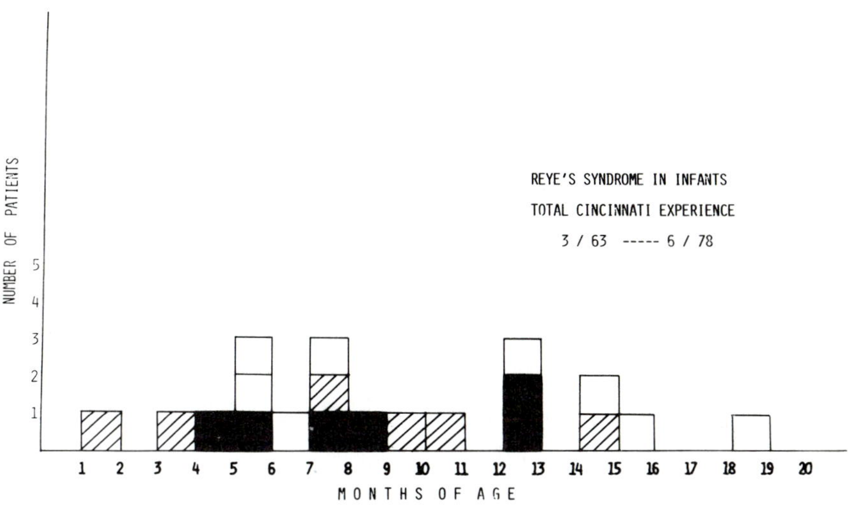

Figure 8

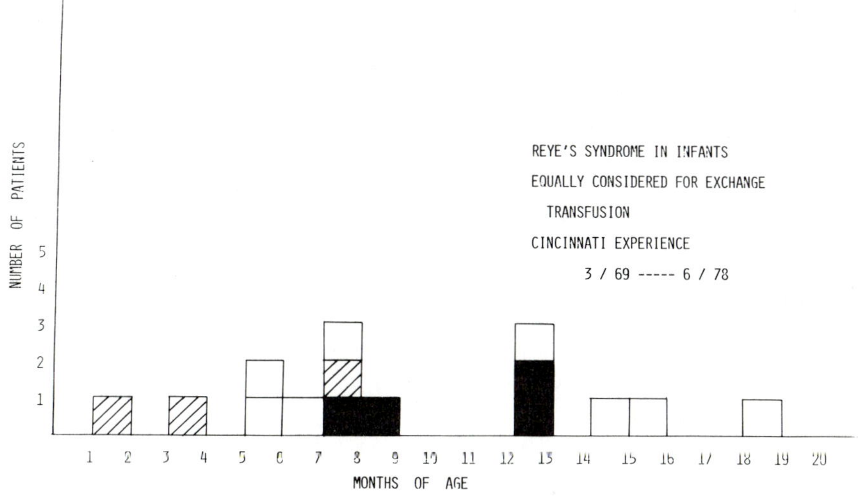

Legend as in Figure 5 and 6

Figure 9

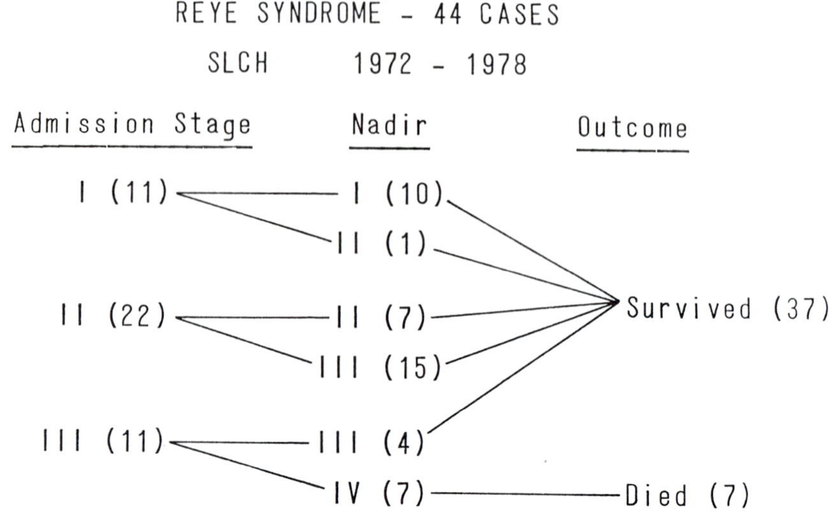

Table III

COMPARISON OF GRADING SYSTEMS IN REYE'S SYNDROME FROM FOUR CENTERS

Degree of Severity	Mild	Moderate	Severe	Brain Dead
Grade Used:				
Schubert, Partin (11)	1	2	3 , 4	5
Huttenlocher (14)	-	1	2 , 3	4
DeVivo, Keating, Haymond (15)	1	1	2 , 3	4
Lovejoy, Smith, Bresan (13)	1	2	3 , 4	5

From 1966-1971, 11 patients were seen, 7 of whom died.
From 1972-1978, 44 patients were seen, 7 of whom died.
All of the latter group of forty-four patients were

treated by the St. Louis group using early elective endotracheal intubation, hypertonic glucose, and intermittent infusion of mannitol. Using this regime, a survival rate of 84% has been achieved. Three patients have residual neurologic abnormalities but have preservation of intellectual function so that they are in school performing at grade level. One has mild ataxia and two have a rapid push of speech with running of words together and failure to modulate the rate at which they speak. (5,16). Similar to our results all patients presenting in what corresponds to our stage I and II survived, patients in our stage III survived but of patients in our stage IV 7 of 11 died. Thus treatment by exchange transfusion, or by elective endotracheal intubation and intensive supportive care, produces an increase in survival to 85-90% compared to the original stated survival of 10% (1) and the estimated present nationwide survival in the United States of 50% (18).

What does exchange transfusion remove or replace? Certainly ammonia and free fatty acids turn over much too rapidly to be significantly affected by exchange transfusion. Exchange may be removing an unidentified exogenous or endogenous toxin or providing albumin binding sites. Relatively dramatic awaking may occur in stage III patients with relapse after several hours suggesting that exchange transfusion may be removing a mitochondrial toxin. Dr. Aprille's work suggests the possibility of such a toxin but further studies of this and other potential toxins are needed(17).We have noted a fall in intracranial pressure concomitant with exchange transfusion in some of the patients in whom intracranial pressure has been monitored as described by Berman, et al, but the falls have not been consistent (19) and clinical improvement is not consistently related to such a change in pressure. Since coma may be present without elevated pressure this fact is not unexpected.

Other treatments presently or previously in use for Reye's syndrome are listed below.

TREATMENTS PROPOSED FOR REYE'S SYNDROME

```
 1 - Intravenous glucose - observation (3,7)
 2 - Exchange transfusion (2,3)
 3 - Intensive support - elective intubation (6,7)
 4 - Intracranial pressure monitoring and
       control (19,20)
 5 - Osmotic agents (mannitol, glycerol)(7,19,20,21)
 6 - Intermittent ventricular CSF drainage (20)
 7 - Peritoneal dialysis (22)
 8 - Blood ammonia reduction (14)
 9 - Corticosteroids (20)
10 - Citrulline - ornithine (23)
11 - Total body washout (24)
12 - Charcoal hemoperfusion (25)
13 - Intravenous Levadopa (26)
14 - Intravenous Pentobarbital(27)
15 - Massive cranial decompression (10)
```

Of these the first, i.e., early recognition, hospital admission and intravenous glucose, is certainly the most important. More severely ill patients should be admitted to an emergency care facility and treated by either exchange transfusion as described above or by elective intubation, hypertonic glucose and mannitol as described by DeVivo(6,7). Patients in our grade III and above should have intracranial pressure monitored and controlled with an osmotic agent. Monitoring of intracranial pressure deserves a word of caution. A wave of enthusiasm has swept the neurosurgical and critical care medicine literature concerning the value of intracranial pressure monitoring in Reye's Syndrome. The pressure can be monitored through a ventricular catheter, or a subdural Richmond bolt, or a Ladd epidural fiberoptic sensor. Monitoring devices which invade the dura or brain substance may have significant complications of ventriculitis, cerebral hemorrhage, or late porencephalic cysts at the site of the ventricular catheter. The epidural monitor has a fragile fiberoptic sensor and may break when most needed but has the lowest incidence of complication. Our experience with monitoring is limited to 12 patients but it has not improved survival. DeVivo summarized the mortality in

approximately 30 monitored patients described to date
at 40-50% (8). Monitoring should be done with care by
those with experience but still may not alter survival.
Although glycerol has been suggested (21)most experience
is with mannitol and the hepatic metabolism of glycerol
may not be normal in Reye's Syndrome as it is in patients with head trauma. If intracranial pressure cannot be controlled medically, bilateral massive surgical
temporo-parietal decompression of the swollen brain may
be life saving (10). Three patients have been treated
in this way in Cincinnati. All were grade IV and severely ill on admission. One is educable but retarded
with a full scale IQ of 47 and a Peabody Picture Vocabulary Test of 5 yr 11 months at 9 years of age, one
has an expressive aphasia and moderately severe brain
damage, and one has a full scale IQ of 70, a Peabody
Picture Vocabulary test of 5 yr 3 months at 7 years of
age and is attending regular school with a tutor. The
major problem with cranial decompression in our hands
has been timing. Despite prolonged coma our neurosurgical colleague, Dr.Robert McLaurin, maintains the
operation's only value is relief of pressure unresponsive to medical therapy. Even with intracranial monitoring Reye's Syndrome patients may have sudden intractable increases in pressure with herniation and loss of
brain stem function before the operation can be performed. Peritoneal dialysis has been shown to be definitely not effective. Reduction of blood ammonia pre-
sumes that the encephalopathy is hepatic in origin. Ammonia elevation is just one effect of mitochondrial dysfunction, and will usually resolve spontaneously. At
any rate, treatment of ammonia elevation alone may be
disastrous. Corticosteroids have been abandoned for
treatment of Reye's Syndrome by many workers in the
field (8,6). Citrulline and ornithine levels in Reye's
Syndrome are low presumably due to deficiency of urea
cycle mitochondrial enzymes and treatment with either
of these amino acids has been suggested to treat this
deficiency and to reduce elevated blood ammonia (23).
With the demonstrated concomitant reduction of carbamyl
phosphate synthetase as well as ornithine transcarbamylase, such therapy should result in a net increase of
ammonia production. Total body washout, better termed
asanguineous hypothermia perfusion, has been used in six

patients, five of whom survived without neurologic sequelae (25). Further experience with this procedure in stage IV disease is needed. It requires an experienced team which can be rapidly mobilized at the odd hours that Reye's Syndrome patients come to diagnosis. Experience with hemoperfusion is to be presented at this meeting. Intravenous pentobarbital to control increased intracranial pressure has been suggested recently (27). Further experience is needed to advocate such therapy, especially since many patients are comatose without increased intracranial pressure.

Presently then, we continue to advocate early diagnosis, prompt exchange transfusion combined with intensive supportive care and elective endotracheal intubation in children with Reye's Syndrome of our clinical grade III-V. Children in grades I and II must be carefully and continuously observed for progression while being treated with supportive measures. Although difficult and expensive, this combination seems most satisfactory to us at the present time. Hopefully,more specific therapy or, better still, prevention of the disease will result from the multiple research efforts and groups presently studying and treating this disease.

REFERENCES

1. Reye, R.D.K., Morgan, G., and Baral,J. 1963. Encephalopathy and fatty degeneration of the viscera. *Lancet 2*:749.
2. Schubert, W.K., Bobo,R.C., Partin,J.C. and Partin, J.S. Reye's Syndrome 1975. *Disease-A- Month*.
3. Bobo,R., Partin,J.C., Partin, J.S. and Schubert,W.K. 1975. Reye's Syndrome in Cincinnati. Treatment with exchange transfusion. *J.Pediat.87*:881.
4. Strauss, R.A., Kling,T.F.,Levinsohn,M.W. et al. 1976 Facilitation of Exchange Transfusions with Scribner Shunts in Reye's Syndrome. *Am.J.Surg. 131*:772.
5. DeVivo,D.C., Keating, J.P.,Haymond,M.W. 1975. Reye's Syndrome:Result of intensive supportive care. *J. Pediatr.87*:875.

6.   DeVivo,D.C., Keating,J.P. 1976- Reye's Syndrome.
     *Adv.Pediatr. 22:*175.
7.   Boutros,A., Hoyt,J.,Menezes,A. and Bell, W. 1977.
     Management of Reye's Syndrome. A rational approach
     to a complex problem. *Crit.Care Med.5:*234.
8.   DeVivo,D.C. 1978. Reye Syndrome: a metabolic re-
     sponse to an acute mitochonrial insult? *Neurology
     28:*105.
9.   Huttenlocher,P.R. 1972. Reye's Syndrome:relation
     of outcome to therapy. *J.Pediatr.80.*
10. Partin, J.C., Partin,J.S., Schubert, W.K. and Mc-
     Laurin,R.L. 1975. Brain Ultrastructure in Reye's
     Syndrome. (Encephalopathy and Fatty Alteration of
     the Viscera). *J.Neuropathol.Exp.Neurol.34:*425.
11. Schubert,W.K., Partin,J.C. and Partin,J.S. 1972.
     Encephalopathy and fatty liver (Reye's Syndrome).
     IN Popper,H. and Schaffner,F.,editors:*Progress in
     Liver Disease,IV,*New York,Grune & Stratton,Inc.,
     pp 489-510.
12. Plum,F. and Posner,J.B. 1972. The Central Syndrome
     of Rostralcaudal Deterioration,*in Diagnosis of
     Stupor and Coma,* Ed.2, Contemporary Neurology
     Series,Philadelphia, F.A.Davis Co. pp 80-90.
13. Lovejoy,F.H.,Smith,A.L.,Bresnan,M.J.Wood,J.M.,
     Victor,D.I. and Adams,P.C. 1974. Clinical staging
     in Reye's Syndrome. *Am.J.Dis.Child.128:*36.
14. Huttenlocher,P.R. 1972. Reye's Syndrome:Relation
     of Outcome to Therapy. *J.Pediatr.80:*845.
15. DeVivo,D.C., Keating,J.P. and Haymond,M.W. 1975.
     Intensive Supportive Approach to the Management
     of Reye's Syndrome. *IN* :J.D. Pollack,ed. *Reye's
     Syndrome,* Grune and Stratton, N.Y.
16. DeVivo, D.C. 1978. Personal Communication.
17. Aprille, J. R. and Asimakis, G.K. 1978. The
     Effect of Reye's Syndrome Serum on Mitochondrial
     Respiration In Vitro. *Ped.Res. 12:*391/429.

19. Berman, W., Pizzi, F., Schut, L. et al. 1975.The
     effects of exchange transfusion on intracranial
     pressure in patients with Reye's Syndrome.*J.Pedi-
     atr. 87*:887.
20. Venes,J.L., Shaywitz, B.A.,Spencer,D.D. 1978.
     Management of severe cerebral edema in the meta-
     bolic encephalopathy of Reye-Johnson Syndrome.
     J.Neurosurg.48:903.
21. Mickell,J.J., Cook, D.R.,Reigel, D.H. et al. 1976.
     Intracranial pressure monitoring in Reye-Johnson
     Syndrome.*Crit.Care Med.4*:1.
22. Samaha, F.J. 1975. The Role of Peritoneal Dialysis
     in Reye's Syndrome. IN Pollack,J.D. (ed.) Reye's
     Syndrome, New York, Grune & Stratton.
23. Delong,G.R., Glick, T.H., Shannon,D.C. 1974.
     Citrulline for Reye's Syndrome.*N.Engl.J.Med. 290*.
24. Lansky, L.L., Kalavsky,S.M., Brackett,C.E. et al.
     1977. Hypothermic total body washout and intra-
     cranial pressure monitoring in stage IV Reye's
     Syndrome. *J.Pediatr.90*:639.
25. Colon, A.R. 1978. Hemocarboperfusion in Cerebral
     Edema and Hepatic Failure. International Confer-
     ence on Reye's Syndrome, Halifax.
26. Fischer,J.E. and Baldessarini, R.J. 1971. False
     Neurotransmitters and Hepatic Failure. *Lancet 2*:
     75.
27. Marshall, L.F., Shapiro, H.M.,Rauscher,A. et al.
     1978. Pentobarbital therapy for intracranial hy-
     pertension in metabolic coma. Reye's Syndrome.
     Crit.Care Med.6:1.

Supported by the Cincinnati Children's Hospital
Research Foundation and in part by N.I.H. Clinical
Research Centers Grant #RR-00123.

DISCUSSION

Unidentified -   In the children 1 or 2 months of age,
     was there any evidence of a pre-natal or neonatal
     infection?

W.K. Schubert-   No. The infants that ended up retard-
     ed or with brain damage historically were normal.
     There was no evidence of a pre-natal infection on
     physical examination, nor are any included that
     had evidence of a birth defect or other disease,
     except one boy who had ulcerative colitis.

S.   Mayo   -   I wonder if you could briefly outline
     the extent of the awareness campaign carried on in
     Cincinnati?

W.K. Schubert-   Members of the Reye's Syndrome Founda-
     tion Chapter in Cincinnati have been active in put-
     ting up billboards which say "Reye's syndrome....
     what is it? Ask your pediatrician".

          Whenever a Reye's syndrome patient is
     admitted to the hospital, the hospital gets word
     to the newspaper and to the television. Dr.Partin
     has appeared on local television with descriptions
     of the disease.

          Probably the biggest single way is
     through pediatric grand rounds, talking to county
     Medical Societies, local practitioners and to em-
     ergency room personnel. The latter is a very im-
     portant group to inform. There the nurse can say
     to the doctor, "This child may have Reye's syn-
     drome" and thus get the child into the Reye's Syn-
     drome diagnostic category.

B.   Kerzner -   I'd like to know how often you find a
     biopsy that isn't Reye's syndrome when, indeed,you
     expected it to be so?

W.K. Schubert-   We sometimes see biopsies that sur-
prise us. One of the patients, for example, had an
amoebic abscess. Somewhere between 10 and 12 patients had clinical presentations of encephalopathy without the histologic ultra-structural findings that we would consider as diagnostic of
Reye's syndrome. We operate under the protection,
perhaps, of the treatment that we're using. That
is, we don't do the biopsy until everything is
ready for the exchange transfusion and this cor-
rects the blood coagulation abnormalities. Even in
the milder cases, we think that they should be biopsied for the purposes of diagnosis.

D.B. Caplan   - Have you used mannitol in any of the
patients who had normal intracranial pressure but
were still comatose?

W.K. Schubert-   We have used mannitol only on the clinical indication of increased pressure or on indication by the intracranial measurement monitor
that there is increased pressure.

M.M. Thaler   - Just a brief comment on what Doctor
Schubert said about liver biopsy. We don't bother
about using the prothrombin time as a contraindi-
cation for biopsies in Reye's syndrome. As you saw
yesterday, and as Dr. Partin showed in his histological series,there is very little perfusion in
that liver. The sinusoids are collapsed and, in
our experience, even with prothrombin times over
20 seconds there is no hepatic bleeding at all.In
fact,that is a potential pathogenic mechanism,with
fat obstructing the perfusion through liver sinusoids.

W.K. Schubert-   We measure the prothrombin time,but
then we go ahead and do the biopsy anyway. The
biggest single difference between this and fulminant hepatic necrosis is the fact that there isn't
any disseminated intravascular clotting. The real
problems with liver biopsy in children is in patients who have disseminated intravascular clot-

ting.

R.T. Shipman - In the light of Dr. Morin's experien-
     ces of patients with recurrent disease, you surely
     must also have recurrent patients among your large
     group.

W.K. Schubert-   I was very interested in the Montreal
     experience, because our recurrences are limited to
     two children.

HIGH DOSE GLYCEROL THERAPY IN THE
MANAGEMENT OF REYE'S ENCEPHALOPATHY

B. Kerzner, M.D., R. Roberts, M.D.,
J. Craenen, M.D., H.J.McClung,M.D.,
E. Sherard, M.D., M. Hilty, M. D.

Elevated intracranial pressure (ICP) contributes significantly to the mortality associated with Reye's syndrome(1,2,3). Although the magnitude of intracranial pressure need not relate directly to the degree of encephalopathy (4), high pressure is frequently a critical precipitating cause of death. Therefore, in recent years we have evolved a tactical approach for the vigorous management of increased ICP, in the hope that by so doing the prognosis for our severe cases of Reye's syndrome will be improved.

MATERIALS AND METHODS:

Over an 18 month period at Columbus Children's Hospital, Reye's syndrome was suspected in 23 patients and diagnosed in 19. Twelve of the 19 who reached Stage III coma were monitored continually, and analysis of the data from these children is presented here. Our criteria for the diagnosis of Reye's syndrome included elevations of blood ammonia and transaminases and a typical serum amino acid pattern characterized by high concentrations of a number of amino acids, including alanine, lysine and alpha amino-N-butyrate (5). For eight of the twelve cases, histological confirmation was available.

Since we believe that successful therapy depends on accurate, sensitive monitoring of increased intracranial pressure and related physiological parameters, we cooperated with Hewlett-Packard to develop a multichannel computerized recorder to undertake this task. The monitor combines oscilloscopes and digital printers

which allow for continuous representation of ICP,
venous pressure, arterial pressure, a single lead EEG
recording and an electrocardiogram. Intracranial pressure is recorded via a Richmond screw placed on the
dura in contact with the subarachnoid space while arterial and venous pressure are recorded from catheters
placed in the femoral vessels. All recorded information is stored in the computer's memory bank. A
plotter automatically sets out recorded information
allowing the clinician to analyze recalled data and
evaluate responses to particular clinical situations.

Initially, four patients received a low dose of
glycerol (less than 0.2 gms/kg/hr) given continuously
to supress background ICP to less than 30 mm Hg and
mannitol (1-2 gms/kg/dose) was given to control unanticipated elevations in pressure. Mortality with this
initial approach remained high, possibly because too
many unanticipated peaks in pressure were placing the
patients at risk. We therefore resolved to be more
aggressive in our treatment of future patients keep-
ing background pressure below 20 mm Hg with increased
doses of glycerol. A half hour bolus was added to
every two hours of continuous background infusion. Two
groups of patients emerged: four with a milder illness
who received a medium range dose of glycerol 0.2-0.5
mg/kg/hr and four more severely affected cases who
required high dose glycerol therapy of more than 0.5
gms/kg/hr.

RESULTS:

The clinical course experienced by the three
groups is illustrated in Figure 1 in which duration and
outcome are indicated. The therapeutic outcome for the
low dose group was not satisfactory. ICP was difficult
to control in patients 1, 2 and 4, all of whom died
after manifesting profound coma. Patient 2, who had
the most extended illness, ultimately died of renal
failure which developed early as a result of cardio-
respiratory arrest when ICP was most difficult to control. The medium dose group had a relatively mild and
brief illness; their ICP was not difficult to control.
None progressed beyond Stage III coma. Frequently

their mental state improved immediately after receiving boluses of glycerol and recovery was rapid and
complete. Three of the patients in the high dose group
had a protracted course and were intensely ill; at the
conclusion of IV therapy localizing neurological signs
including extraocular palsy, hemiparesis and impaired
memory were evident. However, all have made remarkable
progress and now have only minimal residua. None of
these patients died, but their relatively protracted
course probably reflects the severity of their illness.

FIGURE 1

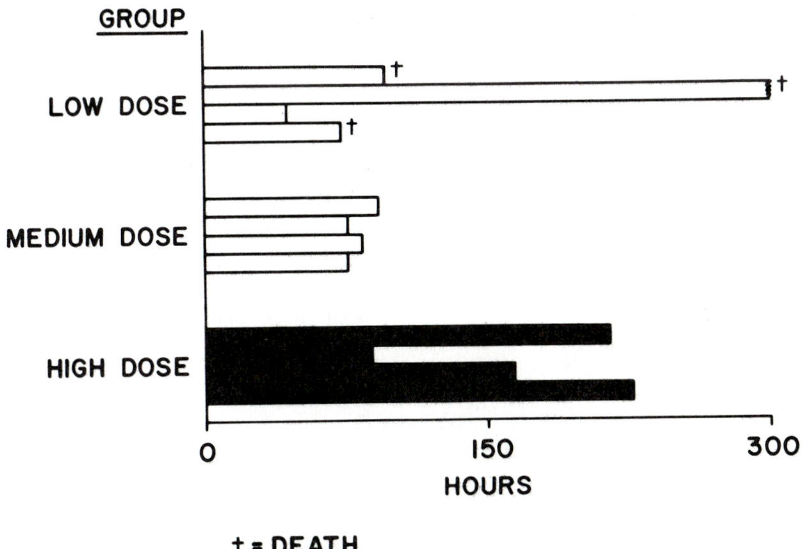

The need for mannitol, which was only given in
response to sudden increases in ICP, diminished in the
medium and high dose groups as reflected by the fact
that the three highest doses of mannitol 0.8, .14 and
.55 gms/kg/hr were employed in the early group of
patients receiving relatively low doses of glycerol.
The most mannitol required by the medium dose group

was 0.6 gms/kg/hr and by the high dose group was 0.7
gms/kg/hr. Equally high serum amino acid values were
found in group I and III, as illustrated in Figure 2,
and lower levels were found in the medium dose group.
The highest mean osmolality per 24 hours achieved for
the total duration of intravenous therapy of all patients in the low dose group was 321 milliosmoles/l.
The highest mean for the medium dose group was 311
milliosmoles/l and the highest mean level of the high
dose group was 389 milliosmoles/l. Three of these
cases reached an osmotic tension of greater than 410.

FIGURE 2

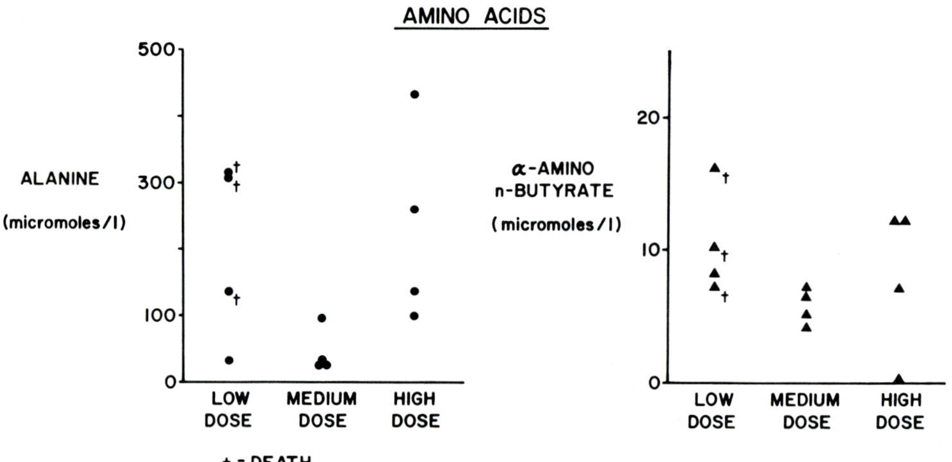

     The mean ICP for the duration of therapy in the
three groups (low, medium, and high) was respectively
24, 21, and 19 mm Hg with the number of peaks above 30
mm Hg in 24 hours being 44, 9, and 4. However many of
the peaks were recorded during the weaning phase of
therapy. Analysis of data through the first 48 hours

of illness shows mean ICP of 24.5, 19.8 and 19.4 mm Hg
with peaks above 30 mm Hg occurring 8, 6 and 3.7 times
in 24 hours.

DISCUSSION:

The degree of coma, the protracted illness and the
high serum amino acid values of the four patients who
received more than 0.5 gms. of glycerol per kilo per
hour suggests that they were as severely affected by
Reye's syndrome as were the three patients, in the low
dose group, who died. We believe that our vigorous
management of the high dose group of patients has been
instrumental in their survival. There can be no doubt
about the effect of glycerol on serum osmolality, because the osmotic tension apparent in the serum of the
high dose group is clearly greater than the other two
groups. Despite osmolality going above 400 in three
patients, all of them have recovered satisfactorily
without significant neurological deficits.

The most confusing aspect of this study is the
fact that mean values for ICP and the number of ICP
peaks above 30 mm Hg for the total duration of therapy
were not convincingly different in the three groups of
patients. However, the values are unduly influenced by
frequent transient pressure peaks occurring when the
therapy was in the process of being discontinued. Possibly a clearer impression of what we have been able to
achieve in terms of altered pressure relates to the
extent of adequate pressure control achieved early in
the illness. In the first 24 hours of glycerol therapy
the mean pressure of the high dose group is indeed
lower than the low dose group, and fewer pressure peaks
are evident in this critical phase of the disease.
From these preliminary data we, therefore, believe that
vigorous control of ICP will improve the survival rate
of severe cases of Reye's syndrome, although such therapy may result in very high serum osmolalities. Because
glycerol will enter the CST over time (6) we presume
that progressively increasing levels of osmotic tension
are actually necessary to maintain a gradient across the
blood brain barrier, which will reverse cerebral edema
until the illness has run its natural course.

High serum osmotic tension may carry its own risks (7,8)
but the hazard is worthwhile if mortality continues to
be reduced.

REFERENCES

1. Evans, H.;C.H.Bourgeois, D.S. Comer, et al. 1970
    Brain lesions of Reye's syndrome. *Arch.Pathol.90:*
    543-546.
2. Bourgeois, C.H.; L.C. Olson, D.S. Comer, et al.
    1971. Encephalopathy and fatty degeneration of the
    viscera: A clinicopathologic analysis of 40 cases.
    Am.J.Clin.Pathol. 56:5, 558-571.
3. Partin, J.C.; J.S.Partin, W.K. Schubert, R. L.Mc-
    Laurin. 1975. Brain ultrastructure in Reye's syn-
    drome (encephalopathy and fatty alteration of vis-
    cera).*J.Neuropathol.Exp.Neurol.* 34, 425.
4. Berman, W.; F.Pizzi, L.Schut, et al. 1975. The
    effects of exchange transfusion on intracranial
    pressure in patients with Reye's syndrome. *J.Pediat.*
    87:6,887-891.
5. Hilty, M.D.; C.A.Romshe, P.V.Delamaster. 1974.Reye's
    syndrome and hyperaminoacidemia. *J.Pediat.84:* 362-
    365.
6. Guisado, R.; A.I.Arieff, S.G. Massry. 1974. Effects
    of glycerol infusions on brain water and electro-
    lytes. *Am.J.Physiol.* 227, 865-872.
7. Arieff, A.I.; H.J.Carroll. 1972. Nonketotic hyper-
    osmolar coma with hyperglycemia; clinical features,
    pathophysiology, renal function, acid-base balance,
    plasma-cerebrospinal fluid equilibria and the ef-
    fects of therapy in 37 cases.*Medicine 51:2,73-94.*
8. Gerich,J.E.; M.M.Martin, L.Recant. 1971. Clinical
    and metabolic characteristics of hyperosmolar non-
    ketotic coma. *Diabetes 20:4,* 228-238.

DISCUSSION

G.D. Gall -   Could you tell me if glycerol crosses
the blood barrier in significant quantities?

B.Kerzner   -   This problem has recently been discussed by Rottenberg et al (*Neurology* July 1977).
   They have described a diminishing effect of intravenous glycerol,presumably based on the development of a reverse osmotic gradient. Reversal of
   the gradient could be the result of glycerol cross-
   ing the blood brain barrier, and animal studies on
   brain matter and CSF clearly show that glycerol
   can enter the brain substance. An alternative explanation is the generation of osmoles within the
   brain, in response to hypertonic states; this occurs in fishes and has been experimentally demonstrated in rats. These 'idiogenic' osmoles probably result from the release of amino acids within
   the neurocytes.

J.C. Partin -   As doctors become more adept at managing their sick patients, more of the patients survive. With more patients living, we must address
   the quality of survival. Drs. Donald O'Grady and
   Bob Brunner, our clinical psychologists, began a
   study of 40 patients who have survived Reye's syndrome for more than one year. Interpreting the results turns out to be a complex problem, indicating the need for orderly and quantitative psycho-
   metric analysis.

B.Kerzner   -   I agree.

THE ABSENCE OF SYSTEMIC COMPLICATIONS
ASSOCIATED WITH THE USE OF INTRAVENOUS
LEVODOPA IN PATIENTS WITH SEVERE REYE'S
SYNDROME.

H.J. McClung, M.D., B. Kerzner, M. D.,
M. Hilty, M. D.,   C. Romshe, M. D.,
and E. Sherard, M.D.

The encouraging reports of levodopa in the treatment of hepatic encephalopathy (1,3) have led to the suggestion that it might also be efficacious in Reye's Syndrome (4). As a preliminary phase of this investigation, we evaluated the safety of levodopa given intravenously to 6 patients with Reye's Syndrome in Stage III coma or deeper.

Our rationale for beginning the study of levodopa in Reye's Syndrome encephalopathy is based upon previous work in which we demonstrated that patients with Reye's Syndrome had depressed hypothalamic levels of dopamine and elevated levels of octopamine (5). These results were within the range previously reported from the brains of patients with chronic hepatic encephalopathy (2,6). We also evaluated the ability of the brain to take up administered levodopa and found that this was normal but that, at least in the pre-terminal phase of the illness, the levodopa did not seem to be converted to dopamine (5). We were left with the question whether this lack of enzymatic conversion represented an enzymatic defect in Reye's Syndrome, or whether it reflected a state of brain death. Because of this dilemma and numerous other neuropharmacological questions about Reye's Syndrome,we developed a protocol evaluating the effect and pharmacology of levodopa in patients with Reye's Syndrome in which the first phase is a study of the drug's safety.

METHODS AND MATERIALS

The diagnosis of Reye's Syndrome was established by the usual clinical and laboratory criteria. All patients had a viral illness followed by severe vomiting and then alterations in consciousness. Laboratory confirmation included the characteristic pattern of serum amino acids (7), elevated liver enzymes (SGOT, SGPT), elevated blood ammonia and, when possible, a liver biopsy.

When informed consent was given by the parents the patients were placed in a double blind, prospective trial. After 24 hours of this trial, if the attending physician or parents so requested, the patient could receive known levodopa for the remainder of the comatose period. This experimental plan has been approved by our hospital's Human Subjects Committee and the Neuropharmacology Branch of the FDA, and is supervised under the first author's IND-12,119. Levodopa or matched placebo is dispensed in a coded fashion by our pharmacy. Patients were given 2.5 mg/kg of drug by slow intravenous push every 4 hours. All patients were classified as Stage III coma or deeper (8). All patients were closely monitored for increased intracranial pressure with an intracranial pressure monitor and were treated intensively with osmolar diuretics if the pressure rose above acceptable limits. Vital signs for this study were recorded on cassette tape after instantaneous computer processing, and were later charted as time profiles. The accumulated data was analyzed with a student's "t" test. Levodopa and matched placebo vials of diluent were supplied by Hoffman-LaRoche.

RESULTS

During the deeper stages of coma, none of the six patients had any objective symptoms or signs of having received levodopa during the intravenous push of the drug or in the immediate 15-minute period afterward. The expected symptoms were nausea, vomiting, or sweating. During the time when these patients were awakening from their coma, several of them did experience

nausea in the immediate post-infusion period. None of
the expected signs of drug administration occurred.
Cardiovascular parameters of heart rate, mean arterial
pressure and venous pressure were unaffected by the infusion.(Table 1). Our two objective measures of CNS
function, the epidural pressure and percentage of EEG
which was delta wave were also unaffected (Table 2).

TABLE 1

Cardiovascular 15-Minute
Response To Intravenous Levodopa

	Heart Rate (beats/min.)	Mean Arterial Pressure (mm Hg)	Venous Pressure (mm H_2O)
Levodopa	+0.2 ± 1.2 (39)	-1.1 ± 0.8 (42)	+1.2 ± 1.7 (29)
Placebo	-2.6 ± 1.5 (9)	+1.7 ± 3.2 (9)	+1.7 ± 1.1 (7)
P	NS	NS	NS

TABLE 2

15-Minute Response to Intravenous Levodopa

	Epidural Pressure (mm Hg)	% Delta Wave on EEG
Levodopa	-0.1 ± 0.7 (42)	+0.3 ± 0.5 (13)
Placebo	-0.3 ± 1.0 (10)	-5.9 ± 7.0 (3)
P	NS	NS

DISCUSSION:

Reye's Syndrome can be compared and contrasted to
hepatic coma(9). In this regard,obvious differences exist,such as liver pathology,the time course of the illness,and the usual absence of jaundice in Reye's Syndrome. The similarities between the two conditions,how-
ever,are striking and include the raised liver enzymes
and ammonia,the predisposition for hypoglycemia, the
occurance of cerebral edema, and the progression through
stages of coma. In addition, both conditions are typi-
fied by similar neurotransmitter profiles(5). Because
the pathogenesis of Reye's Syndrome encephalopathy is
not fully delineated,it seems logical to use hepatic coma as an initial pathogenetic model (10).

Recent literature on the pathogenesis of hepatic coma has explored the possibility that a major contributor
to the coma is an imbalance among the neurotransmitter
substances within the brain. In particular,the dopame-
nergic system has been found to be deranged. Dopamine
and norepinephrine are extremely low in the brains of
patients with liver coma,while partially synthesized
components of these catechols circulate in high levels
and are deposited in increased amounts in basal ganglia
of the brain (1-3,6). The normal sequence of synthesis
of dopamine and norepinephrine are shown in Figure 1.
Phenylalanine is hydroxylated to tyrosine and again,hy-
droxylated to levodopa. Levodopa is the compound of
this series which most easily crosses the blood brain
barrier. From this point,side chain reactions occur.The
l-aromatic amino acid decarboxylase converts levodopa
to dopamine, and dopamine-B-hydroxylase converts it to
norepinephrine. The final step is completed as phenylethanolamine N-methyl-transferase N-methylates norepinephrine to epinephrine.

Current thinking holds that invertebrate and bacterial biochemical systems do not usually complete the
second hydroxylation of tyrosine to levodopa, but rather perform the side chain reactions on either phenylalanine or tyrosine to produce their neurotransmitter
substances(11). (Figure 1). The products of such reactions are found in only tiny amounts in normal

FIGURE 1

Biochemical Relationships of the Synthesis of Normal
And "False" Neurotransmitters in the Dopaminergic System

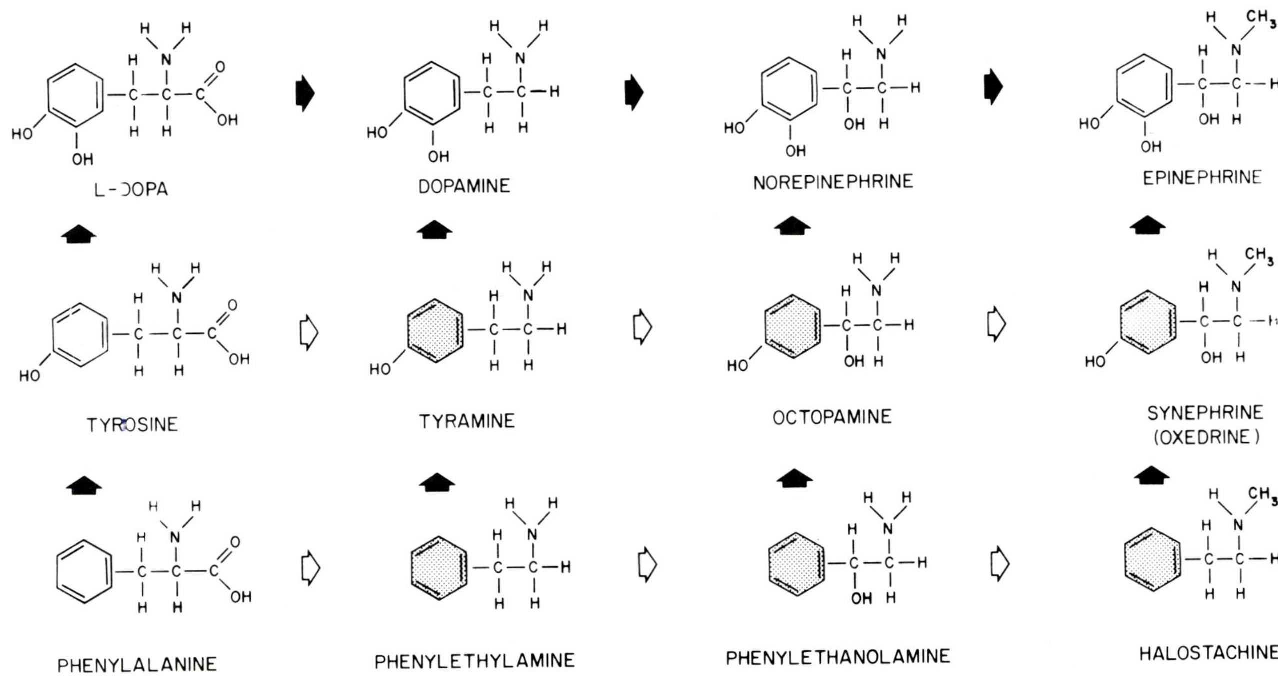

mammals and are rapidly hydroxylated to more acceptable
products or are degraded in the liver by monoamine oxidase degradation pathways.

In liver failure, it is speculated that either large
amounts of blood by-passes the liver, or the liver is
so severely affected that it cannot carry out these detoxification reactions. Bacteria in the intestine are
constantly producing the "incomplete" catecholamines
which then circulate freely, cross the blood brain barrier and become attached to neural endplates. In this
location they are not appropriately released for neural
synaptic transmission and thus have been labeled, false-
neurotransmitters. Particularly, tyramine, octopamine
and phenylethanolamine have been implicated in hepatic
coma (12-16) while halostachine is thought to be a contributor to staggers in sheep (17).

With this background, it is natural to see if additional levodopa might in some way reverse the clinical
picture of hepatic coma. While the results have not been
uniform, numerous reports now claim therapeutic benefit in improving the awake-pattern on EEG or the clinical stage of coma in liver coma patients (1-3,18).Based
upon these assumptions, levodopa has been used in
Reye's Syndrome patients and preliminary reports suggest that it may have a beneficial effect (4).

Exploration of the pharmacology and pharmacokinetics
of levodopa along with the important questions regarding the ability of this drug to alter the coma or clinical course of the illness are in progress. In the
meantime, it can be confidently stated that the intravenous form of levodopa can safely be studied in patients with severe Reye's Syndrome.

REFERENCES

1. Parks,J.D.,Sharpstone,P.,Williams,R. 1970. False
    neurotransmitters and hepatic coma.*Lancet 2*:1341-3.
2. Fischer,J.E.,Baldessarine,R. 1971. False neuro-
    transmitters and hepatic coma.*Lancet 2*:75-79.
3. Fischer,J.E.,James,J.H.,1972.Treatment of hepatic
    coma and hepatorenal syndrome.Mechanism of action
    of L-dopa and aramine.*Am.J.Surg.123*:222-230.

4.   Crocker,J.F.S.,MacDonald, R.G.,Ozere, R.L., 1973.
     Levodopa in Reye's Syndrome.*Clin.Res.21*:1033.
5.   Lloyd,K.G.,Davidson, L.,Price,K.,McClung,H.J.,Gall,
     D.G. 1977. Catecholamine and octopamine concen-
     trations in brains of patients with Reye's Syndrome
     Neurology 27:985-988.
6.   Dodworth, J.M., James, J.H., Cummings, M.G.,
     Fischer, J.E. 1974. Depletion of brain norepine-
     phrine in acute hepatic coma. *Surgery 75*:811-820.
7.   Hilty, M.D., Romshe,C.A., Delamater,P.V. 1974.
     Reye's Syndrome and hyperaminoacidemia. *Pediatrics
     84:* 362-365.
8.   Sherard, E.S., Cooper, R.F. 1975. Multiphasic
     diagnosis of Reye's Syndrome in *Reye's Syndrome,*
     Ed.J.D.Pollack,Grune & Stratton,New York,27-38.
9.   Partin,J.C. 1977. Hepatic encephalopathy and Reye's
     Syndrome. *Pediat.Ann.6:*346-354.
10. Zieve,L.,Nicoloff,D.M. 1975. Pathogenesis of hepa-
     tic coma. *Ann.Rev.Med.26*: 143-157.
11. Axelrod,J.,Saavedra,J.M. 1977. Octopamine. *Nature
     265:* 501-504.
12. Capocaccia,L., Cangiano,C.,Attili,A.F.,Angelico,M.,
     Cascino, Fanelli,F.R. 1977. Octopamine and ammonia
     plasma levels in hepatic encephalopathy.*Clin.Chim.
     Acta 75:* 99-105.
13. Chase,R.A.,Trewby,P.N.,Davis,M.,Williams, R. 1977.
     Serum octopamine,coma,and charcoal haemoperfusion
     in fulminant hepatic failure.*Eur.J.Clin.Invest.7:*
     351-354.
14. Smith, A.R.,Rossi-Fanelli,F.,Ziparo, V., James,J.H.
     Perelle,B.A.,Fischer,J.E. 1978. Alterations in
     plasma and CSF amino acids,amines and metabolites
     in hepatic coma.*Ann.Surg.187:* 343-350.
15. Zoghbi,F.,Emerit,J.,Fermanian,J.,Bousquet,O.,
     Legrand,J.C.,Sarrazin,A.,Desgrez,P. 1977. Compara-
     tive study of urinary excretion rates of parahy-
     droxymandelic acid,homovanillic acid,vanylmandelic
     acid in cirrhotic patients with and without enceph-
     alopathy. *Biomedicine 27*:37-40.

16.   Bloch, P., Delorme,M.L.,Rapin,J.R., Granger,A.,
      Boschat,M.,Opolon,P. 1978. Reversible modifica-
      tions of neurotransmitters of the brain in experi-
      mental acute hepatic coma. *Surg.Gyn.Obst.146:*551-
      558.
17.   Aasen,A.J.,Culvenor,C.C.J., Finnie,E.P., Kellock,
      A.W.,Smith,L.W. 1969. Alkaloids as a possible
      cause of ryegrass staggers in grazing livestock.
      Aust.J.Agric.Rec.20· 71-86.
18.   Chajek,T.,Friedman,G.,Berry,E.M., Abramsky,O.1977.
      Treatment of acute encephalopathy with L-dopa.
      Postgrad.Med.J. 53: 262-265.

DISCUSSION

J.F.S. Crocker - We had some primary interest in L-
      Dopa with Reye's patients, but the biggest
      problem was getting enough patients to do a
      control study to prove that we had accomplished
      anything. How long would it take you to get con-
      trol data with L-Dopa in Reye's syndrome, with
      your current caseload?

H.J. McClung   - About three years.

A.R. Colon   - We've measured neurotransmitters in
      CSF in 10 patients in hepatic coma who've under-
      gone hemocarboperfusion and, in looking at epin-
      ephrine, norepinephrine, dopamine, Serotonin and
      total catecholomines, we've had no significant
      changes either way with the use of the hemocarbo
      perfusion. If anything, some of the total epine-
      phrines have gone up a slight amount in the CSF,
      but it's been an insignificant change.

H.J. McClung   - This,of course, goes right back to the
      point that I made about doing cerebral spinal
      fluids studies and, at the moment, I must con-
      fess that I am a bit discouraged. As you know,

there is a tremendous gradient of neurotransmitter substance from the ventricules down to
where we normally do an L.P so that, if you take
sequential samples of fluid, you will have almost 100% difference in the first sample to the
second to the third to the fourth, and it's extremely difficult to know how to interpret this
data.

REYES SYNDROME (RS) IN MICHIGAN

W.D. Engle,M.D.,J.V. Baublis,M.D.,T.E. Duff,M.D.,
N.M. Rosenberg,D.O.,R.P. Tucker,M.D.,G.W. Kindt,M.D.,
R.C. Kelsch,M.D. and R. Weeks,PhD

Encephalopathy has long been recognized as a serious
complication of infectious disorders of childhood (1,2).
In 1963 Reye, Morgan, and Baral (3) observed that certain
clinical and pathophysiological features in patients
with encephalopathy were consistently associated with
fatty degeneration of the viscera. Subsequently, the
clinico-pathologic entity of "encephalopathy with fatty
degeneration of the viscera" in children has been
referred to as Reye's syndrome (RS). RS is recognized
as a frequently fatal neurologic illness which can occur
with dramatic frequency during outbreaks of influenza
(4). Sporadic cases of RS are observed in patients
recovering from chickenpox and other common viral diseases (5).

Uncertainty regarding the interrelation of factors
which precipitate RS as well as a fragmentary grasp of
its pathogenesis have led to empiric recommendations of
various therapeutic regimes (6-9). Cerebral edema is a
major clinical feature of RS and has been a constant
finding at autopsy (10) underscoring the importance of
increased intracranial pressure (ICP) in the death of
patients with RS. We examined survival and the frequency
of neurologic complications among patients with RS as
predicted by the patient's condition at the time of
admission, i.e., level of coma, grade of electroenceph-
alographic (EEG) abnormality (12), and the blood ammonia
concentration (NH_3). The outcome of a management
protocol, which was basically supportive and included
continuous monitoring and controlling ICP of patients

with RS, was compared with the outcome of earlier management protocols which did not make use of continuous
monitoring.

MATERIALS AND METHODS

The medical records of children who experienced
sixty-eight episodes of RS during the period 1969-1977
were reviewed. Patients in this study were referred to
Mott Children's Hospital (MCH) from throughout Michigan.
However, the majority lived in the southeastern part of
the state. Patients were excluded from the study if
they showed evidence of drug intoxication, meningitis,
or viral encephalitis. RS was diagnosed on the basis of
the following criteria:

1. A characteristic biphasic clinical course that
included apparent viral disease followed by protracted
vomiting and an altered state of consciousness.

2. Laboratory confirmation of hepatic dysfunction
on the basis of two or more of the following test results: (a) SGOT and SGPT levels twice normal or greater. (b) Prothrombin time prolonged two seconds or more
compared to the normal control value. (c) A blood
ammonia concentration at least twice the normal control
value.

None of the patients with these findings had to be
excluded on the basis of a conflicting histopathologic
diagnosis. Specific information was obtained from
medical records concerning the date of admission, the
outcome of the illness, the patient's sex and age, and
the patient's clinical status on admission described
by: 1. Stage of coma (11). 2. Grade of EEG abnormality (12). 3. Blood ammonia concentration (13,14).

Prior to 1974, management consisted of routine
supportive measures such as ventilatory support, fluid
and electrolyte maintenance, antibiotic treatment of
purulent infections, and the administration of osmotic
agents for any perceived increase of ICP. A few patients
were treated with additional measures reported to be
of benefit in patients with RS such as glucose/insulin
infusions (6), peritoneal dialysis (7), and exchange

transfusion (8,9). Since 1974 the principal goal of our
management protocol was to maintain and preserve
cerebral perfusion. This goal was pursued by a multi-
disciplinary management team in a consistent manner who,
in addition to routine measures, employed an ICP monitor
(15) in a nonrandom fashion for patients admitted in
coma (Stage III) or who deteriorated to a comatose state
subsequent to admission. Continuous ICP monitoring was
used in these patients in order to promote the judicious
use of osmotic agents such as urea and mannitol (1G/kg/
dose), and of hypothermia (90°-92°F), hyperventilation
(PCO_2 - 20-25mm), and fluid restriction (2/3 maintenance).

RESULTS

During the study period, there were sixty-eight
admissions to MCH which met our criteria for RS. Thirty-
eight episodes of RS occurred in males and thirty episodes were observed in females. One girl who survived an
episode of RS at the age of four years without sequellae,
succumbed a year later during a second episode. Death
occurred in a nine year old black female, the only non-
Caucasian in the study group.

TABLE 1. SEX OF THE PATIENT AND SURVIVAL IN RS

	MALE		FEMALE		TOTAL	
	NO.	(%)	NO.	(%)	NO.	(%)
SURVIVORS	24	(63)	22	(73)	46	(68)
NON-SURVIVORS	14	(37)	8	(27)	22	(32)

The survival rate for patients hospitalized with
RS was 68 percent. Survival was more frequent in
female (73 percent) than male (63 percent) patients
(Table 1). Although RS occurred throughout the year,
over half of the episodes of RS occurred during the first
quarter of the year, January through March (Figure 1).

In 1974, there was a pronounced increase in the

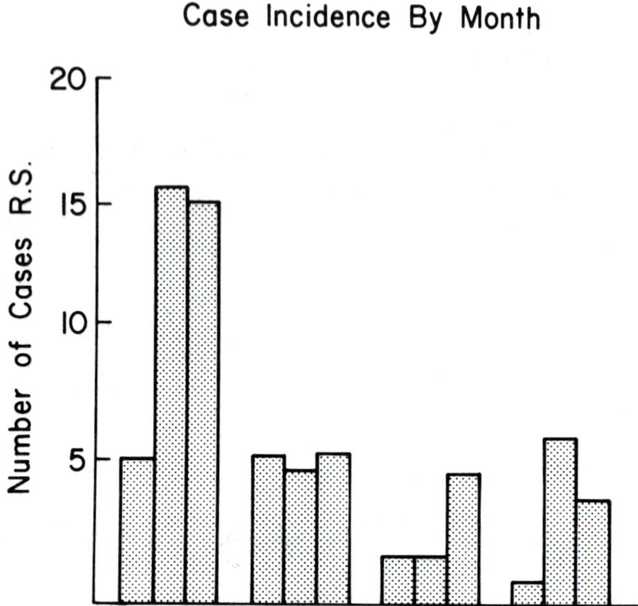

Figure 1. Case Incidence by Month

number of patients admitted to MCH with the diagnosis
RS (Figure 2). Prior to this time, the survival of
patients with RS was 57 percent. Since 1974, the survival rate of 69 percents suggests that there has been
a trend toward improved survival (.05>p<.10 chi square).

     The level of coma at the time of admission appear-
ed to vary inversely with the survival rate of patients
with RS (Table 2). Only five of the seventeen patients
who were beyond Stage III at the time of admission survived. In contrast, 40/50 patients admitted in Stage
III or a lesser stage of coma survived (p=.0015 chi
square). Indications of the adverse implications of
deep coma at the time of admission were evident from
the poor quality of survival. Three of the five patients

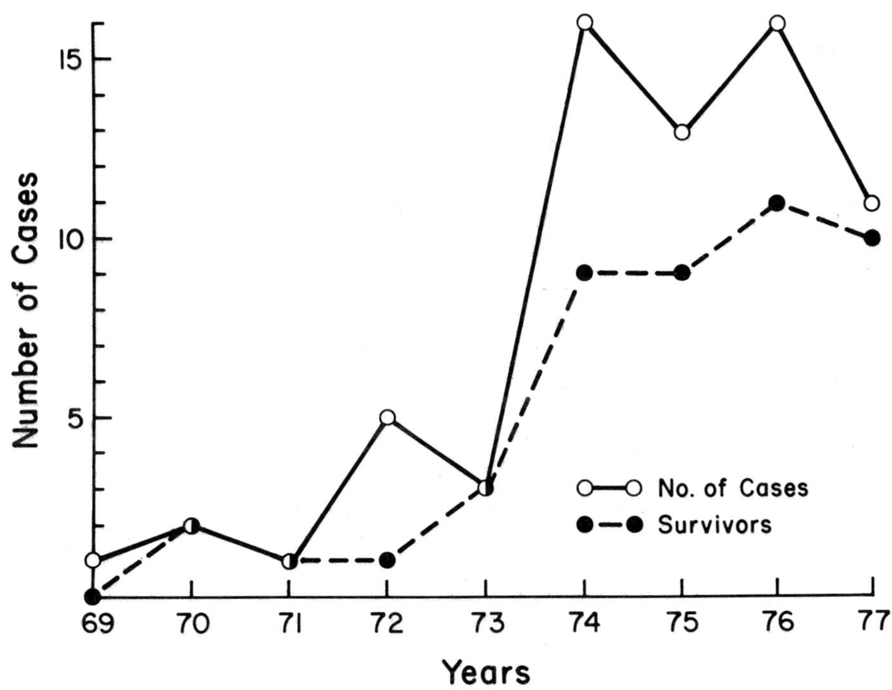

Figure 2.

who survived despite admission in severe coma (Stage IV-V) have severe neurologic sequelae.

Prior to the introduction of continuous ICP monitoring in 1974, 6/13 patients admitted in Stage I or II deteriorated to Stage III, and four of these patients died. Since the inception of the monitoring program, 8/18 patients admitted in these mild levels

TABLE 2.   STAGE OF COMA ON ADMISSION AND
           SURVIVAL IN RS

	I	II	III	IV	V
SURVIVORS	5	21	14	4	1
NON-SURVIVORS	1	3	6	6	6
TOTAL	6	24	20	10	7

of coma deteriorated but with only one fatality. Improved survival was also apparent among patients admitted in more severe stages of coma. Five of sixteen patients admitted in Stage III, IV, and V who were managed without an ICP monitor survived, while fourteen of the twenty-one patients managed with an ICP monitor survived. In addition to enhanced survival, the quality of survival appears generally improved. Severe neurologic sequelae were observed in two of the five patients managed without a monitor, whereas only three of fourteen patients managed with the monitor experienced such complications.

The grade of EEG abnormality in patients with RS appeared to run parallel to the depth of coma and was also predictive of outcome (Table 3). Among patients with EEG grades of 2 and 3, 30/37 survived, whereas only 6/17 of those admitted with an EEG of grade 4 or 5 survived (p=.004 chi square). Among the six surviving patients with grade 4 or 5 abnormalities at admission, only two made a complete neurologic recovery. Hence, stage of coma and grade of EEG abnormality both were predictive of morbidity and mortality.

The blood ammonia level in a patient with RS may reflect the extent of urea cycle dysfunction and consequently the severity of the metabolic pathology. The

TABLE 3.   GRADE OF EEG ABNORMALITY ON ADMISSION
           AND SURVIVAL IN RS

| | EEG GRADE | | | |
	2	3	4	5
SURVIVORS	6	24	6	0
NON-SURVIVORS	0	7	9	2
TOTAL	6	31	15	2

$(NH_3)_b$ of RS patients varied directly with the depth of
coma and grade of EEG abnormality. There was however a
high degree of variance noted within each stage and
grade (Figure 3.).

The mean $(NH_3)_b$ concentrations for patients within
a given clinical stage of RS were significantly higher
among the non-survivors (Figure 4). Likewise, when
NH_3 levels within a given EEG category were compared,
higher values were noted among the non-survivors. Regardless of the stage of coma or grade of EEG abnormality, 33/38 of those patients with an admission NH_3
level 270 µg/100 ml. survived while only 10/21 of those
with a level 270 µg/100 ml. survived (p=.0024). Furthermore, only four of the ten surviving patients with an
admission $(NH_3)_b$ 270 µg/ml. recovered without sequelae
(Table 5).

A modifying influence on survival of patients
whose disease was judged severe on the basis of a
$(NH_3)_b$ in excess of 270 µg/100 ml. could also be
shown. Such patients appeared to have a poor prognosis
despite the stage of coma or grade of EEG determined at
admission. Sixty percent of the patients in this category who were managed with the aid of the ICP monitor
survived whereas only 17 percent of those patients
not monitored survived (p=.09 by Fisher).

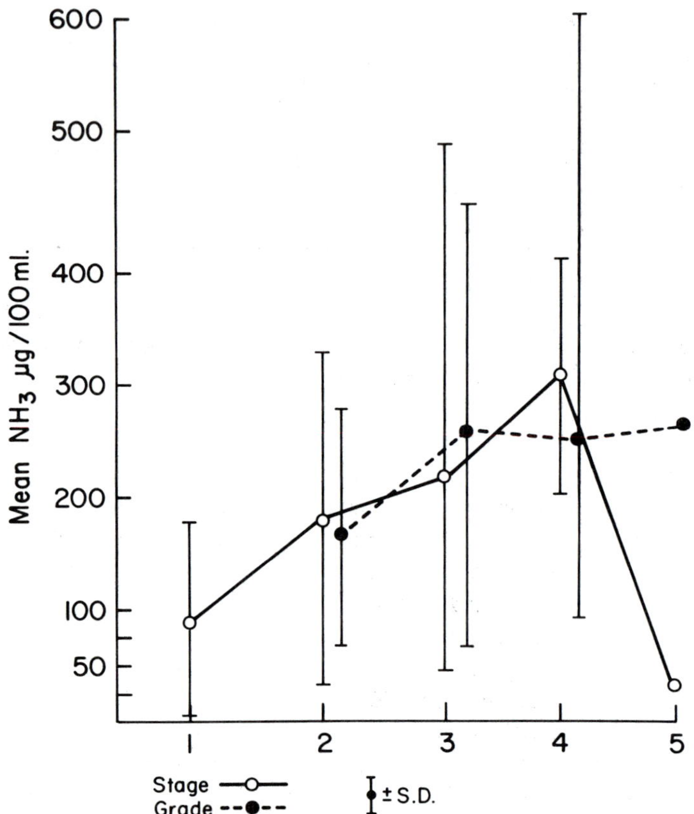

Figure 3.   Mean Admission NH_3 Levels, Stage and Grade

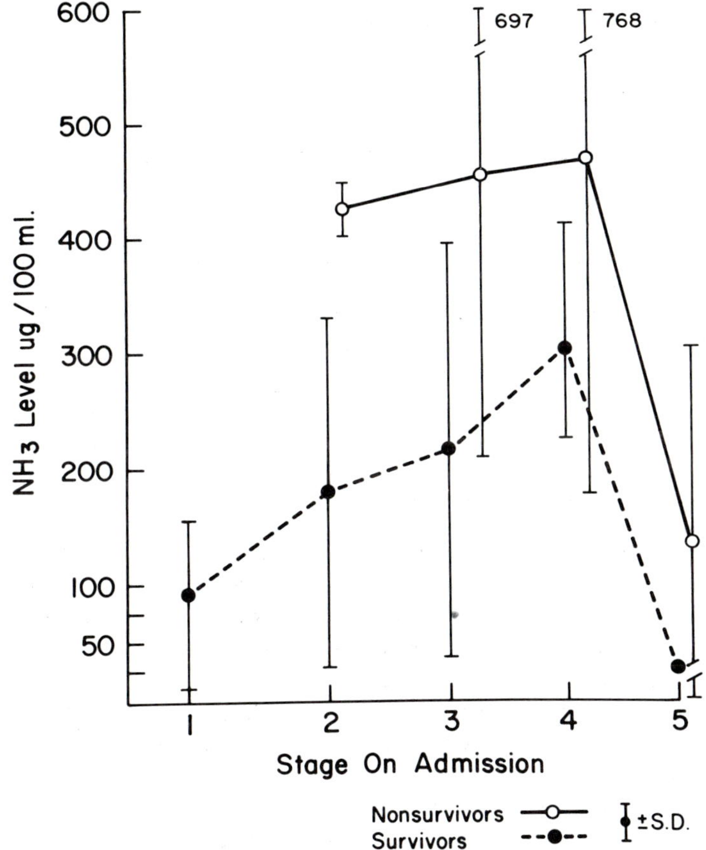

Figure 4. NH$_3$ Levels and Survival Within Each Stage

Since there are theoretical reservations regarding
the administration of urea to patients with impaired
urea cycle enzyme function, we examined the outcome of
RS in patients who received this drug. Thirteen of the
twenty patients admitted in severe coma (Stages III-V)
who received urea to control apparent brain edema survived while only six of the seventeen patients in this
category who did not receive urea survived (Table 4)
(p=.07 chi square).

TABLE 4.   UREA ADMINISTRATION AND SURVIVAL IN
           STAGES III-V.

	UREA		NO UREA	
	NO.	(%)	NO.	(%)
SURVIVAL	13	(65)	6	(35)
NO SURVIVAL	7	(35)	11	(65)

An effect on survival was not apparent when patients
were grouped according to the use of mannitol. Nine of
twenty patients in Stages III-V who received the latter
drug survived while 10/17 of those patients at this
level of coma who did not receive mannitol survived.
Furthermore, of the thirteen Stage III patients who received mannitol, only seven survived, whereas all seven
of the patients in this category who did not receive
mannitol survived. It is interesting to note that four
of these seven patients who did not receive mannitol did
indeed receive urea to control an ICP crisis!

Of the forty-six patients who survived acute
episodes of RS, an eleven year old boy discharged without apparent neurological residue died suddenly at home
several days following discharge with no discernible
cause of death at autopsy. Another patient, a thirteen
year old boy, had sustained severe neurological sequelae
as a consequence of RS and died six months following
discharge. Eight additional patients were left with
neurologic complications ranging from esotropia to

to severe psychomotor retardation with seizures
(Table 5).

TABLE 5.   SEQUELAE OF RS

						RESIDUAL DEFECTS
CLINICAL CHARACTERISTICS ON ADMISSION						
Case #	Sex	Age	Stage	Grade	NH_3	
1	M	5 mo.				Seizures, delayed development
2	F	9 mo.	IV	4	180	Seizures, M.R.
3	F	18 mo.	V	3	30	Seizures, M.R.
4	F	18 mo.	II	4	620	Seizures, M.R.
5	F	3 yrs.	III	4	32	Seizures, M.R.
6	F	5 yrs.	IV	3	400	M.R. (improving)
7	M	9 yrs.	III	4	320	Esotropia
8	M	11 yrs.	II	3	110	Unexpected death after discharge
9	M	13 yrs.	II	3	270	Severe M.R., subsequent death
10	M	15 yrs.	III	3	480	Aphasia, emotional component
ENHANCED SUSCEPTIBILITY						
11	M	5 yrs.	II	–	130	Second episode survived

TABLE 5. SEQUELAE OF RS. (continued)

ENHANCED SUSCEPTIBILITY

Case #	Sex	Age	Stage	Grade	NH_3	RESIDUAL DEFECTS
12	F	4 yrs.	II	3	-	Second episode death
13a*	F	14 yrs.	II	4	440	Death
13b	M	11 yrs.	I	-	40	Normal
14a*	F	8 yrs.	IV	4	910	Death
14b	M	11 yrs.	II	-	-	Survived

* designates pair of siblings affected with RS

Hence significant sequelae could be documented for 19.5 percent of the patients in this series. Those patients two years of age or less appeared to be particularly vulnerable to neurologic sequelae. Five of our eleven patients in this age group died and four of the six survivors sustained severe brain damage (Table 5). Although patients of this age represented only 16 percent of the series, they accounted for 44 percent of the sequelae.

In addition to death and neurologic sequelae, our study suggests an enhanced susceptibility to RS among children of some patients' families. A four year old girl was seen at MCH with RS on two occasions, thirteen months apart. She succumbed during the second episode. One year after his initial episode of RS at MCH, a five year old boy was successfully managed during a second episode of RS at his community hospital. Two families were identified in which more than one child appeared to be susceptible to RS. In one family, both siblings became ill simultaneously and one died. In the other family, an eleven year old male was admitted, to another hospital, one year following the death of his sister due to RS at MCH.

DISCUSSION

The etiology, diagnosis, and treatment of RS have been recently reviewed. Despite some advances, the disease is not well understood and continues to be associated with a high fatality rate. Davidson (16) et al challenged the early view that patients either recovered completely from RS or succumbed. They were able to identify significant psychological and neurological impairments in a substantial number of survivors.

We have examined the frequency and quality of survival in our series of patients on the basis of stage of coma, severity of EEG abnormalities, and extent of hyperammonemia found at the time of admission to MCH. In general, the frequency of survival was inversely related to these indices. In this respect our results are in agreement with those of Lovejoy et al (11) who reported survival in only two patients who progressed beyond Stage III and both remained in coma. We found that 5/17 patients beyond Stage III coma survived and three of these survivors sustained severe neurologic damage.

The blood NH_3 concentration has been observed to be of considerable importance as a contributing factor in the encephalopathy of RS (13,14). In the experience of Glasgow et al (14) the blood NH_3 concentration was directly related to the level of consciousness and survival. On the other hand, they noted considerable variation among their patients and some of those with severely impaired consciousness had $(NH_3)_b$ in the normal range. Their experience is consistent with the relationship between $(NH_3)_b$ and the stage of coma in patients from our series. Thaler (17) had suggested that either an inherited or induced defect in NH_3 metabolism may be present in patients with RS. It would appear that a disturbance of the urea cycle on the basis of a lesion within the hepatic mitochondria could be instrumental in initiating the hyperammonemia of RS.

Arterial blood hyperammonemia can be readily detoxified in the brain at levels below 300 µg/100 ml (18).

Our results support this finding as we noted a significant increase in the fatality rate among patients with NH_3 concentration in excess of 270 µg/100 ml. Three of ten patients who survived despite this level of hyperammonia had severe neurologic sequelae. The average blood NH_3 concentrations for nonsurvivors in Stages II-IV were similar. Within each stage the mean ammonia level for nonsurvivors was considerably higher than that for survivors (Figure 4). Some patients in Stage V coma had lower blood NH_3 concentrations than anticipated on the basis of this trend. Shannon et al (18) observed a normal venous blood NH_3 level in one of their nonsurvivors despite an extremely high arterial blood level. On the basis of the arterial-venous difference observed in this patient, they felt these results suggested a net cerebral uptake of NH_3 by the brain. We are unable to comment on this possibility in our Stage V patients since arterial-venous differences could not be determined from the available data. Such unanticipated levels of NH_3 could be observed early in the chronology of RS if the accumulation of neurotoxic substances such as short-chain fatty acids initiated a severe encephalopathy and death occurred prior to dysfunction of the urea cycle (19). The metabolic dysfunctions of RS appear transient. It is also possible that blood NH_3 levels may have fallen from elevated levels prior to the hospitalization of some of our patients.

We might anticipate a favorable influence on survival of patients with RS from an established protocol which can provide consistent management of a series of patients. This benefit would be augmented by thoughtful modification based upon increasing experience with RS. Continuous monitoring of ICP in patients with RS has become recognized as a valuable adjunct to therapy. Bruce et al (20) monitored twenty-four patients over a three year period and attributed only two of ten deaths to elevated ICP. We have compared results obtained with our present management protocol, which includes continuous monitoring of ICP, to results obtained with "historical controls" who were matched for severity but admitted in the years predating our ICP monitor use in RS. The monitoring provided a consistent objective method for anticipating catastrophic episodes of elevated ICP. Our confidence in this management protocol is supported by an improved survival rate among patients admitted in coma (Stages III-V).

Continuous monitoring of ICP during management of RS made it possible to insure the use of osmotic agents during documented episodes of elevated pressure in the presence of ambiguous clinical signs. It also obviated the routine scheduled administration of these agents in the absence of specific indications - a procedure which might predispose to overdosage. The prolonged administration of hypertonic agents might complicate the tenuous clinical state of the patient. Empirically, we have been most impressed with the response of RS patients with severe encephalopathy to urea.

Theoretical reservations could be raised regarding the use of urea in RS patients with an elevated serum NH_3. If evaluation of risks and benefits warranted, the adverse influence of urea on the $(NH_3)_b$ might be obviated with measures such as vigorous bowel cleansing (21). Among our patients, there was a trend toward greater survival among those patients in Stage III-IV coma who received urea to control ICP. When survival rates were compared in patients grouped on the basis of the use of mannitol or steroids, no apparent differences were observed. For this reason, we have continued with the judicious use of urea as an integral part of our management of the severe encephalopathy of RS.

Increasing experience with RS has convinced us that survival is possible despite the presence of severe clinical and metabolic derangements in patients at the time of admission. Furthermore, a good quality of survival is not precluded by the presence of such findings upon admission. On the other hand, we have observed that one can be misled by the patient's level of consciousness in the emergency room. Patients admitted in milder stages of coma sometime have deteriorated to a point where their management becomes difficult and death or serious brain damage has resulted. It is on the basis of this risk of deterioration that we recommend that patients with RS are most appropriately

managed in centers with the capability for managing
brain edema in conditions such as closed head injuries
and encephalopathy with continuous direct ICP monitoring.

The poor prognosis for patients with RS who have
deteriorated beyond Stage III at the time of admission
has been addressed by a program of community education
which promotes: 1. Awareness of the early signs and
symptoms of RS by parents. 2. Sensitivity among
physicians to the appropriate concerns of parents with
children who manifest the early signs and symptoms of
RS. 3. Appropriate action by the family doctor to
confirm an impression of RS. 4. Prompt referral of the
patient with RS to a center staffed and equipped to provide intensive care to children with increased ICP.

REFERENCES

1. Brown, C.L. and Symmers, D. 1925. Acute serious
    encephalitis. *Amer J Dis Child 29:* 174.
2. Brain, W.R., Hunter, D. and Turnbull, H.M. 1929.
    Acute meningoencephalitis of childhood. *Lancet 1:*
    221.
3. Reye, R.D.K., Morgan, G., and Baral, J. 1963.
    Encephalopathy and fatty degeneration of the viscera.
    Lancet 2: 749.
4. Reynolds, D.W., Riley, H.D.Jr., LaFont, D.S.,
    Vorse, H., Stout, L.C. and Carpenter, R.L. 1972.
    An outbreak of Reye's Syndrome associated with
    influenza B. *Journal of Pediatrics 80:* 429.
5. Turel, Jr., A.P., Levinsohn, M.W., Derakhshan, I.,
    and Gutierrez, Y. 1975. Reye Syndrome and Cerebel-
    lar Intracytoplasmic Inclusion Bodies. *Arch.
    Neurol. 32:* 624.
6. Brown, R.E., Madge, G.E. and Schiller, H.M. 1971.
    Observations on the pathogenesis of RS. *S. Med.
    J. 64:* 942.
7. Samaha, F.J., Blau, E. and Beradinelli, J.L. 1974.
    Reye's Syndrome: Clinical diagnosis and treatment
    with peritoneal dialysis. *Pediatrics 53:* 336.

8. Huttenlocher, P.R. in J. D. Pollack, ed.: Reye Syndrome. New York, Grune and Stratton (1975), 391.
9. Bobo, R.C., Schubert, W.K., Partin, J.C. and Partin, J.S. 1975. Reyes Syndrome: Treatment by exchange transfusion with special reference to the 1974 epidemic. *Cincinnati Ohio J. Ped. 87:* 881.
10. DeVivo, D.C. and Keating, J.P.: Reyes Syndrome in Advances in Ped. vol 22: 175 Yearbook Med. Pub.1976.
11. Lovejoy, F.H., Smith, A.L., Bresnan, M.J., Wood, J.M., Victor, D.I. and Adams, P.C. 1974. Clinical Staging in Reyes Syndrome. *Am J Dis Child 128:*36.
12. Aoki, Y. and Lombroso, C.T. 1973. Prognostic value of electroencephalography in Reyes Syndrome. *Neurology 23:* 333.
13. Huttenlocher, P.R., Schwartz, A.D. and Klatskin, G. 1969. Reyes Syndrome: Ammonia intoxication as a possible factor in the encephalopathy. *Pediatrics 43:* 443.
14. Glasgow, A.M., Cotton, R.B., Dhiensiri, K. and Kaen, K. 1972. Reye's Syndrome: Blood ammonia and consideration of the nonhistologic diagnosis. *Amer J Dis Child 124:* 827.
15. Kindt, G.W., Waldman, J., Kohl, S., Baublis, J. and Tucker, R.P. 1975. Intracranial pressure in Reye's Syndrome: Monitoring and control, *J.A.M.A. 231:* 822.
16. Davidson, P.W., Willoughby, R.H., O'Tuama, L.A., Swisher, C.N. and Benjamin, S.D. Neurological and intellectual sequelae of Reyes Syndrome: A preliminary report. In J.D. Pollack, ed. Reyes Syndrome, New York, Grune and Stratton, 1975 (55-60).
17. Thaler, M.M., Hoogenraad, N.J. and Boswell, M. Reyes Syndrome due to a novel protein-tolerant variant of ornithine-transcarbamylase deficiency. *Lancet 2:* 438, 1974.
18. Shannon, D.C., DeLong, R., Bercu, B., Glick, T., Herrin, J.T., Moylan, F.M.B., and Todres, I.D. 1975. Studies on the pathophysiology of Encephalopathy in Reyes Syndrome: Hyperammonemia in Reyes Syndrome. *Pediatrics 56:* 999.

19. Brown, R.E., Madge, G.E., Trauner, D.A. and
     David, R.B. 1972. Lipid and Lipoprotein studies
     in Reye's Syndrome. *Virginia med. mth. 99: 622.*
20. Bruce, D.A., Berman, M.D. and Schut, L. in
     Barness, L.A., Advances in Pediatrics, Vol. 24,
     1977, Chicago, Year Book Medical Publishers, Inc.,
     (233-290).
21. Wolpert, E., Phillips, S.F. and Summerskill, W.H.J.
     1971. Transport of urea and ammonia production in
     the human colon. *Lancet 2:* 1387.

ACKNOWLEDGEMENTS

The excellent care provided by nurses of the Mott
ICU and the Mott Isolation Ward for these patients.

DISCUSSION

J.R. Aprille - With respect to your relapse cases;did
     some children suffer the antecedent viral illness
     the second time,and was it the same viral antece-
     dent as on the first occasion?

J.V. Baublis - In one case, Influenza A was experienced
     at approximately one year after an attack of Influ-
     enza B. In another case,chicken pox was responsi-
     ble for the second attack,and the first attack was
     initiated by an undifferentiated respiratory dis-
     ease.

M.R. Hurley - In the sibling pairs that had it later,
     did they both live?

J.V. Baublis - In one pair of siblings, the sister was
     admitted a year prior to the brother. They both
     experienced an A Victoria infection; the sister
     was the first affected,and she died. In the second
     pair of siblings again, there was one death and
     one survival.

M.R. Hurley - From Doctor Hilty's paper,all their
sibling pairs survived and they had it associated
with the same type of infection. In hemolytic
uremic syndrome where there seems to be a clustering,the patients do reasonably well, whereas those
who get it in a family one, two, three years apart
have a very lethal disease.

J.V. Baublis -The sharing of familial susceptibility
leaves us with the possibility of a genetic link.
However,the fact that the susceptibility seems to
extend for a finite period in time makes me favor
something environmental.

Q. Ghanem - Regarding the Intercranial Pressure
Monitoring (ICP), how many cases have you so far
managed using ICP, and have you been able to correlate the information from the ICP against EEG
activity?

J.V. Baublis -The ICP monitor should not be looked at
as a substitute for the EEG. The EEG is essentially a useful diagnostic tool. Together with staging
of disease, blood ammonia, and other evaluations,
it enables us to identify a subgroup of patients
who are going to be in urgent need of intensive
care. I don't think I can compare the two of them
quite directly.

SECTION III

BIOCHEMISTRY, CYTOLOGY AND TOXICOLOGY

LIVER AND MUSCLE ULTRASTRUCTURE IN REYE'S SYNDROME

John C. Partin, M.D., Kevin Bove, M.D.,
Jacqueline S. Partin, M.S., Wm. K. Schubert, M.D.

INTRODUCTION

During the four years since the last major
symposium on Reye's syndrome (1), we have extended our
experience with the ultrastructural pathology of Reye's
syndrome to the study of 99 liver biopsy proven cases.
The ultrastructural pathology of these 99 cases has
been compared with the liver ultrastructure of about
30 children who were suspected by various physicians
to be suffering Reye's syndrome because they presented
signs of cerebral disease and hepatic dysfunction, but
who ultimately proved to have some other condition.
These observations, in turn, have been interpreted in
the light of our experience with about 2300 diagnostic
liver biopsies performed at the Cincinnati Children's
Hospital during the past 15 years.

The ultrastructural changes of the liver in Reye's
syndrome appear to represent a specific biochemical
injury which involves the mitochondria in an important
way. In liver biopsies obtained during the first 3 or
4 days after the onset of vomiting and before extensive
glucose infusion or exchange transfusion, the liver
ultrastructural changes are highly characteristic of
the disease — they are truly diagnostic in the sense
pathologists use the term. The liver lesion can heal
rapidly, however, and glycogen stores return promptly
when glucose is infused. The obvious signs of liver
mitochondrial injury can disappear after two or three
days of treatment even in children who are comatose
and dying because of encephalopathy or cerebral edema.

Because of the rapidity with which the liver can heal,
biopsy tissue for diagnostic and biochemical study
should be obtained soon after admission.

During the past four years we have considerably
expanded our knowledge of the liver lesion in neurological stage I patients. It is now quite clear that
it is dangerous to consider all stage I cases as "mild"
or even early cases of the disease, because about one-
third of neurological stage I cases have changes in
liver ultrastructure as severe as those encountered in
comatose patients. The finding that many apparently
"mild" cases have severe hepatic involvement justifies
the policy, discussed elsewhere in this volume, of
treating all neurological stage I patients with glucose
infusions until <u>normal appetite has returned</u>.

The observation of severe liver injury very early
in the evolution of encephalopathic signs strengthens
the argument that liver injury may be central to the
pathogenesis of Reye's syndrome; on the other hand, as
originally described by both Reye (2) and Dvorackova
(3), there is clear evidence of involvement of muscle
as well as liver and brain in the disease. We have
been able to study the ultrastructural pathology of
needle biopsies of muscle during the acute encephalopathy and after recovery. Many of the changes found in
the hepatocyte are found, to a lesser degree, in the
skeletal muscle cells.

CASE MATERIAL

The Cincinnati Children's Hospital is the sole
pediatric referral center and pediatric primary care
hospital for the city of Cincinnati and Hamilton County,
Ohio. It is also the principal pediatric referral
center for southwestern Ohio, northern Kentucky and
southeastern Indiana. Because of the regional nature
of the hospital and because of a high level of awareness of Reye's syndrome by physicians and parents, it
is likely that we have examined and treated most of
the cases occurring in a region populated by about 1.9
million people. Virtually all patients present with
the triad: prodromal respiratory illness (including

chicken pox), vomiting, and elevation of serum glutamic-
pyruvic transaminase (SGPT) without jaundice. Many
patients have prolonged plasma prothrombin times, elevated creatine phosphokinase (CPK) and increased pre-
treatment blood ammonia concentrations. In spite of
the ready availability and frequent use of the SGPT and
blood ammonia determination, we have been unable to
detect "subclinical" or non-vomiting cases of Reye's
syndrome.

MATERIALS AND METHODS

Initial diagnostic liver biopsies are performed
within a few hours after admission before exchange
transfusion. All biopsy specimens are examined by
electron microscopy and histochemistry as well as in
standard paraffin sections. The details of tissue
processing have been published before (4), but it is
worth reiterating the importance of certain steps in
processing tissue for electron microscopy. We process
all tissues immediately. The appearance of the mitochondrial matrix and other organelles is considerably
affected by the buffer used in the fixation process.
We use Millonig's phosphate buffer with 0.54% dextrose
and calcium chloride in the preparation of the 3%
glutaraldehyde fixative, which is adjusted to pH 7.35.
We use the same buffer without calcium chloride to
prepare 1% osmium tetroxide. We always fix tissue
in the osmium fixative alone as well as glutaraldehyde
followed by osmium post fixation, because mitochondrial
pleomorphism is much more pronounced in tissue fixed
in osmium alone. All fixatives are made fresh each
Monday morning and stored at $4^{\circ}C$. Purified glutaraldehyde stock solution is obtained from Ladd Research
Industries in nitrogen filled ampoules. The ampoules
are stored at $4^{\circ}C$.

The Menghini liver biopsy sample is aspirated into
physiological saline and expelled onto a large circle
of Whatman No. 1 filter paper, and then transferred
with a miniature spatula to a sheet of dental wax where
it is sliced and transferred to pools of ice cold fixative. The whole process takes 30 to 90 seconds under
usual circumstances.

Muscle Biopsy. Vim-Silverman needle biopsies were obtained from the gastrocnemius-soleus group at the time of initial liver biopsy and after recovery in 18 cases of Reye's syndrome. The needle biopsy tissue was processed in a manner similar to liver tissue. Total CPK, and its 3 isoenzymes were obtained on serum from 16 of the 18 muscle biopsied patients and 10 additional cases of Reye's syndrome.

LIGHT MICROSCOPY

Light microscopy of liver sampled before therapy typically reveals diffuse transformation of the normally polygonal hepatocytes into more or less clear cells that are usually swollen, but sometimes partially collapsed, variably glycogen depleted and engorged with microvesicular lipid best demonstrated along with glycogen content in appropriately treated frozen sections. Histochemical activity of certain enzymes such as succinate reductase and cytochrome oxidase is depressed; the activity of others such as acid and alkaline phosphatase, DPNH reductase, and alpha-glycerol phosphate reductase is unaltered.

The amount of glycogen depletion and the severity of cell swelling in early biopsies correlates roughly with the severity of the encephalopathy at the time the sample is obtained. The amount of lipid is more difficult to estimate and of much less value; oxidative enzyme depression is usually severe, regardless of the clinical state, a finding that supports the hypothesis that mitochondrial membranes have been injured. Unfortunately, near normal stainable glycogen and minimal cell swelling may be early findings in the liver of a few patients who deteriorate rapidly, a fact that discourages the use of histochemical criteria to predict outcome. Such studies do, however, provide reliable bases for distinguishing Reye's syndrome from disorders that may mimic it.

LIVER ULTRASTRUCTURE IN STAGE I (NON-COMATOSE) CASES

The hepatic changes in non-comatose children can be divided into three classes: morphologically "early"

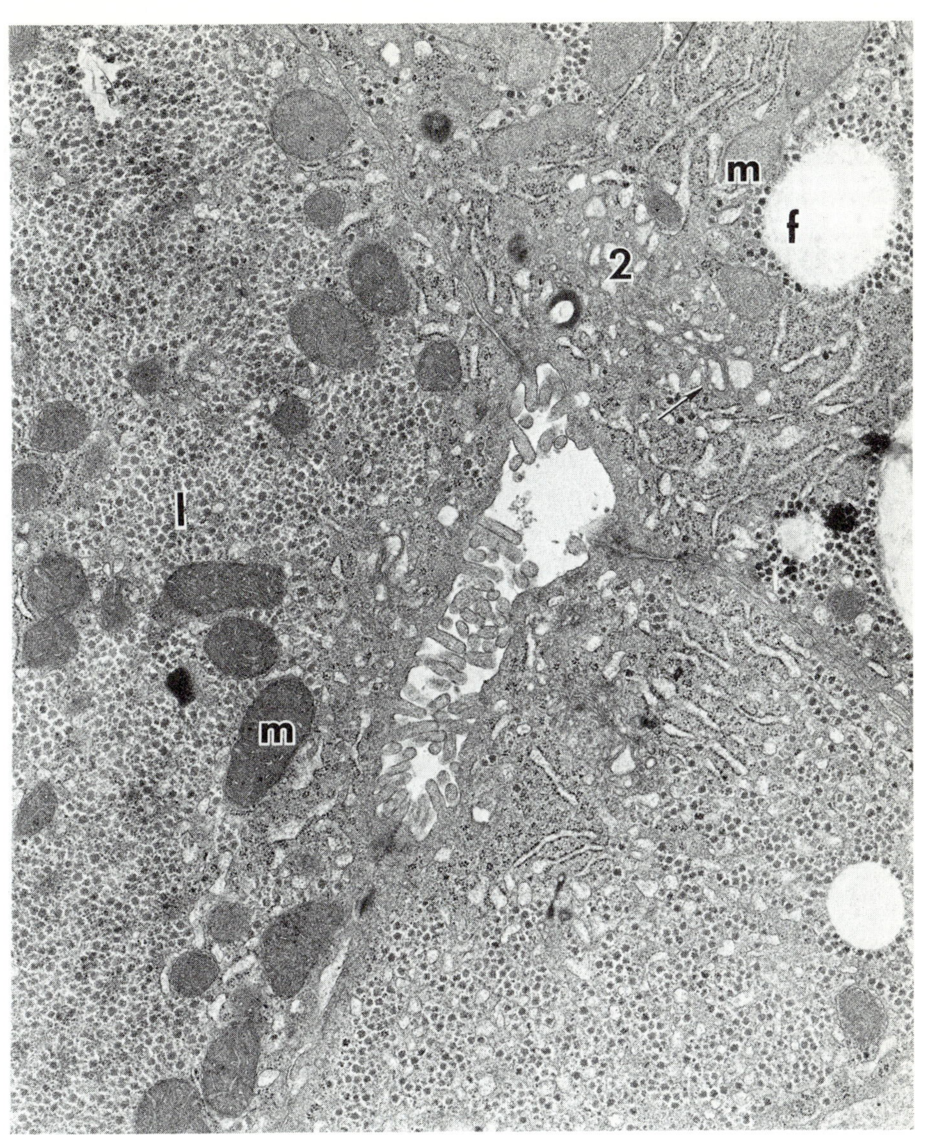

Figure 1.   Portion of 3 liver cells from a mild stage
I patient. Mitochondria in cell marked 1 are
normal. The mitochondria of cell 2 show early
matrix expansion and the adjacent bile canaliculus is slightly dilated. Throughout the
figures m = mitochondria, f = triglyceride
droplets, small single arrow indicates Golgi
saccules. Mag. 15,400x.

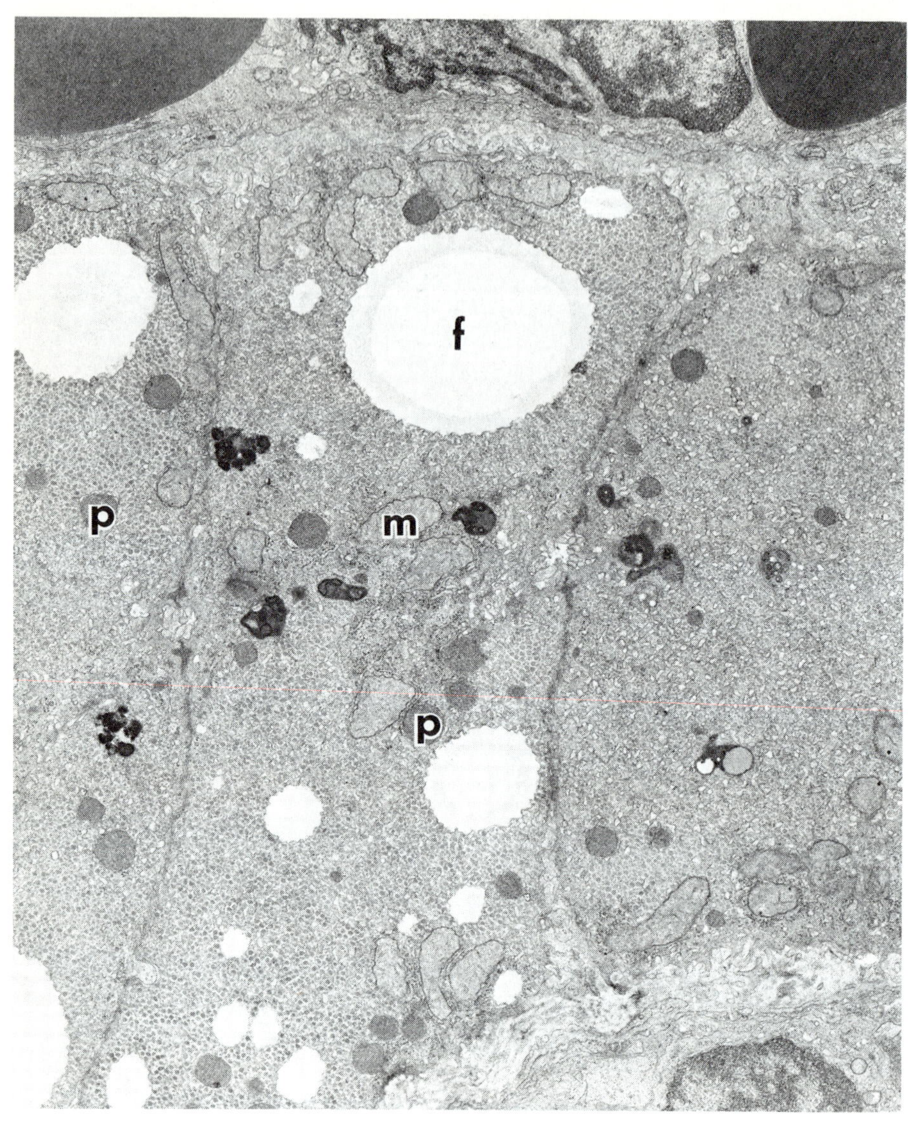

Figure 2.   Typical hepatocytes in mild stage I cases.
All mitochondria exhibit matrix rarefaction
and most have lost matrix dense bodies.
Large peroxisomes, p, are evident. Glycogen
is abundant. Mag. 10,600x.

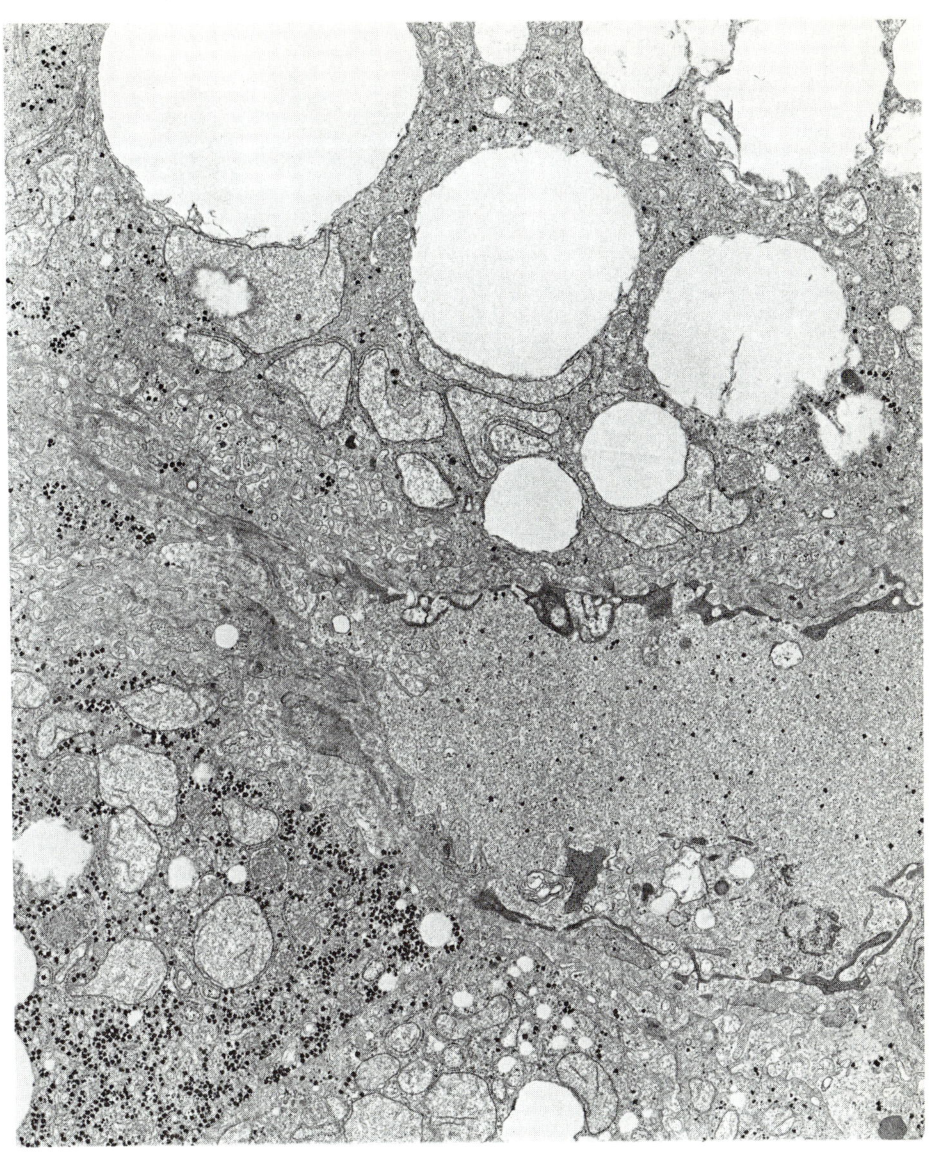

Figure 3.   Portion of 3 hepatocytes and a sinusoid
            from a neurologic stage I child whose liver
            was severely affected. All mitochondria
            show marked matrix expansion. The uppermost
            cell demonstrates severe loss of glycogen
            and abnormal peroxisomes. Mag. 10,100x.

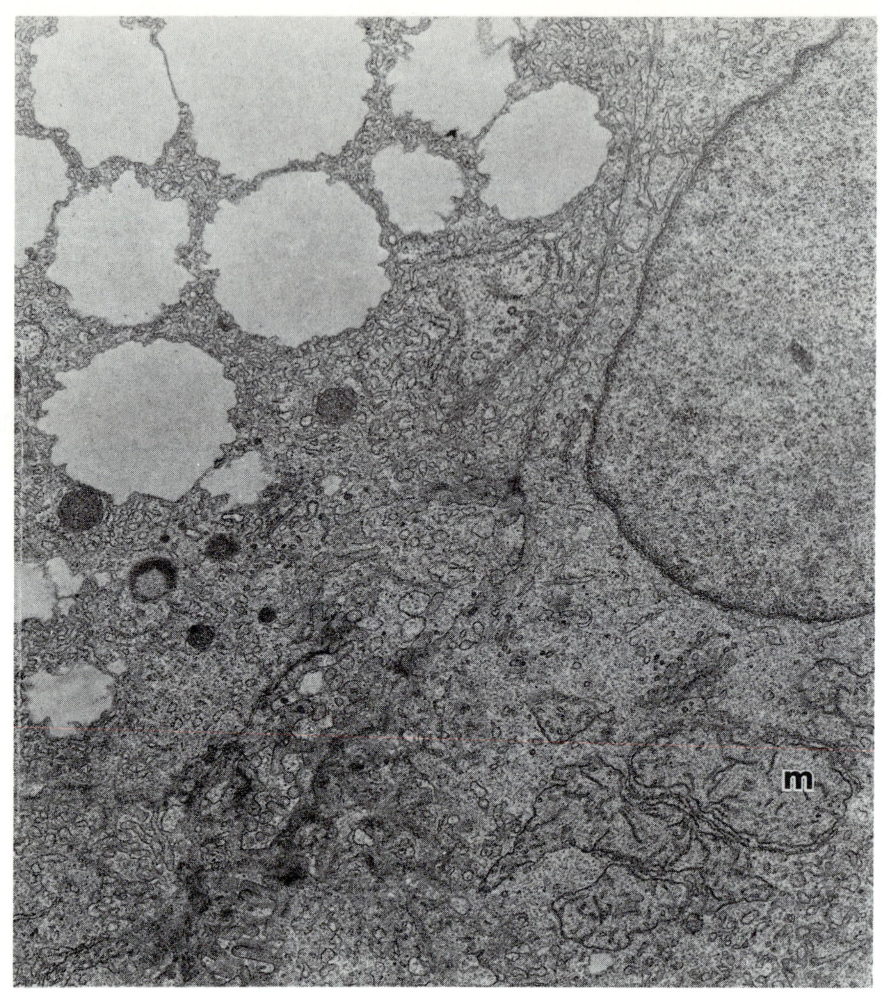

Figure 4. Portion of two liver cells and a bile canaliculus from a fatal varicella associated
case of Reye's syndrome, neurological stage
IV. One cell contains many small fat droplets, Golgi devoid of pre-beta lipoprotein
particles and hypertrophy of the smooth endoplasmic reticulum. The second cell contains
several pleomorphic mitochondria which exhibit marked matrix change and loss of matrix
dense bodies. Glycogen is virtually absent
from both cells. The bile canaliculus is
dilated and filled with cellular debris.
Mag. 17,000x.

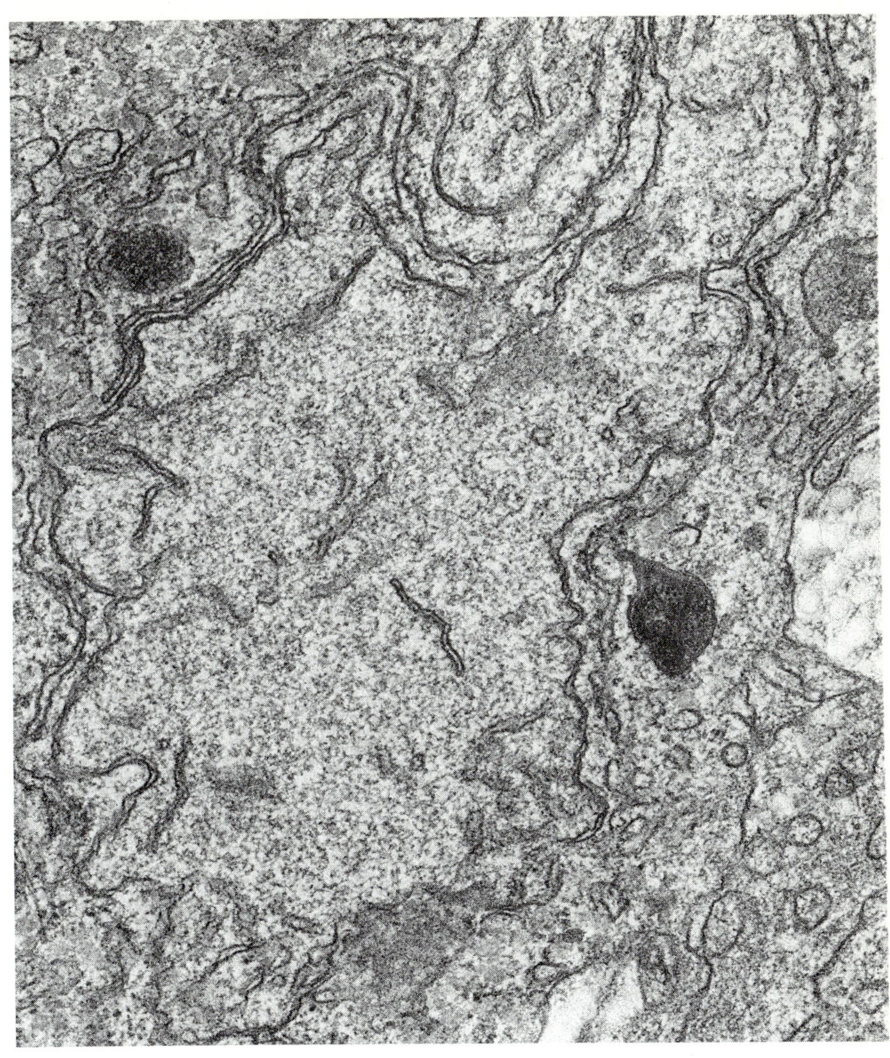

Figure 5. Same patient as Figure 4. Highly
pleomorphic mitochondrion with highly disorg-
anized matrix substance. Mag. 70,000x.

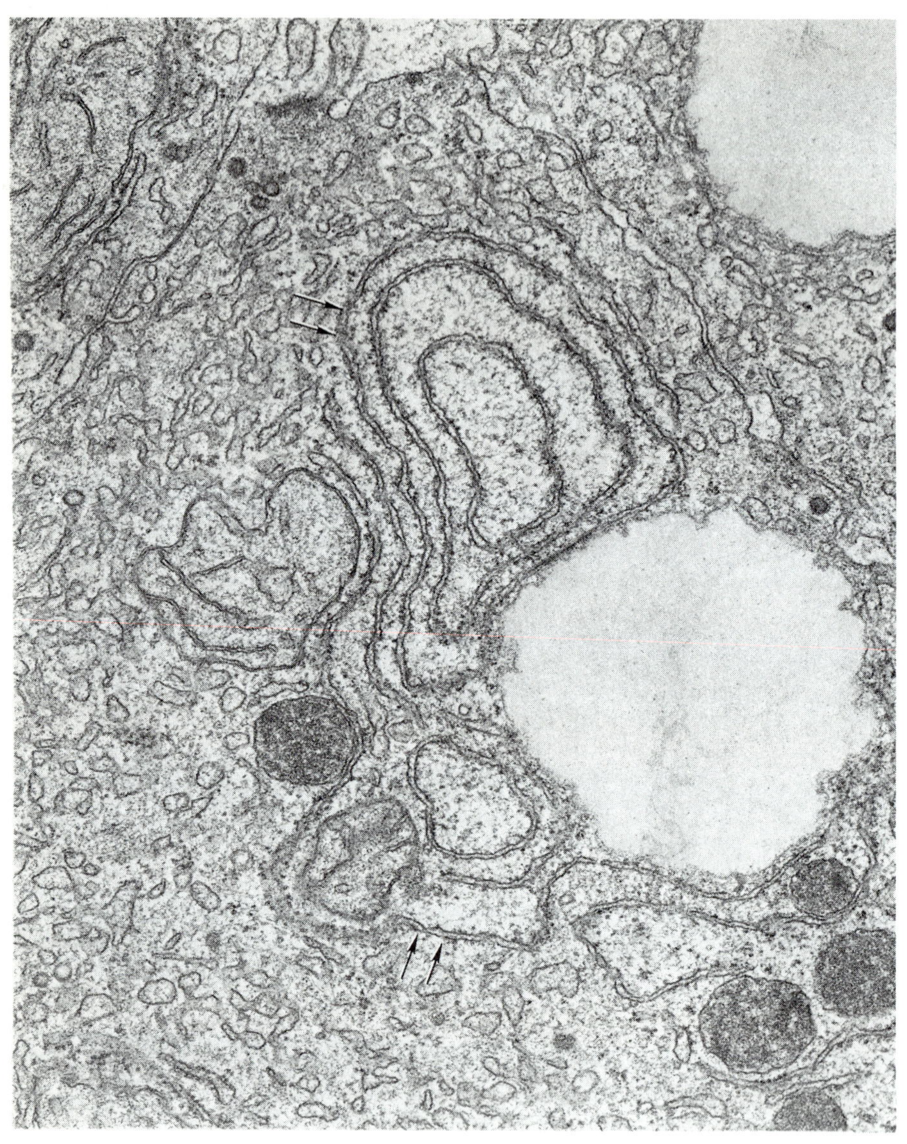

Figure 6.   Same patient as Figure 4.   Rough endoplasmic
            reticulum, double arrows.   Mag. 38,000x.

changes, changes which cannot be distinguished from
those encountered in comatose children, and a group in
which the liver lesion appears to be healing.

In biopsies which seem to represent the earliest
stage of hepatic injury, mitochondria exhibit mild but
definite matrix expansion and early pleomorphism. Mitochondrial matrix dense bodies are absent from some, but
not all mitochondria, and the degree of mitochondrial
involvement varies from cell to cell and sometimes within individual cells. Glycogen is reduced but there is
considerable variability from cell to cell in the degree of deglycogenation. There is a progressive increase
in smooth endoplasmic reticulum. Peroxisomes are first
increased in number and then, in more severely affected
cases, exhibit a watery alteration of their matrix. In
the milder specimens, there is abundant triglyceride
within the smooth endoplasmic reticulum and in small
non-membrane bounded cytoplasmic droplets. Golgi saccules contain abundant pre-beta lipoprotein particles
in the mild cases, but as the mitochondrial alteration
progresses and deglycogenation proceeds, the Golgi
saccules cease to contain fat transport particles.

Although jaundice is not present in Reye's syndrome, histological evidence of mild cholestasis has
been observed in "late" liver biopsies (5,6). Examination of liver biopsy samples from stage I patients
demonstrates that there is progressive mild to moderate
dilatation of bile canaliculae and, in more severely
affected samples, swelling and loss of some microvilli
and the accumulation of amorphous material in the
canalicular lumina.

Probably due to the combined effect of triglyceride accumulation, increase in smooth endoplasmic reticulum, increase in cytoplasmic water and an increase
in mitochondrial volume, there is progressive increase
in total liver cell volume and a consequent compression
of sinusoids.

Except for an increased prominence of sinusoidal
Kupffer cells, inflammation is minimal or absent in
early liver biopsies.

Nuclear changes consist of loosening of nucleolar structure and, in a day or two, a burst of mitotic activity. An inventory of the ultrastructural changes is shown in Table I.

TABLE I

Mitochondrial Changes
    Matrix expansion
    Progressive loss of matrix dense bodies
    Mitochondrial pleomorphism
    Matrix disorganization
    Gross swelling, outer membrane rupture (late)

Cytoplasmic Changes
    Glycogen depletion
    Smooth endoplasmic reticulum increase
    Triglyceride accumulation in endoplasmic
      reticulum
    Peroxysome increase → alteration
    Decreasing Golgi VLDL content
    Watery expansion of cytosol
    Increased lysosomes
    Increasing cell volume

Canalicular Changes
    Progressive dilatation
    Microvillus alteration
    Luminal accumulations

Nuclear Changes
    Nucleolar "skein"-ing
    Mitotic burst during early recovery
    Nuclear swelling and disorganization of
      chromatin in fatal cases

LIVER ULTRASTRUCTURE IN COMATOSE PATIENTS (STAGE III, IV, V)

The ultrastructural pathology of the liver lesion during the first two or three days after the onset of encephalopathy with coma has been well described (1, 4,7). The severity of the mitochondrial lesion and the degree of glycogen depletion parallel the severity

of encephalopathy and, while in most cases, the hepatic
injury looks as if it should be reversible, we have
encountered a few cases in which the liver appeared to
be irreversibly injured at the time of admission. In
these severely affected cases, there is extreme disorganization of the mitochondrial matrix and virtual
absence of glycogen in many hepatocytes. The cisternae
of rough endoplasmic reticulum does not become dilated,
but the organelle is found arranged in concentric
lamellae and the ribosomes appear to be in the process
of becoming detached.

ULTRASTRUCTURAL PATHOLOGY OF SKELETAL MUSCLE

     In keeping with the observations of Roe, Sidbury
and co-workers (8), total CPK was elevated in the
serum of the 26 children whose admission samples were
examined. The average value was 88 Bioscience units,
and the total CPK ranged from slightly elevated to more
than 300 times normal. Skeletal muscle derived isoenzymes accounted for more than 95% of the total CPK
in most children. Fourteen patients also had elevations
of cardiac derived isoenzyme ranging from 1 to 25% of
the total.

     Most of the muscle biopsies demonstrated definite
ultrastructural changes when compared to recovery
biopsies. Glycogen was reduced, triglyceride increased
and the sarcoplasmic reticulum was somewhat dilated
with a loss of intraluminal substance.

     Two types of mitochondrial alteration were en-
countered. The first, affecting the majority of mitochondria, consists of moderate matrix swelling which
produces mitochondrial profiles that are too smooth
and which present slight to moderate alterations of
matrix density. The second type of mitochondrial
alteration consists of frank disruption of mitochondrial
matrix. This kind of injury was associated with frank
myolysis and disorganization of myofibrils and myo-
filaments.

     Thus, skeletal muscle shares with liver and brain
a process which results in triglyceride accumulation,

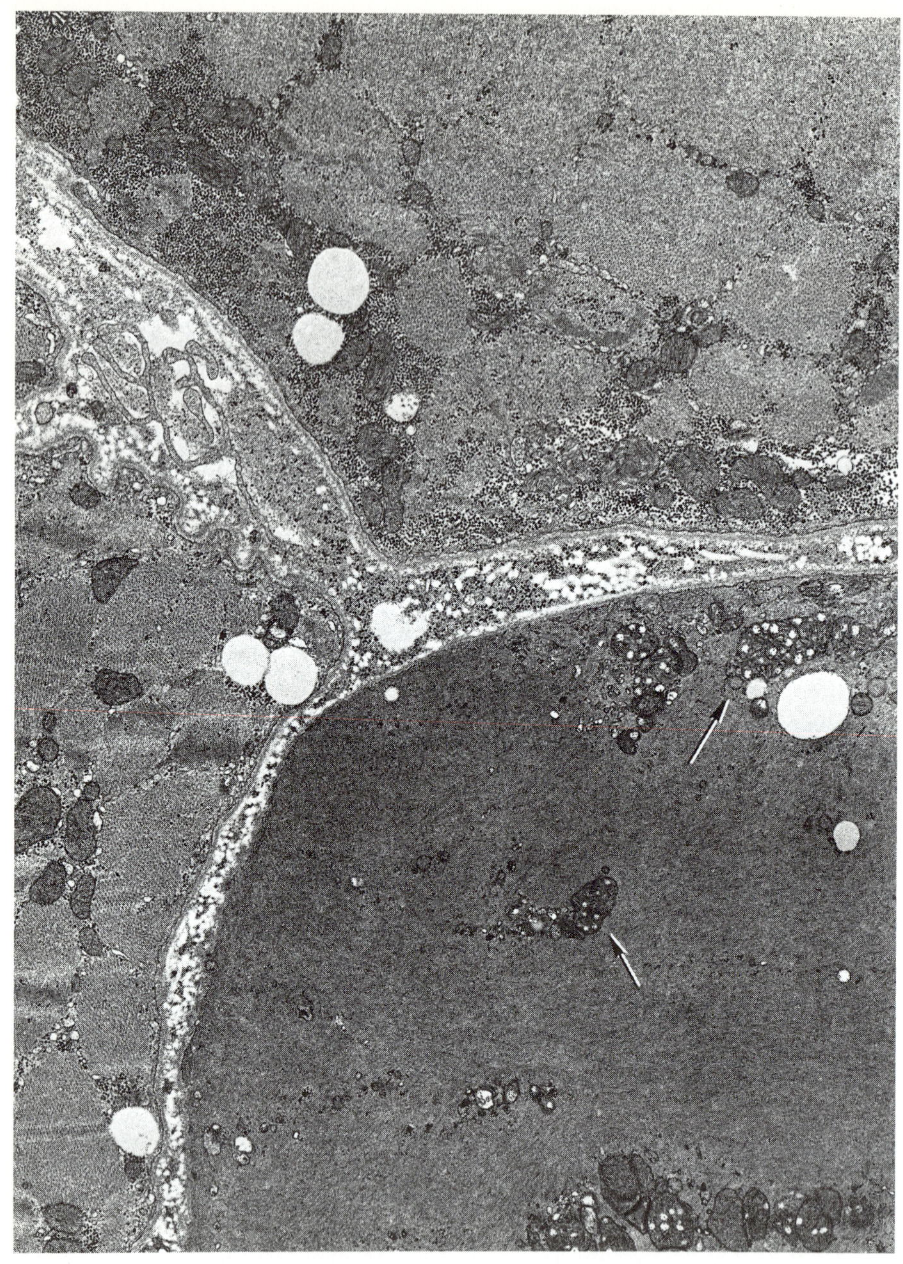

Figure 7. Portion of three skeletal muscle cells. One
cell demonstrates disorganization of myofibrils and myo-
filaments. Glycogen is lost. Some mitochondria(arrow)
have dilated intracristal spaces. Such cells are in the
process of dissolution or myolysis. Mag. 12,800x.

deglycogenation and mitochondrial injury. Unlike the
process in hepatocyte and neuron in which all mitochondria seem equally susceptible to injury, the muscle
cell seems to possess a major population of mitochondria which are relatively resistant to matrix alteration
and a smaller population which are quite susceptible
to it.

CONCLUSIONS

Reye's syndrome is a distinct disease entity both
at the clinical level and at the level of ultrastructural pathology. The ultrastructural changes are so
constant in character that one may hypothesize a single
mechanism of injury or injury to a specific cellular
process which is necessary for normal mitochondrial
metabolism in liver, muscle and brain.

REFERENCES

1. Partin, J.C. 1975. Ultrastructure in Reye's
    syndrome, p. 117. *In* J.D. Pollack (ed.), Reye's
    Syndrome. Grune and Stratton, New York.
2. Reye, R.D.K., G. Morgan, and J. Baral. 1963.
    Encephalopathy and fatty degeneration of the vis-
    cera: A disease entity in childhood. *Lancet ii*:
    749.
3. Dvorackova, I., V. Vortel, M. Hrock. 1966. Enceph-
    alitic syndrome with fatty degeneration of viscera.
    Arch. Path. 81: 240.
4. Partin, J.C., W.K. Schubert, J.S. Partin. 1971.
    Mitochondrial ultrastructure in Reye's syndrome
    (Encephalopathy and fatty degeneration of the
    viscera). *New Engl. J. Med. 285*: 1339.
5. Brown, R.E., and G.E. Madge. 1975. The pathology
    of Reye's syndrome: An overview, p. 77. *In* J.D.
    Pollack (ed.), Reye's Syndrome. Grune and Strat-
    ton, New York.
6. Bove, K.E., A.J. McAdams, J.C. Partin, J.S. Partin.
    1975. The hepatic lesion in Reye's syndrome.
    Gastroenterology 69: 685.

7.   Iancu, T.C., W.H. Mason, H.B. Neustein. 1977.
     Ultrastructural abnormalities of liver cells in
     Reye's syndrome. *Human Path. 8:* 421.
8.   Roe, C.R.C., L.B. Schonberger, S.H. Gelbach, L.A.
     Wies, J.B. Sidbury, Jr. 1975. Enzymatic alter-
     ations in Reye's syndrome: Prognostic implicat-
     ions. *Pediatrics 55:* 119.

Supported by a grant from the National Foundation-
March of Dimes, The Cincinnati Children's Hospital
Research Foundation, and N.I.H. Clinical Research
Centers grant #RR-00123.

Acknowledgement: This work would have been impossible
without the support of the Children's Hospital Medical
Center housestaff, especially Doctors Alan Gober and
Fred Suchy and Gastroenterology fellows, Michael
Farrell, James Heubi, and Donna Volk.

DISCUSSION

Unidentified - How many patients do you find are such
      bad bleeders that you can't biopsy them?

J.C. Partin - Our patients generally have prolonged
      Prothrombin Times, many of which are corrected
      by Vitamin K. They do not have clinically sig-
      nificant bleeding problems. Under the circum-
      stances that we have been doing these biopsies,
      we have been prepared to do exchange transfu-
      sions. If you run into a patient who has evi-
      dence of disseminated intervascular coagulation,
      or clinical evidence of bleeding, one must look

hard at the diagnosis. Now obviously, some patients who have also received large quantities of Aspirin may have some bleeding problems related to the Aspirin.

K.L. Bick -   In your liver studies, have you had any opportunity to determine if cells located centrally in the lobule are more sensitive to these early changes, and has it been possible to make a lobular correlation?

J.C. Partin - Well, in a general way the ultrastructural changes are very uniform throughout the lobule. If you take comatose patients, there are differences in the degree of deglycogenation from one cell to the next. In a general survey, you don't get the impression that there is a marked zonal difference in the severity of the injury. In the grade one patients, we haven't examined the material in sufficient detail to be able to answer your question. I suspect, based on the histochemical studies, that there will be some zonal changes, but it is going to require a stereological semi-statistical analysis to show this really firmly.

J.D. Pollack - Do changes in the smooth endoplasmic reticulum (E.R.) occur at the same frequency and the same time as changes in the mitochondria?

J.C. Partin: - The smooth endoplasmic reticulum is markedly proliferating in the patients who have severe mitochondrial injury. In the group of mild patients, there seemed to be a proportionate increase in the severity of the mitochondrial injury and increasing smooth endoplasmic reticulum. So,again, with the caveat we have not done morphometric studies which might be necessary to find some mild differences. The smooth E.R. and mitochondrial lesion go hand in hand. One factor that you have to cope with is the progressive loss of glycogen which unmasks the endo-

plasmic reticulum. So,it's much harder to get a
quantitative idea of how much endoplasmic reticulum is there in a grade 1 patient who still
has relatively abundant glycogen. I almost think
if one wanted to study that aspect, one would
want to do comparative ultrastructural and biochemical studies where one would be measuring
some enzyme activities specific for the smooth
endoplasmic reticulum.

D.B. Tower -   I'm not too familiar with this area.
How many other conditions do you see these mitochondrial changes in?

J.C. Partin -   These mitochondrial changes have not
been encountered in any other disease except
Reye's. Based on our experience, if one does
not use electron microscopy as a discriminator,
one might confuse - on clinical grounds - certain patients who have hepatopathy and encephalopathy due to causes other than Reye's syn -
drome. One such group are those presenting with
infection associated liver injury. These patients may have some triglyeride accumulation
and zonal changes, including necroses, but none
have had changes in the mitochondria resembling
Reye's syndrome. As a matter of fact, frequently
liver biopsies from this class of patient have
densification of the mitochondrial matrix and
increased numbers of dense bodies. A second
class of patient which can cause clinical confu-
sion are infants presenting with metabolic defects and fatty livers. While some of these patients have truly panlobular microvesicular fat,
we have found none who have the mitochondrial
changes of Reye's syndrome.

D.B. Tower   Changes similar to this (I won't say
they are identical because I am not that familiar with the details) are seen in the experimental animal model of alkyltin intoxication, in
which the earliest changes are in the mitochondria.

J.C. Partin   -   In the liver?

D.B. Tower   -   I don't know whether that means any-
            thing or not, but that's why I asked the ques-
            tion because I didn't think these changes occur
            very commonly. The other question I had was:
            do you see any changes in glycogen in the astro-
            cytes in the central nervous system?

J.C. Partin   -   I think Jackie Partin is going to al-
            lude to these things in the central nervous sys-
            tem. Do you know about the liver in the alkyltin
            intoxication? We do not, and it would be a good
            study to do.

D.B. Tower   -   Not for sure.

J.R. Lamontagne -I'm curious; do you see these changes
            in the muscle cells in Reye's syndrome attri-
            buted to Herpes Zoster, or is it characteris-
            tic of Influenza B?

J.C. Partin   -   I haven't studied any patient with
            Zoster. We do have some muscle biopsies from
            chicken pox patients that we can't distinguish
            from the non-chicken pox patients. I have stud-
            ied an epidemic of Influenza B myopathy which
            occurred in the spring of 1977. None of these
            patients had elevated transaminases or ammonias.
            We did not do liver biopsies on any of them,
            therefore. We did do muscle biopsies and the
            muscle biopsy changes in the influenza myopathy
            are very similar to the changes I have shown you.
            That's the only other viral syndrome that I have
            studied.

J.R. Lamontagne -Have you ever done serial sections on
            the liver cells to look and see how different
            the mitochondria are structurally?

J.C. Partin   -   You mean, have we done serial recon-
            structions?No, we have not done that.

BRAIN ULTRASTRUCTURE IN REYE'S SYNDROME;
ACUTE INJURY AND REPAIR

Jacqueline S. Partin, M.S., A. James McAdams, M.D.
Robert L. McLaurin, M.D., Wm. K. Schubert, M.D.
and John C. Partin, M.D.

In Dr. Reye's original description of encephalopathy and fatty degeneration of the viscera, a pathological change always seen at necropsy was brain swelling, "sufficient to produce obvious flattening of the cerebral convolutions, but it never reached a degree sufficient to produce herniation of tissue, and only rarely was any flattening of the pons and medulla or coning of the cerebellum apparent" (1).

Clinical and ultrastructural observations make it seem possible that Reye's patients died of a metabolic encephalopathy complicated by developing cerebral edema. Subsequent experience has shown that potentially fatal brain swelling complicates a proportion of Reye's Syndrome cases. The sophisticated intensive care facilities available for the treatment of Reye's Syndrome in the United States probably allow certain patients to remain alive long enough to develop even more profound brain swelling than that described in Reye's group of cases.

One of us had previously developed the use of extensive craniectomy with wide excision of the dura for the treatment of the cerebral edema complicating the metabolic encephalopathy due to lead poisoning in children (2).

In February of 1974, we treated a child with Reye's Syndrome who appeared to be dying of brain

swelling in spite of intensive measures to control
cerebral edema. This child was treated by craniectomy
with wide excision of the dura and survives with good
quality of life. Brain biopsies obtained at the time
of craniectomy were studied by light and electron
microscopy (3).

In 1975, two additional children were treated by
craniectomy for intractable cerebral edema, and they
also received cortical biopsies. After recovery, at
the time of bone flap replacement, brain biopsies were
obtained from all three children (4). This series of
biopsy specimens has allowed us to define the ultrastructural changes in the brain in Reye's Syndrome both
during the acute stages of the encephalopathy and
during the process of recovery.

Table I gives the admission blood chemistry values
of all three children. All three were graded clinical
grade 4 on admission, but patients #1 and #2 had been
in other hospitals for 15 hours and 30 hours, respectively. Patient #1 had been treated for salicylate
intoxication and Patient #2 for a suspected Compazine
reaction. Menghini needle liver biopsies performed on
all three patients were white and fatty, and subsequently were shown to have the typical morphological,
histochemical and ultrastructural changes of Reye's
Syndrome. All three children were also treated with
intensive supportive care and exchange transfusion, and
all three survived. Patient #1 is educable and attends
a slow learners' class. Patient #2 is more severely
brain damaged: her speech consists of 2 to 3 word
sentences and she is unable to do any school work.
Patient #3 is enrolled in a regular elementary school
class and appears to be close to her pre-illness level
of intelligence, although she had vertical nystagmus
that persisted for some time after recovery.

Light and electron microscopy of acute biopsies of
all three patients revealed similar alterations; injury
of neuronal mitochondria, astrocyte swelling, and
myelin bleb formation.

TABLE I: INITIAL BLOOD CHEMISTRY VALUES

	Patient #1 6 yrs	Patient #2 15 yrs	Patient #3 5 yrs
SGOT (Normal < 32)	176 IU	402 IU	386 IU
SGPT (Normal < 36)	344 IU	634 IU	584 IU
Total Bilirubin	1.3 mg%	1.4 mg%	0.8 mg%
Glucose	122 mg/dl	35 mg/dl	48 mg/dl
Ammonia (Normal < 125 µg/dl)	----	731 µg/dl	760 µg/dl
CPK-T (Normal $\leq$ 2.5 units)	24 units	188 units	1378 units

Neuronal somata of all acute biopsy specimens showed similar changes, consisting of a usually electron dense cytoplasm, extensive dispersement of ribosomes, dilatation of rough endoplasmic reticulum and a severe alteration in mitochondria (Figure 1). Pleomorphic, irregular outline of the mitochondrial outer membrane and matrix rarefaction, without cristal alteration were seen in all neurons. In addition, fusion of pleomorphic mitochondria with lysosomal bodies was a common occurrence, particularly in Patient #3. All specimens showed an increased number of dense residual bodies in the neuronal somata.

Both somata and processes of astrocytes were swollen; they contained normal mitochondria, variable amounts of alpha or beta glycogen and, frequently, vacuolated endoplasmic reticulum cisternae. Oligodendrocytes were normal.

Neurites, or neuronal processes filled with degenerative mitochondria and residual bodies were commonly found in acute biopsies of all three children (Figure 1).

[1] Total Creatine Phosphokinase levels done by Bioscience Laboratories, Inc.

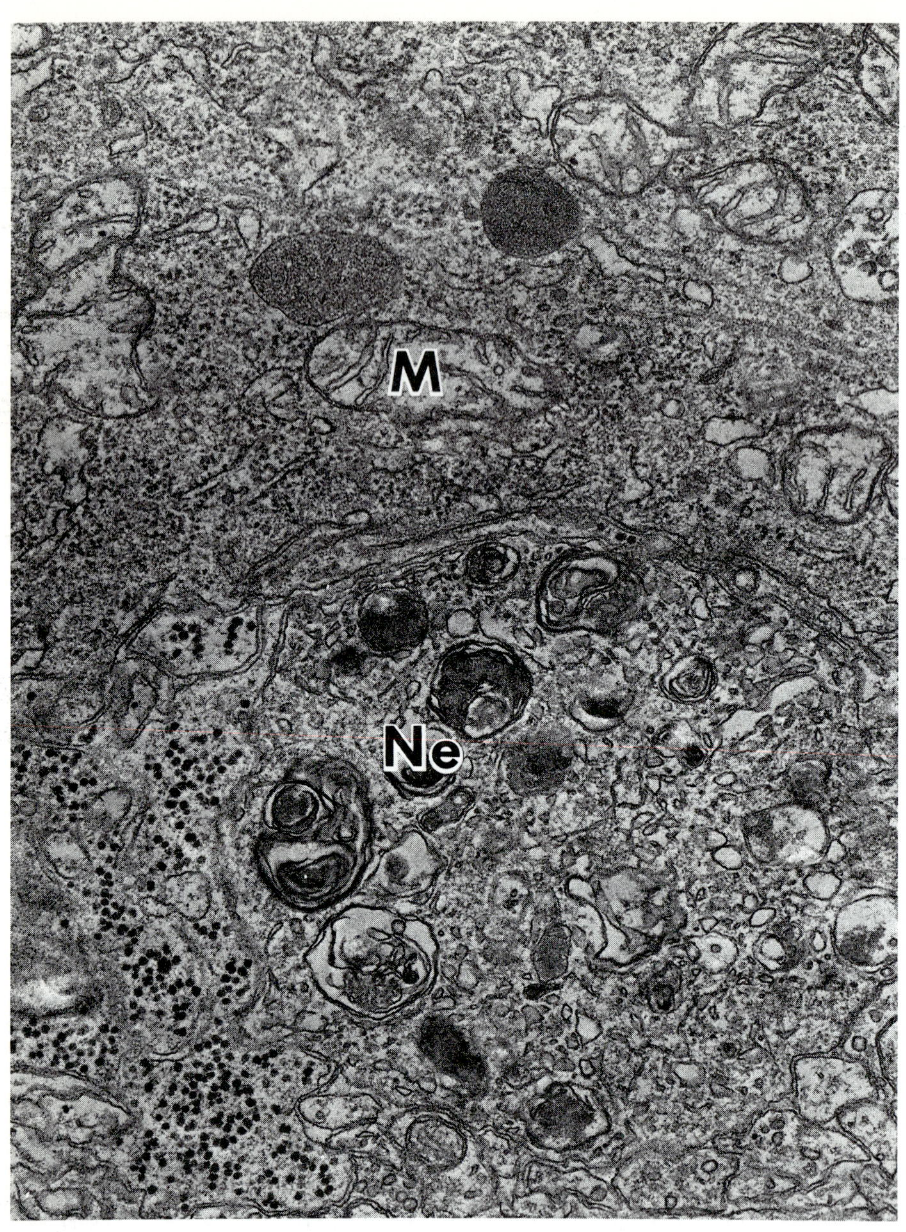

Figure 1. This micrograph illustrates part of a neuron in which mitochondria (M) are pleomorphic and ribosomes are dispersed. A large neurite (Ne) containing degenerating organelles and an astrocyte process with glycogen granules are also seen in this field. Patient #1, acute phase biopsy. Mag. 34,000x.

Myelinated fibers in which myelin lamellae were split, with the formation of large fluid-filled blebs, were seen throughout all the acute biopsies (Figure 2). The splits were at the intraperiod line, usually occurred in the outer lamellae of the sheath, and the large blebs protruded into the neuropil. Myelin periodicity was unaffected in other areas of the same sheath. Axonal changes varied from no alteration to accumulation of organelles or even complete loss of axon cylinders, with collapse of the myelin sheath. Extracellular myelin ovoids were seen in acute biopsies of two of the three patients.

Patient #2 had sustained a respiratory arrest and was in shock on admission to CHMC, and ultrastructural evidence of ischemia in addition to the alterations of Reye's Syndrome could be recognized in her cortical biopsy tissue. Specific changes which we attribute to ischemia were necrotic neurons, other neurons with swollen and rounded mitochondria, which occasionally showed disruption of the outer membrane, and in some mitochondria, the appearance of amorphous electron dense matrical inclusions. Additional ischemic alterations were greatly swollen post-synaptic dendritic terminals and a mild hydration change in some myelinated fibers.

Follow-up biopsies were obtained at varying intervals after recovery (Table II).

TABLE II

	Acute Biopsies: Hours After First CNS Signs	Recovery Biopsies: Days After Original Illness
Patient #1	43 hrs.	586 days
	72 hrs.	---
Patient #2	51 hrs.	54 days
	75 hrs.	75 days
Patient #3	53 hrs.	43 days
	77 hrs.	---

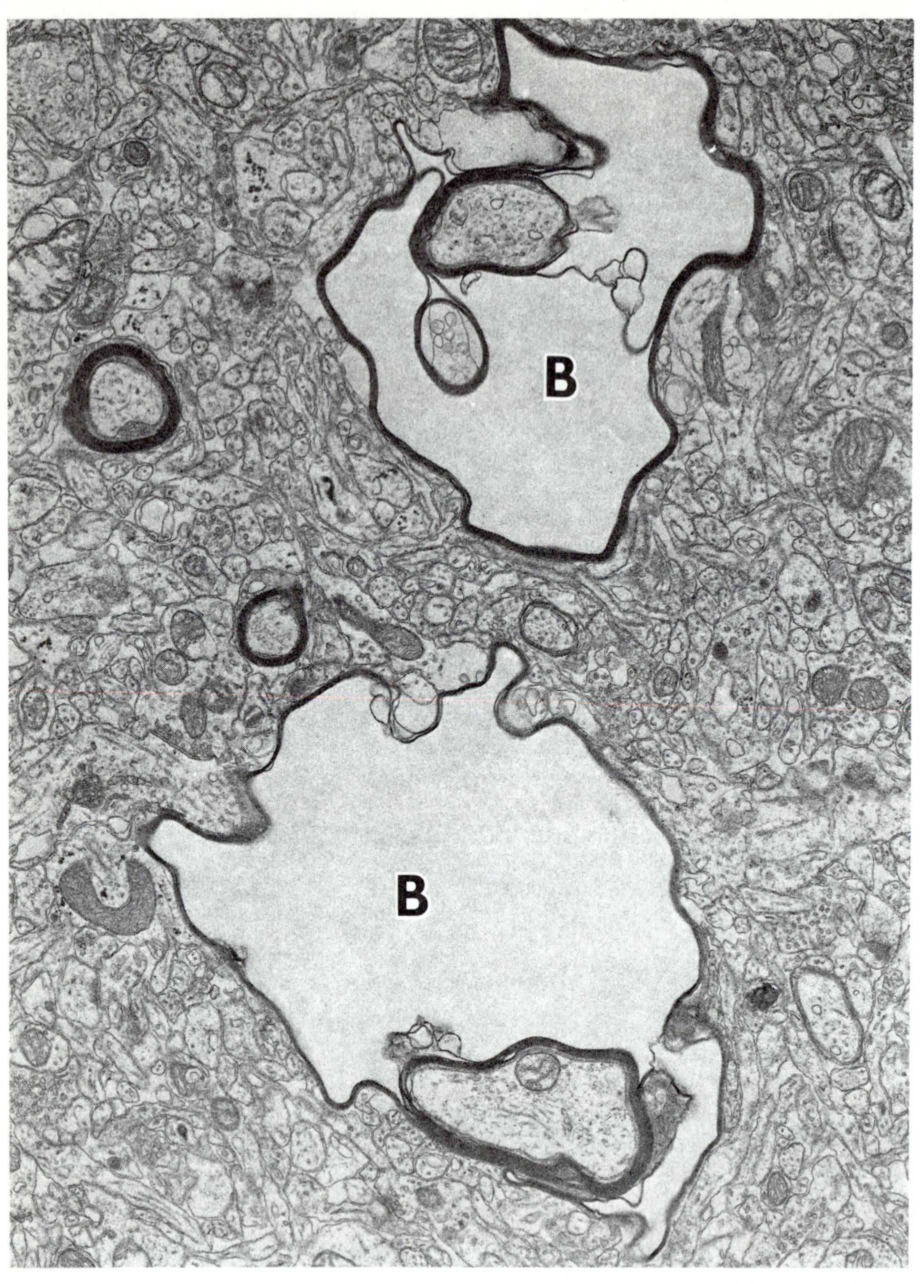

Figure 2. A micrograph from a second-day acute phase biopsy specimen from Patient #3 illustrates two axons with greatly ballooned myelin sheaths (B). Surrounding neuropil appears normal.   Mag. 14,000x.

Patient #1, because of severe pulmonary complications, did not undergo restorative surgery until more
than a year and a half after her original illness. At
this time, except for mild vacuolar change, little
evidence of injury or repair was appreciated by light
microscopy. Ultrastructurally, the only neuronal finding was the presence of numerous dense residual bodies
in the perikarya. Astrocytes occasionally contained
phagocytic vacuoles or large residual bodies. More
numerous residual bodies were present in microglia.
Not uncommonly, in the neuropil, myelin ovoids or re-
generating myelin sheaths were evidence of healing of
a pathological process.

Only in Patient #2 was there evidence of significant neuronal loss. This occurred particularly in
layers 3,5 and 6, and recovery biopsies demonstrated
astrocytic gliosis, microgliosis and rarefaction of the
neuropil in these zones. These findings were interpreted as probably due to the early hypoxic injury
rather than to Reye's Syndrome specifically. Surviving
neurons contained increased numbers of organelles, including increased numbers of rough endoplasmic reticulum cisternae, enlarged Golgi apparati and large areas
of cytoplasm occupied by polyribosomes. Reactive prot-
oplasmic and fibrous astrocytes were numerous. They
contained many dense residual bodies as well as an
occasional phagocytic vacuole. Microglia, filled with
dense residual bodies, were widespread throughout the
biopsy specimens, but more abundant in the zones of
neuronal loss. Throughout the neuropil, in both
Patient #2 and Patient #3, frequent myelin ovoids gave
evidence of loss of axons (Figure 3). Surviving myelinated processes showed widespread Wallerian degeneration, presence of frequent myelin ridges and axo-
plasmic sequestration.

Patient #3 had a less severe hospital course and
underwent replacement of bone flaps sooner than the
other two, thereby allowing us a view of earlier re-
parative processes. Neurons, as in the previous child,
contained increased numbers of organelles. Proto-
plasmic astrocytes were reactive, with a great increase
in numbers of organelles and cytoplasmic density, and

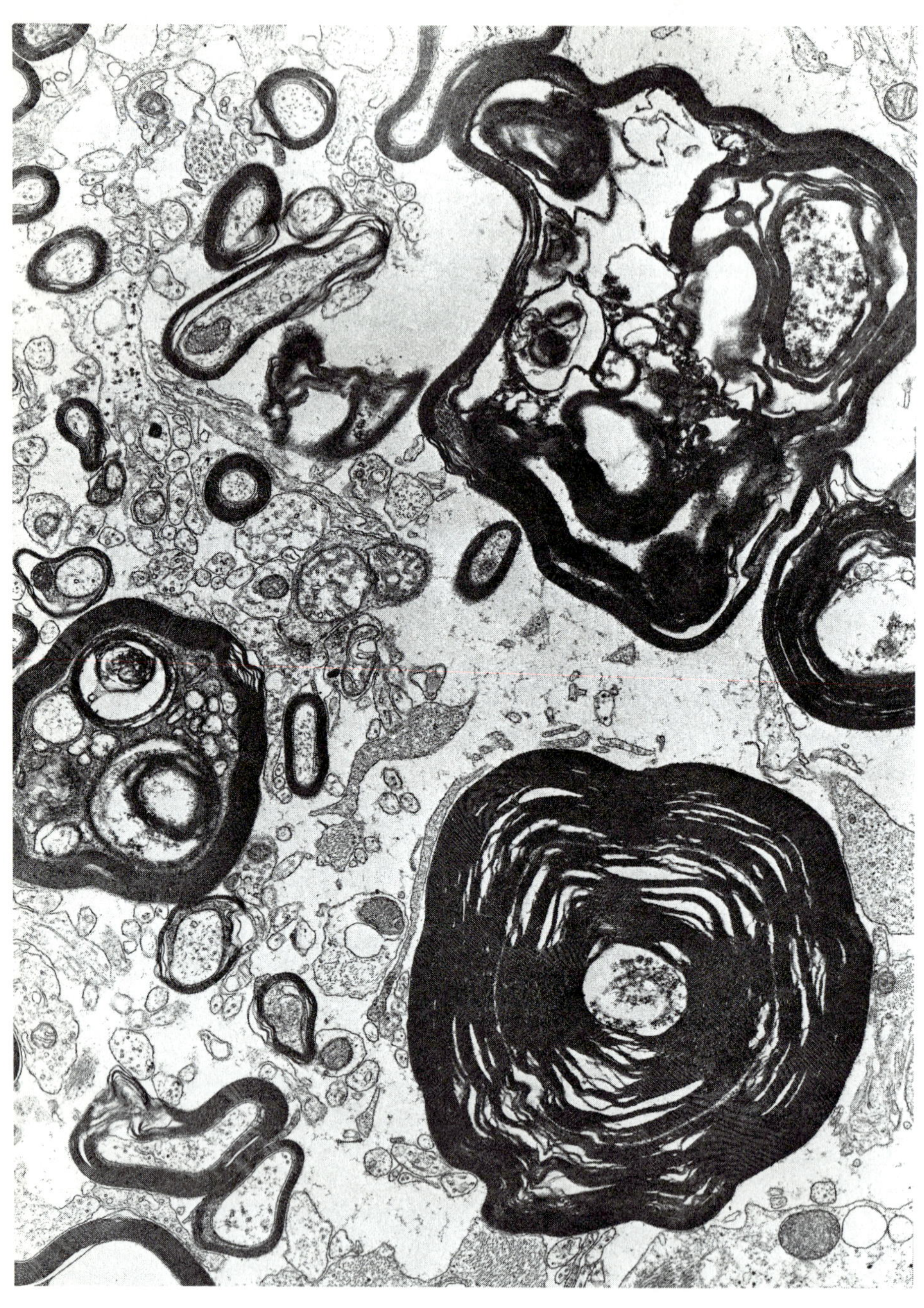

Figure 3. During the recovery phase, myelin ovoids,
some containing degenerating axon cylinders, are
widespread. Patient #3. Mag. 15,000x.

a few fibrous astrocytes were seen. Alterations of
oligodendrocytes were striking in that they had increased cytoplasm, increased numbers of microtubules,
numerous residual bodies and many free lipid droplets.
It has been previously reported that, in conditions
involving destruction of myelin without subsequent
invasion of macrophages, glial cells can exhibit phagocytic activity (5), and this process is evident in this
specimen in particular. As in the previous two patients, frequent myelin ovoids, myelin ridges, axo-
plasmic sequestration of axonal organelles and regen-
erating myelin sheaths were all seen.

Study of brain ultrastructure from these three
patients who had differing degrees of ischemic injury
during the acute phase of their illness allows us to
make certain speculations concerning the pathophysiology of the brain injury in Reye's Syndrome.

Myelin ovoids, or collapsed myelin sheaths from
which axons are lost, as well as Wallerian degeneration
of some large axons, are evidence that injury to the
neuron cell body has occurred, but do not specify the
kind of injury, ischemic or toxic. The mitochondrial
alteration seen in Reye's Syndrome in the brain appears
to be characteristic if not specific. A specific
injury to neuronal mitochondria could result in decreased energy production and failure of affected
neurons to maintain their trophic influence on the
sheaths myelinating their axons. Experimentally, myelin sheaths degenerate and collapse from an axon
severed from its cell body before recognizable degeneration of the axon has occurred (5). It is possible
that with neuronal mitochondrial injury there is a
movement of water into susceptible myelin lamellae.
Simultaneous injury to hepatocyte mitochondria resulting in an increased circulating ammonia level may be a
contributing factor to fluid accumulation in astrocytes.

This proposal is supported experimentally by
studies showing that the known toxins resulting in
myelin bleb formation, hexachlorophene, triethyltin,
isoniazide and cuprizone, are agents affecting mito-

chondrial function, although _in_ _vivo_ ultrastructural
alterations may not be apparent.

In summary, the ultrastructural evidence suggests
that the encephalopathy of Reye's Syndrome may be due
to a metabolic injury closely related to or perhaps
the same as the injury which is manifest in the liver
and skeletal muscle. The biochemical and ultrastructural evidence is compatible with the hypothesis that
the mitochondrion is the principal site of injury. The
organelle pathology is not that of ischemia, ammonia
intoxication or hypoglycemia, and appears to be highly
characteristic of the disease.

REFERENCES

1. Reye, R.D.K., G. Morgan, and J. Baral. 1963.
    Encephalopathy and fatty degeneration of the vis-
    cera: A disease entity in childhood. _Lancet ii_:
    749.
2. McLaurin, R.L., and J.B. Nichols, Jr. 1957. Ex-
    tensive cranial decompression in the treatment
    of severe lead encephalopathy. _Pediatrics 20_:
    653.
3. Partin, J.C., J.S. Partin, W.K. Schubert, and R.L.
    McLaurin. 1975. Brain ultrastructure in Reye's
    Syndrome (Encephalopathy and fatty alteration of
    the viscera). _J. Neuropathol. Exp. Neurol. 34_:
    425.
4. Partin, J.S., A.J. McAdams, J.C. Partin, W.K.
    Schubert, and R.L. McLaurin. In press. Brain
    ultrastructure in Reye's Syndrome II: Acute
    injury and recovery processes in three children.
    J. Neuropathol. Exp. Neurol.
5. Cook, R.D., and H.M. Wisniewski. 1973. The role
    of oligodendroglia and astroglia in Wallerian
    degeneration of the optic nerve. _Brain Res. 61_:
    191.

Supported by the Cincinnati Children's Hospital
Research Foundation and in part by N.I.H. Clinical
Research Centers grant #RR-00123.

DISCUSSION

D.B. Tower   -   Can you tell us how old these children
were?

J.S. Partin -   I'm sorry; I forgot that. 6 years, 15
years, and 5 years, and they were all girls.

G.D. Gall   -   The question is raised by both Partin
papers as to whether this is a generalized mitochondrial damage throughout the body, or is it
liver specific? We have published a paper looking
at enzymes involved in gluconeogenesis and Kreb
cycle in liver tissue from patients with Reye's,
and showed that the mitochondrial enzymes are
depressed. This is what one would expect from looking at the other report studies on urea cycles,
that there is a generalized mitochondrial injury
of the liver mitochondria. We have also looked at
brain tissue and muscle tissue. The numbers are
small but, when you look at mitochondrial enzymes
involved in the Kreb cycle in brain tissue and
muscle, they're normal compared with controlled
material obtained in exactly the same fashion. So
we're not able to show,at least biochemically,the
mitochondrial injury in the brain or in the muscle.

J.S. Partin -   Are you looking at homogenates of tissue?

G.D. Gall   -   Yes.

J.S. Partin -   I think that one of the major differences in the liver and the muscle and brain is
that there is a much greater homogeneity of mitochondrial types in the liver. In the brain, we
find that the neuron mitochondria are definitely
abnormal, whereas the astrocyte mitochondria are
not. Two fibre types are in the muscle; one has
different mitochondria than the other and they

function differently.

H.J. McClung - Have you had an opportunity to correlate
       any residual neurologic dysfunction with your
       pathology?

J.S. Partin - Well, we have only done the three chil-
       dren,and they all have some degree of residual
       brain damage. This correlates very well with the
       ischemic injury much more than anything else. All
       three cases were clinical Grade 4 when they were
       admitted to the hospital; but, two of them had had
       ischemic episodes before the craniectomies were
       done so I think that the neurological sequela cor-
       relate very well with their ischemic periods.

L.O'Tuama   - The so-called blood brain barrier sys-
       tem, in particular the choroid plexus,have been
       viewed as possible sites for regulation of CNS el-
       ectrolyte metabolism and it would seem that their
       dysfunction might be well open to a disorder of
       cerebral edema as a common manifestation,and I
       just wondered if you were aware of any systematic
       studies that have been done of the function of
       the barrier tissues, particularly the choroid ple-
       xus,pathologically in this entity?

J.S. Partin - There have been some indications that
       they may be morphologically altered, but our ex-
       perience is not large enough to make comment on
       this.

D.B. Tower -   Let me comment on the problem of the mi-
       tochondria. In the human brain there are far less
       neurones per unit volume than there are in smaller
       brains, like rodents'. Less than 20% of the total
       cells will be neurones,and the rest of them will
       be astrocytes and oligones. So that,if only the
       neuronal mitochondria are involved, you will not
       necessarily see this. Now I have a question; did
       you see regeneration of myelin sheaths in your 15-
       year-old patient?

J.S. Partin   - Yes, we did.

D.B. Tower   - Because that's a very remarkable obser-
                vation.

J.S. Partin   - We certainly did. There is a great in-
                crease in ologodendrocyte activity in all
                three of the children, and large cytoplas-
                mic masses, increased organelles, and re-
                generating sheaths.

INCREASED PHOSPHORYLATION OF A PLASMA
MEMBRANE COMPONENT OF THE FAT CELL IN
REYE'S SYNDROME

Ellen S. Kang, M.D., and Ronald E. Gates, M. D.

Excessive lipolysis is a prominent feature of
Reye's Syndrome and is believed to account, in part,
for the accumulation of neutral fat in the liver (1).
Ordinarily, this process is highly regulated by the
complex interplay of the polypeptide hormones and the
catecholamines which utilize the second messenger system to mediate their intracellular effects (2). Markedly abnormal increases in the concentrations of the
lipolytic and antilipolytic hormones have not been observed in this disorder, although plasma levels of the
most potent lipolytic hormones, the catecholamines,
have not yet been reported in Reye's Syndrome(3).

To explore the possibility that a circulatory factor with hormone-like activities could be present in
the blood of these patients and account for the excessive lipolysis observed, the effect of Reye's plasma on
the lipolytic response of isolated fat cells from the
epididymal fat pads of Sprague-Dawley rats was examined.
The addition of 300 μl of plasma (EDTA) to 2 x 10^5
cells in a total volume of 1 ml showed a slight increase
in glycerol released in 30 minutes in Reye's samples
(Figure 1) compared to normal control plasma. However,
a similar increase was noted in sick controls (children with a flu-like illness without a Reye's sequela.)
Thus, a factor which could mimic the lipolytic hormones
in plasma cannot account for the enhanced lipolysis
seen in the disorder.

The possibility was, therefore, considered that an
intrinsic abnormality may be present in the target tis-

LIPOLYTIC ACTIVITY OF PLASMA IN RAT FAT CELL ASSAY
(30 MINUTE INCUBATION)

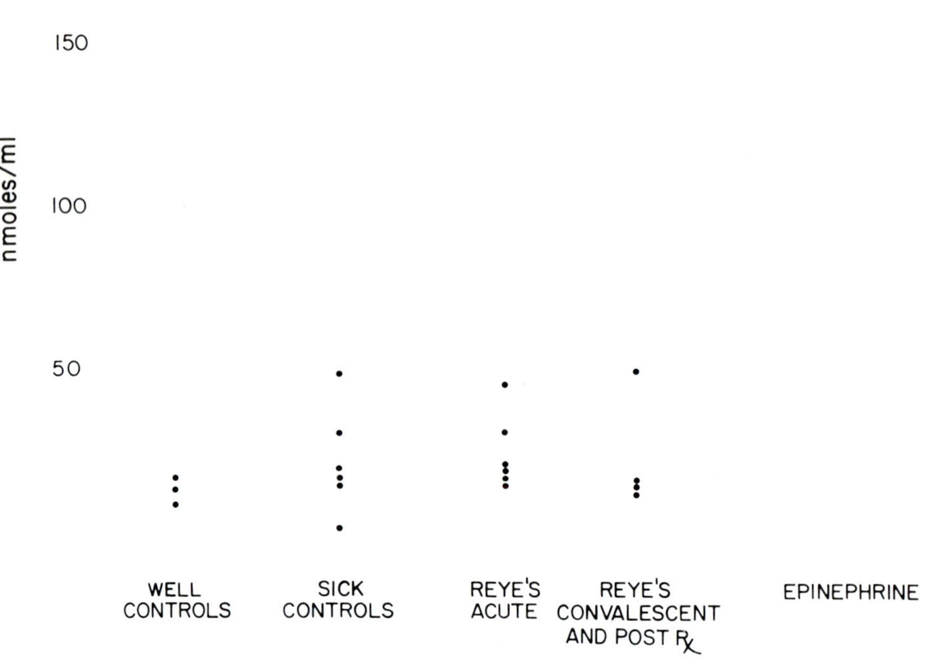

Figure 1. Isolated fat cells in Krebs-Ringer
bicarbonate buffer, pH 7.4, 4% albumin,
cell number 2×10^5/ml, 37°C., flushed
with 95% O_2, 5% CO_2.

sue, allowing for an exaggerated response to normal sti-
muli. We focused particularly on the plasma membrane of
the fat cell because these cells obtained from patients
at post mortem exhibit a peculiar responsiveness to
glucagon in Reye's syndrome, and there is evidence that
the plasma membrane of another tissue, muscle, may also
be involved in this disorder as reflected by the appearance of cytoplasmically located enzymes of muscle
in the plasma compartment of many patients. Isolated

fat cells from adipose tissues obtained at autopsy from Reye's and control subjects exhibit responsiveness to epinephrine at concentrations of 10^{-5}M (see Table 1). Cells from Reye's #1 show a response to glucagon, a finding not evident in 2 controls and probably within the limits of error for the method in a third control. Glucagon responsiveness has not been found in human fat cells by other investigators (4).

Classically, the polypeptide hormones and the catecholamines bind to specific receptors located on the plasma membranes of receptive cells. This event triggers the synthesis of cyclic AMP from ATP by the membrane-bound enzyme adenylate cyclase. The raison d'être for cyclic AMP is the activation of protein kinase by binding to the regulatory subunit of the protein kinase complex, resulting in the dissociation and activation of the catalytic subunit of this enzyme (Figure 2). The catalytic subunit catalyzes the transfer of the terminal or γ-PO$_4$ of ATP onto appropriate seryl or threonyl peptides in ester linkage. The resulting phosphorylated enzyme or protein is activated or inactivated in the phosphorylated form. Protein phosphatases reverse this process, thus adding still another factor in the multiple steps involved in the regulation and transmission of hormone effects (5).

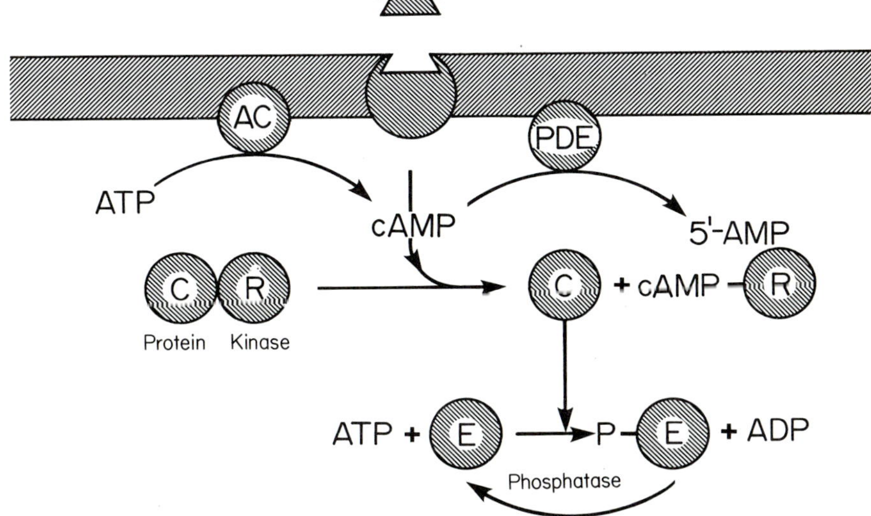

TABLE 1.

LIPOLYTIC RESPONSES OF HUMAN FAT CELLS
OBTAINED AT AUTOPSY

Subject	Age (Years)	Hours Post Mortem	Response to Hormone in NMoles/ML of Glycerol Formed			
			$\underline{E}$	$\underline{G}$	ACTH	TSH
REYES 1	15	8	7.5	15.5	5.5	15.5
*REYES 2	8	6	12.5	Not Done	Not Done	Not Done
CONTROL 1	29	5	190	0	0	0
CONTROL 2	57	$3\frac{1}{4}$	6	0	0	0
**CONTROL 3	54	4 3/4	7	2	0	Not Done

Incubation 90 min., 37°C, KRB-4% Albumin in 95% O_2, 5% CO_2, corrected for basal lipolysis.
Cell # 15 x 10^4 in 1 ml except for:* = 5 x 10^4 and **=26 x 10^4
E=Epinephrine 4 x 10^{-4}M   G=Glucagon 3 x 10^{-8}M   ACTH 20u/ml   TSH 0.2u/ml

   Adipose tissue treated with collagenase according to
Rodbell's method(6) leads to the recovery of viable,in-
tact and hormonally responsive cells. Cells were thus
prepared from fresh biopsied subcutaneous fat from Reyes
and control subjects.Solubilization of intact cells with
sodium dodecyl sulfate (SDS) and electrophoresis,using
a gradient of acrylamide 7.5-17.5% on a Laemmli slab of
10 cm height,followed by Coomassie staining, results in
a characteristic protein pattern (Figure 3). Approximate
molecular weights of these proteins can be determined by
comparison with pure standard of known molecular weights
which are coelectrophoresed.

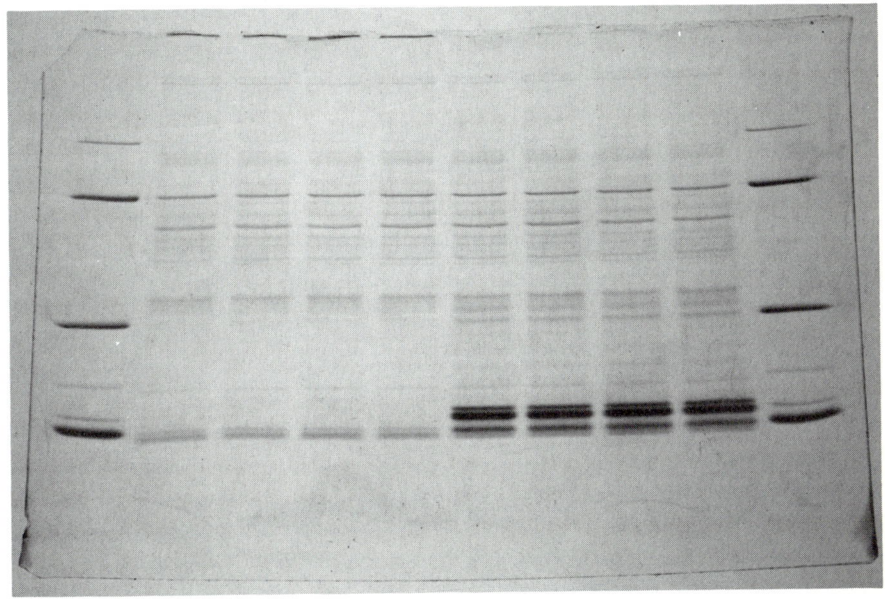

Fig.3. Outer lanes represent molecular weight markers
   from the top of the gel to the bottom: β-galactosidase
   130,000,bovine serum albumin 68,000, carbonic anhyd-
   rase 29,000 and cytochrome C 14,200 daltons. Lanes 2-5
   are intact cells while Lanes 6-9 are intact cells
   plus histone.

When control cells are incubated with ATP labeled
in the γposition, the uptake of label is most prominent in two components with molecular weights of approximately 63,000 and 57,000 daltons (Figure 4). The
addition of cyclic AMP in uM concentrations results in
the increase in labeling of these two components.

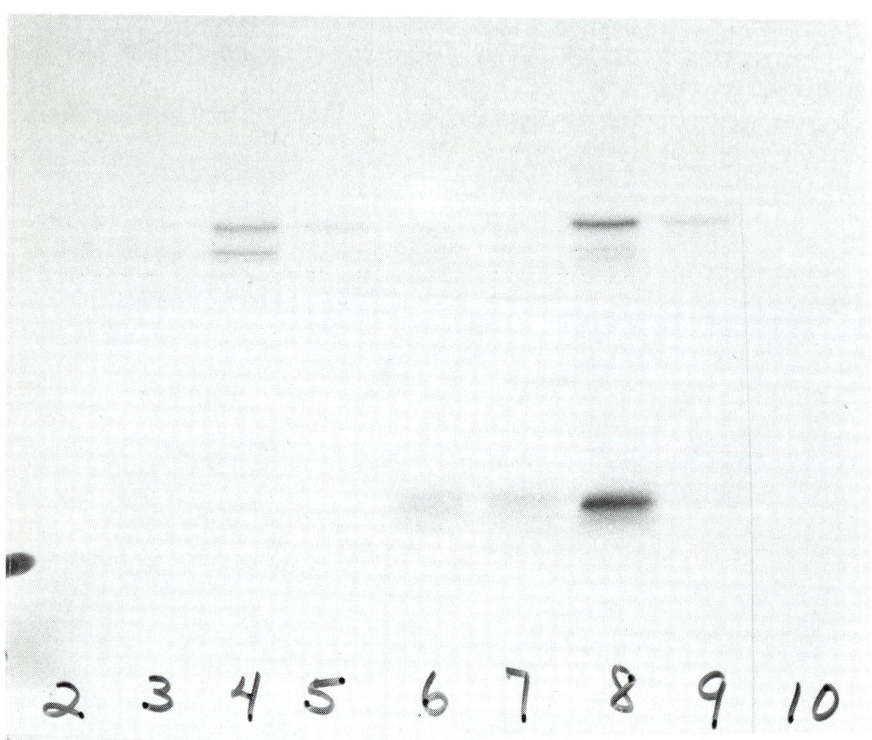

Figure 4. Radioautograph of dried gel:

Lanes 2 & 3 are cells alone.
Lane 4 is cells plus cyclic AMP.
Lanes 6 & 7 are cells plus histone.
Lane 8 is cells plus histone and cyclic AMP.

Incubation in Krebs-Ringer bicarbonate
buffer, pH 7.4, containing 2.5mM (γ -^{32}P)
ATP, 10 µCi, 30° for 2 min., flushed with
95% O_2, 5% CO_2 . Cyclic AMP when present was
2 µM. Histone was 100 ug/ml.

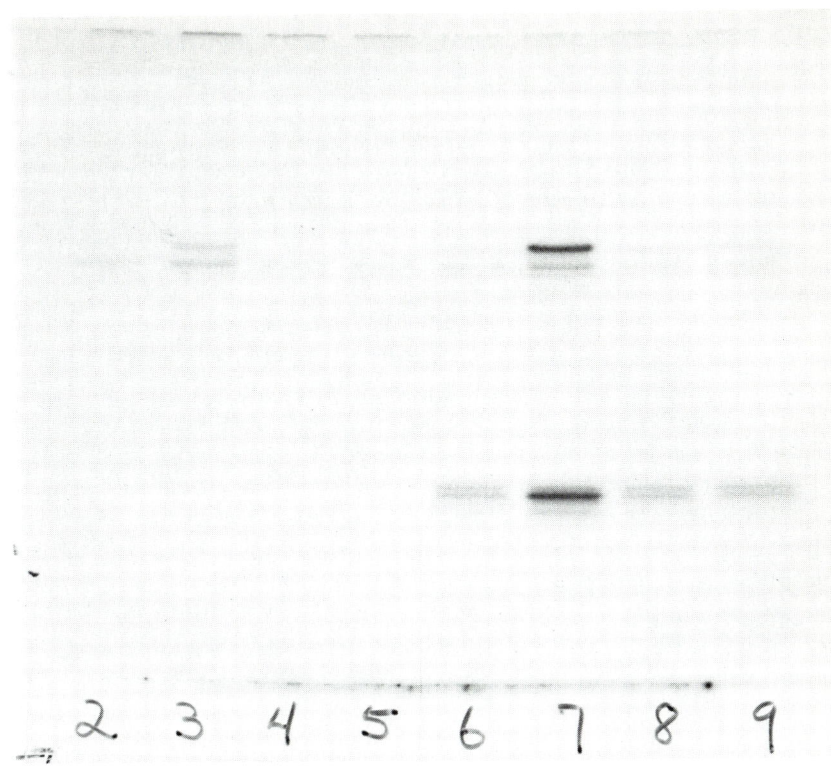

Figure 4B. Radioautograph of dried gel:
         Lane 2 is cells plus cyclic AMP.
         Lane 3 is cells plus cyclic AMP.
         Lane 6 is cells plus histone.
         Lane 7 is cells plus histone and cyclic AMP.
         Incubation conditions as in Figure 4A.

The addition of histone, a substrate for protein kinases, results in the incorporation of label into histone. Since histone is too large to penetrate the intact cell and protein kinase activity is not present in
the infranatant of such preparations, this observation
indicates that kinase activity is located on the surface of the human fat cell.The addition of both histone and cyclic AMP results in a marked enhancement of
label incorporated into histone, as well as the 63,000
molecular weights component.

A similar pattern is seen in fat cells from a
Reye's syndrome subject, except for an increase in the
intensity of the labeling of the 63,000 molecular weight
component in the presence of cyclic AMP and histone.
Densitometric scans of these gels were obtained using
an Ortec densitometer. Ratios of radiographic densities
under basal and combined cyclic AMP and histone additions were compared for Reye's and control cells and
are presented in Table 2. Considerably greater increase in label incorporation into the 63,000 and 57,000
components is seen in Reye's than in control cells when
both cyclic AMP and histone are added to intact cells.
Cell homogenates were also compared for total kinase
activity. Preliminary results indicate an enhancement
of label incorporated into histone (the added substrate)
in Reye's than in control samples.

These findings indicate the presence of a kinase
within the plasma membrane of the fat cell with unusual
properties in Reye's syndrome. Histone is known to dis-
sociate the regulatory and the catalytic subunits of
protein kinases (7), thereby enhancing the activation
of protein kinase activity. The increased incorporation
of label into the 63,000 and 57,000 molecular weight
components in the presence of both cyclic AMP and histone indicates that this enzyme in Reye's fat cells is
more susceptible to dissociating influences than cells
from control subject. Whether the homogenate findings
reflect the activity of the same enzyme or intracellular enzymes cannot be differentiated from the studies.
The question should be raised as to whether this finding is unique to fat cells. Since phosphorylation of

TABLE 2

INTEGRATED AREAS OF DENSITOMETRIC SCANS OF RADIOAUTOGRAPHS OF
SOLUBILIZED FAT CELLS EXPOSED TO (γ-32P) ATP FOLLOWED BY SDS-PAGE

	Area of 63,000 Dalton Component	Fold ↑ Above Basal	Area of Histone Region
Control Basal	4		
+cAMP	21	(5.2)	
+Histone	0.5		16
+cAMP and Histone	34	(8.5)*	74(4.6)
Reye's Basal	2		
+cAMP	11	(5.5)	
+Histone	5	(2.5)	22
+cAMP and Histone	44	(22)*	58(2.6)

ATP 12.5 uM, 2 Min at 30° C.

enzymes by protein kinases either activates or inacti-
vates them, the possibility of accounting for inhibition of enzymes via this mechanism is highly possible.
This has particular significance in so far as the enzyme pyruvate dehydrogenase is concerned.This enzyme
pyruvate dehydrogenase,is a mitochondrially-located enzyme, and has been sufficiently characterized to establish that it is phosphorylated by protein kinase
which results in <u>inactivation</u> of the enzyme, whereas
activation requires the dephosphorylation of this enzyme by a protein phosphatase (8). Pyruvate dehydrogenase has recently been shown to be markedly inhibited
in Reye's syndrome (9). In view of our findings of an
unusual protein kinase effect in Reye's fat cells,the
possibility should be considered that enzymes such as
pyruvate dehydrogenase may be inactive secondary to exaggerated kinase effects.

ACKNOWLEDGEMENT
     This work was supported by USPHS NIH Grants HD11657
and GR RR05423. We thank Drs. Robert Boehm,J.T.Jabbour
and E.Wrenn for patient referrals, and Dr.John Griffith
for his support.

REFERENCES

1. Brown,R.E., Madge,G.E. and Schiller,H.M. 1971. Observations on the pathogenesis of Reye's syndrome.
   South.Med.Jnl.64:142-146.
2. Manganiello,V.C.,Murad,F. and Vaughan,M. 1971. Effects of lipolytic and antilipolytic agents on cyclic 3'5' - adenosine monophosphate in fat cells.
   J.Biol.Chem.246:2195-2202.
3. Haymond,M.S.,DeVivo,D.C.,Karl,I.E.,and Keating,J.P.
   Sequential metabolic observations in Reye's syndrome
   In:J.D.Pollack:Reye's Syndrome,pp.215-225, Grune &
   Stratton,Inc.,New York, 1975.
4. Burns,T.W. and Langley,P.E. 1970. Lipolysis by human adipose tissue:The role of cyclic 3' 5'-adenos-
   ine monophosphate and adrenergic receptor sites.
   J.Lab. and Clin. Med. 75:983-997.

5. Rubin,C.S. and Rosen,O.M. 1975. Protein phosphory-
    lation. *Ann.Rev.Biochem.44*:831-887.
6. Rodbell, M. 1964. Metabolism of isolated fat cells.
    I. Effects of hormones on glucose metabolism and
    lipolysis. *J.Biol.Chem.239*:375-380.
7. Corbin,J.D.,Keelye,S.L. and Park,C.R. 1975. The
    distribution and dissociation of cyclic adenosine
    3':5' - monophosphate-dependent protein kinases in
    adipose,cardiac and other tissues. *J.Biol.Chem.250*:
    218-225.
8. Linn,T.C., Pettit,F.K. and Reed, L.J. 1969. Alpha-
    keto acid dehydrogenase complexes. X Regulation of
    the activity of the pyruvate dehydrogenase complex
    from beef kidney mitochondria by phosphorylation
    and dephosphorylation. *Proc.Nat.Acad.Sci.62:Part II*:
    234-241.
9. Robinson,B.H., Gall,D.G. and Cutz, E. 1977. Defici-
    ent Activity of hepatic pyruvate dehydrogenase and
    pyruvate carboxylyase in Reye's syndrome.*Ped.Res.11*:
    279-281.

MORPHOLOGICAL FINDINGS IN THE THYMUS
IN CHILDREN WITH REYE'S SYNDROME

Rosa Beatriz Fuksman de Cherjovsky, M. D.

INTRODUCTION

Inspired by Selye (1) and Henry's (2,3) works on
the accidental involution of the thymus, we conducted a
comparative study of the thymic morphology in children
dying from different causes between the ages of 1 hour
and 5 years.

Four states of uniform thymic involution were identified and it was possible to classify all but three patients in one of these states of uniform involution.
When reviewing the autopsy protocols, we realized the
cause of death in these three children was Reye's syndrome.

We wish to present our observations on the unique
histological changes in the thymus in children dying
with Reye's syndrome.

A total of 217 thymuses were studied histologically. Nineteen of these autopsies were children with Reye
syndrome and 198 were of children dying of other causes.
All thymuses were fixed in 10% formalin,embedded in paraffin and stained with hematoxylin and eosin, Period-
ic Acid Schiff(PAS) and the Gomori technique for reticulum fibres. Tissue was also frozen and stained with
Sudan for lipids.

The morphological classification of thymic pathology was correlated with age, sex, duration of illness,
date, diagnosis, therapy with corticosteroids, and nutritional state.

The following morphological changes were used to

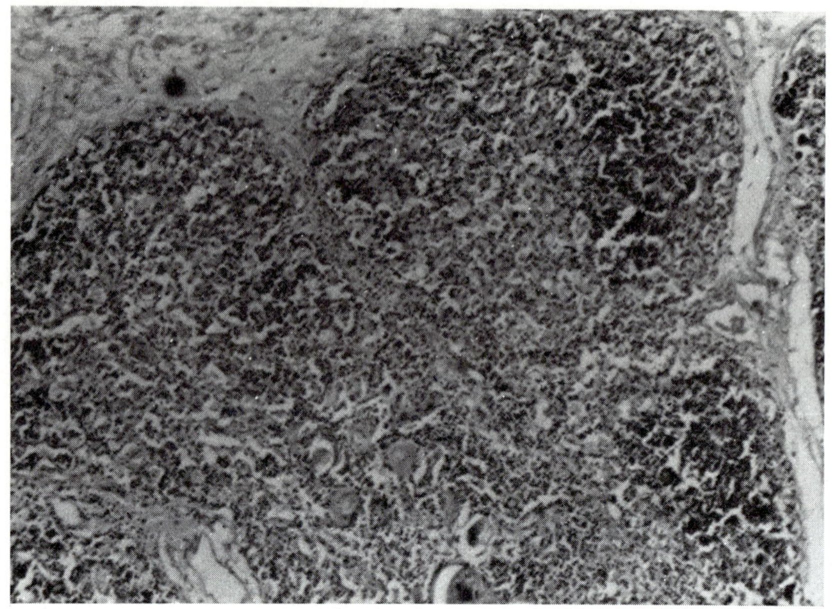

Fig.1.   Grade 1,the periphery of the lobule (cortex)
         is 4 to 5 times denser in lymphocytes than
         the center (medulla).

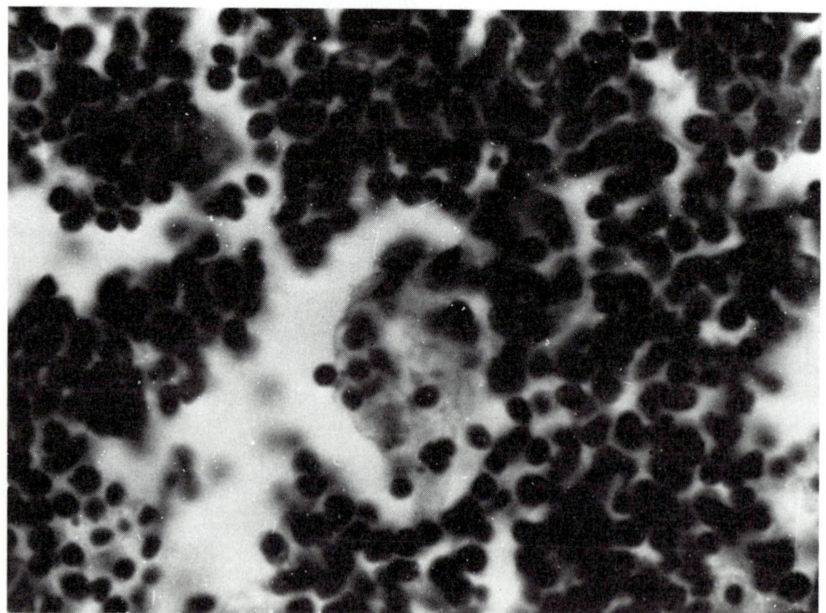

Fig.2.   Cortical cells with macrophagic capacity
         loaded with cellular debris.

classify thymic changes:-
GRADE 1 - (normal thymus-Figure 1) In the cortical zone,
the thymocytes population is 4 to 5 times larger than
in the marrow. Clear spaces without thymocytes may exist between the thymocytes of the cortex. Occasionally,
cells with phagocytic activity (Figure 2) were found.

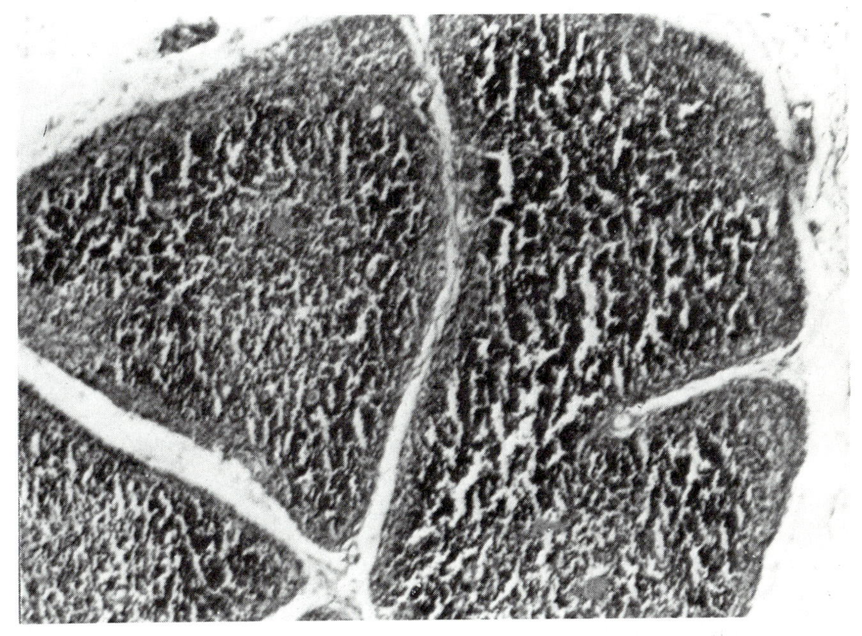

Fig.3. Grade 2, there is a loss of subcapsular
       thymocytes.

GRADE 2 - (Fig.3) There is preservation of the para-
medullary lymphocytes, but a decrease in the number
seen in the subcapsular region of the cortex. The space
left by the absence of thymocytes is occupied by cells
with phagocytic capacity whose vacuolated cytoplasm
(Figure 4) is loaded with PAS positive and sudanophilic
materials.

GRADE 3 - (Fig.5) The number of thymocytes in the cortex and medulla is the same. The last is recognized
only by the presence of Hassal's corpuscles. The number of phagocytic cells are increased.

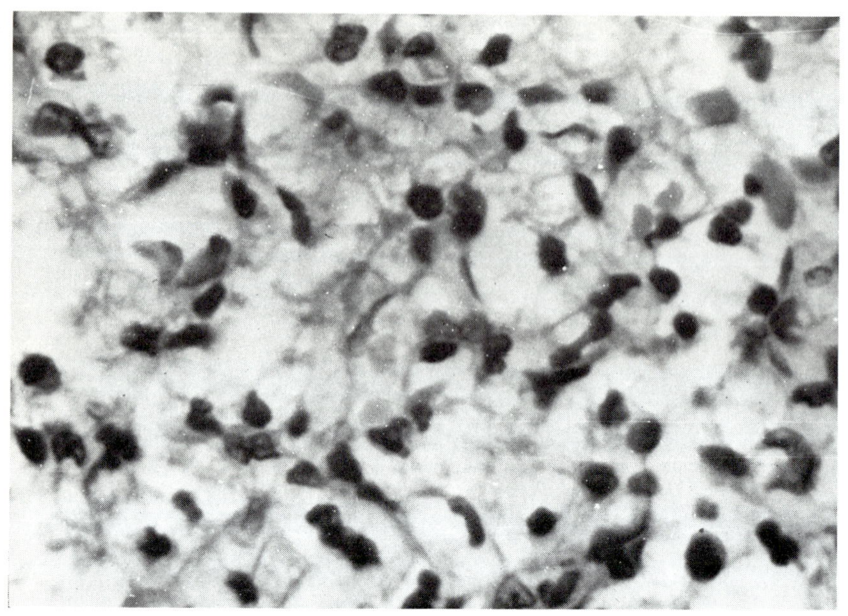

Fig. 4.   Macrophagic cells with vacuolated
          cytoplasm.

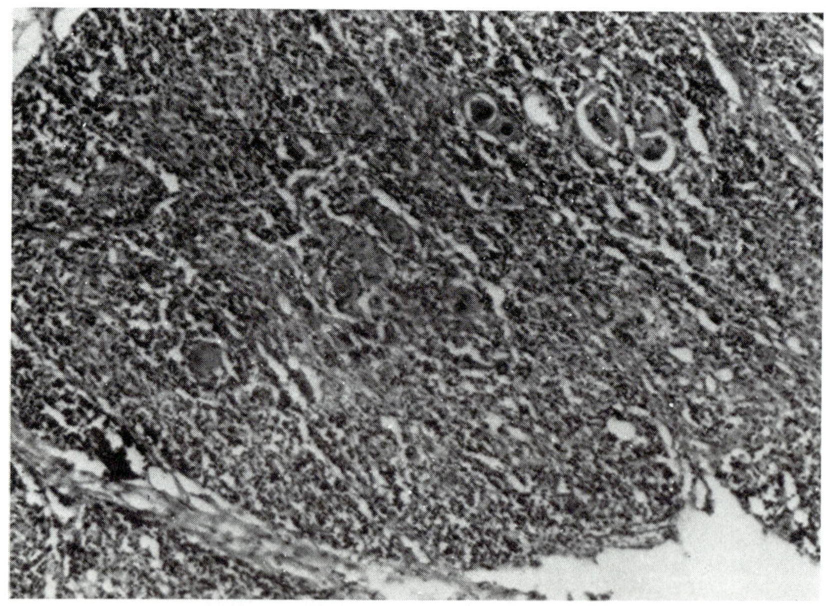

Fig. 5.   Grade 3. There is the same proportion
          of thymocytes in cortex as in medulla.

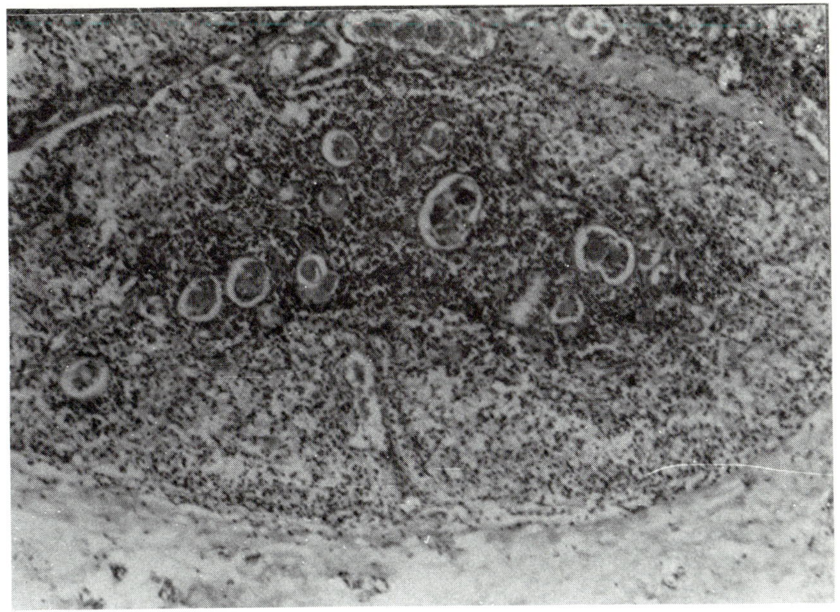

Fig.6.   Grade 4. There are more thymocytes in
         the medulla than in the cortex.

GRADE 4 - (Figure 6). There is an inversion of the
normal thymic appearance, the population of thymocytes
in the medulla is 4 to 5 times larger than in the cortex. Phagocytic cells are increased in number. Together with these microscopic changes, there is a reduction in the weight of the thymus, each lobe is reduced in size and the reticulum content increased.

Comparison of morphological and clinical findings
led to the following conclusions:-

In the well-nourished patients (Eutrophics), the
more advanced the illness, the greater the involution.
Involution appeared to advance more rapidly with sepsis
or corticosteroid therapy. (Graphic 1).

The poorly-nourished patients (Dystrophics) begin
their illnesses with thymic changes of Grade 3; that
is to say, malnutrition is an important factor in accidental involution (Graphic 2).

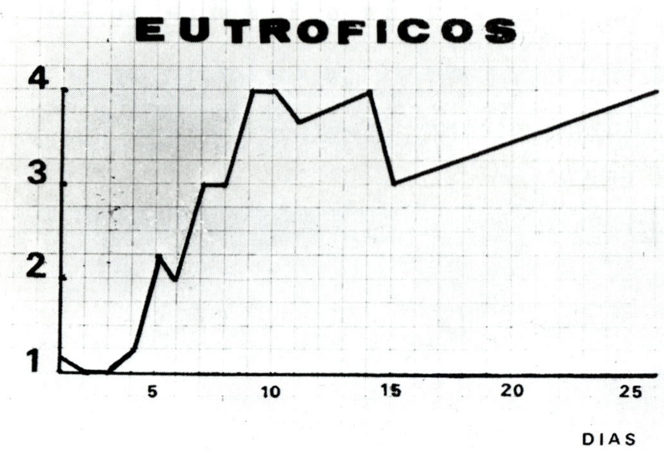

Graphic 1. Involution in Eutrophics

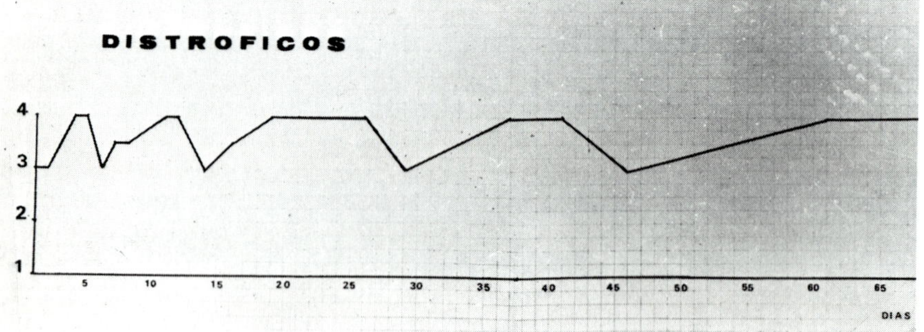

Graphic 2.   Involution in Dystrophics

Prematures of greater than 1.7 kg. birth weight
react to illnesses, corticosteroid therapy and malnutrition in a similar way to the eutrophics. Those prematures weighing less than 1.7 kg at birth have less
thymic involution (Graphic 3).

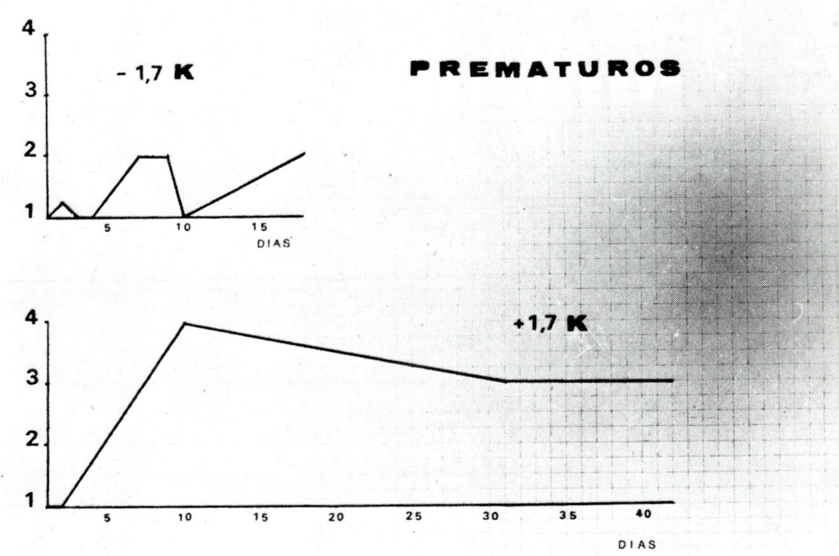

Graphic 3.   Involution in Prematures.

Thymic changes of non-homogeneous nature, with the
morphological changes of varying grades of involution
in different lobes in the same thymus, and even different parts of the same lobe, were called "irregular involution". These were also characteristic of thymocytes
throughout the lobules. (Figures 7 to 10).

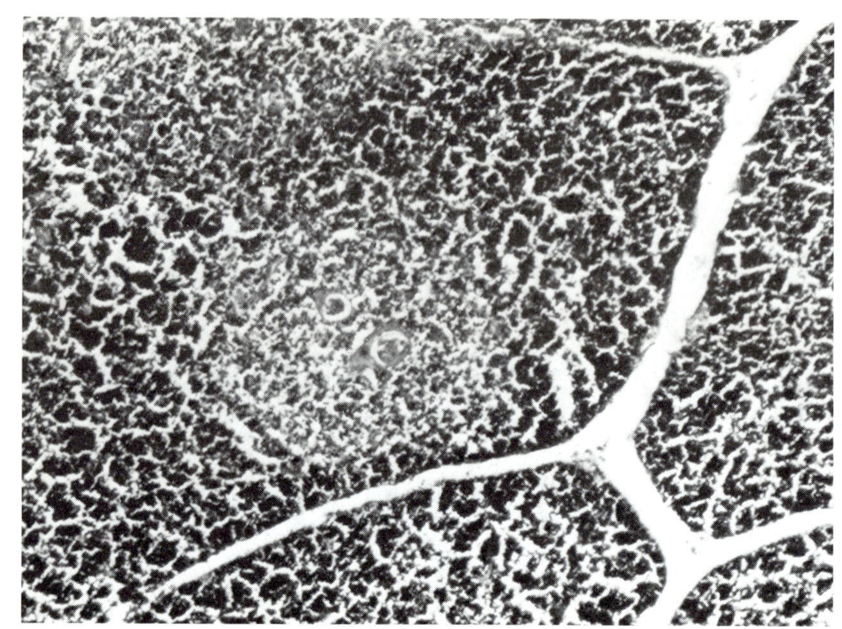

Fig.7

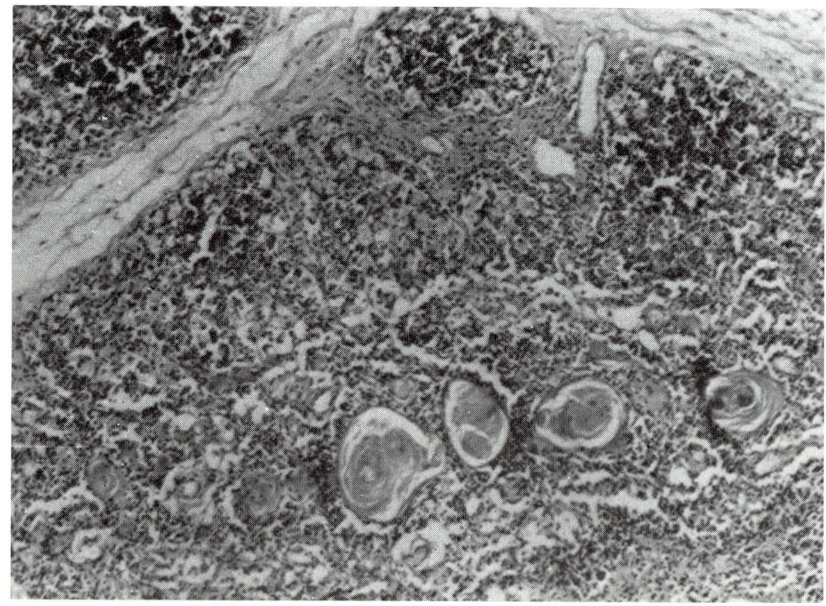

Fig.8

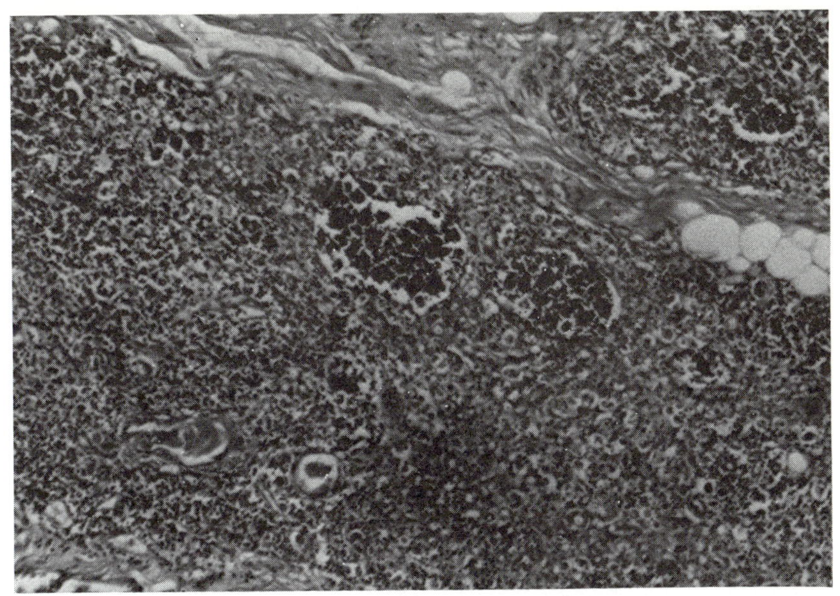

Fig. 9

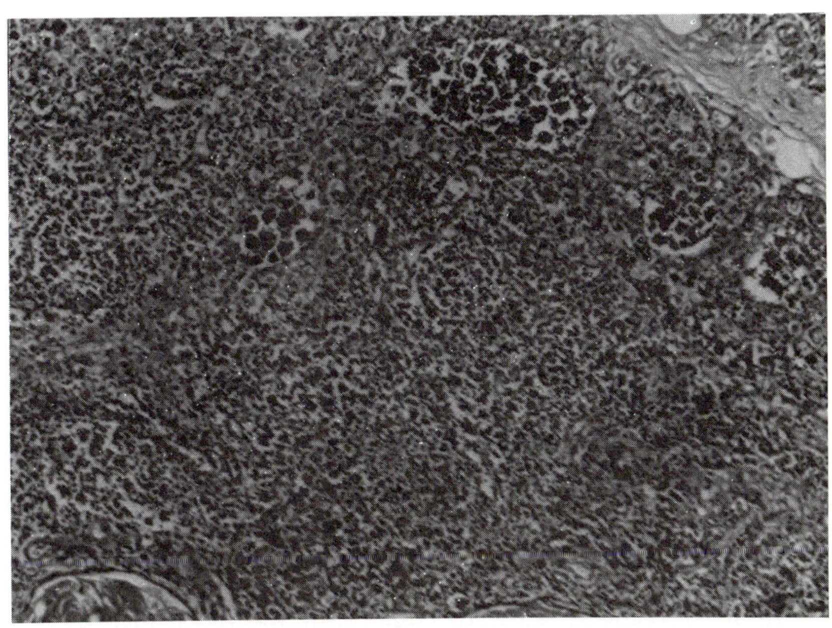

Figs.7,8,9,and 10. Irregular involution;
   images of several grades take place
   in the same lobule.

RESULTS

Thymic changes of irregular involution have been found in 9 of the 19 patients with Reye's syndrome and in 6 of the 198 patients who died from other causes. This observation was statistically significant (p<0.01) (Graphic 4)

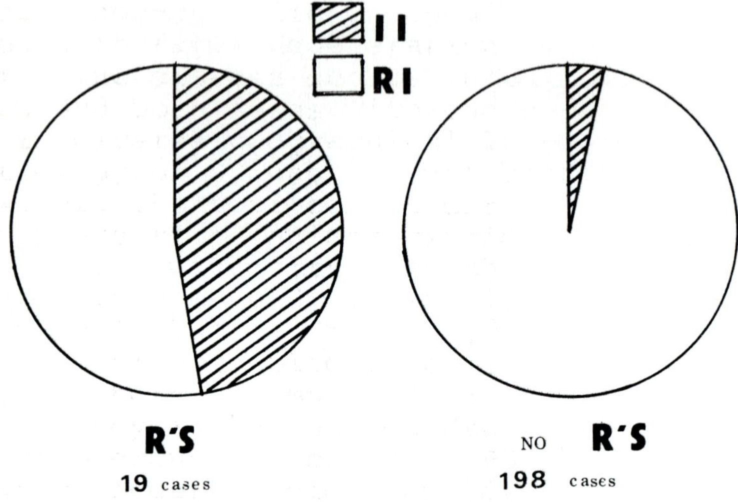

Graphic 4. Cases with Reye's syndrome and
          without Reye's syndrome.
          II: Irregular Involution
          RI: Regular Involution

The cause of death in the six patients without Reye's syndrome is shown in Table 1.

The data of those children dying with Reye's syndrome is presented in Table 11. From its study, we conclude that age, season, sex and nutritional state have no effect on the irregular involution of the thymus. The administration of corticosteroids did appear, however, to have a statistical effect.(Graphic 5).

TABLE I

IRREGULAR INVOLUTION OF THE THYMUS WITHOUT REYE'S SYNDROME

Diagnosis	Age	Corticosteroid Therapy
Maternal Spasm	Newborn	No
Chronic Nreloid Leukemia	5 years	No
Premature	Newborn	Not Known
Premature	Newborn	Not Known
Meconium Aspiration	Newborn	Yes
Infant of Diabetic Mother	Newborn	No

T A B L E   2

Area	Thymus Grade	Duration (days)	Corticosteroid Therapy	Diagnoses	Nutrition	Sex	Age
S.Martin	Ir In	2	-	Pneumonitis	E	F	2 m
"	Ir In	4	+	Pur.meningitis	E	M	12 m
				Fibrinous pleurisy			
				Herpetic pharyngitis			
				Sepsis			
"	Ir In	2	+	Pneumonitis	E	F	10 m
"	1	2	-	Pneumonitis	E	M	6 m
"	1	2	-	Pancreatitis	E	F	19
"	1	2	+	Varicella	E	F	5 m
"	Ir In	1	?	Peribronchitis	E	F	16 m
				Esophagogastritis			
LaPlata	Ir In	2	+	Bronchitis	E	M	9 m
"	1	2	-	Chronic bronchitis	E	M	5 m
"	1	2	-	Bronchopneumonia	E	F	11 m
"	Ir In	2	+	Down syndrome	E	F	12 m
				Bronchopneumonia			
"	1	2	-	Pulmonary edema	E	M	8 m
"	1	3	+	Bronchopneumonia	E	M	5 m
"	Ir In	3	+	Pneumonitis	E	M	4 m
"	1	3	-	Pneumonitis	E	M	5 m
Haedo	1	3	-	Pneumonitis/bronchopneu.	E	F	16 m
"	Ir In	3	-	Supp.adenitis/Dchol.synd.	D	F	17 m
Sask.	4	?	?			?	?
S.Diego	Ir In	?	?			?	?

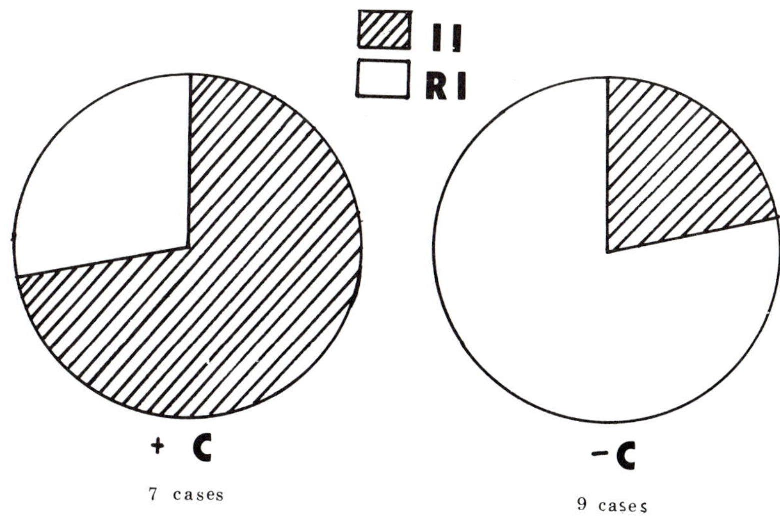

Graphic 5. Cases of Reye's Syndrome with
           corticosteroids (+C) and without
           them (-C).
           II-irregular involution
           RI-regular involution

    Additional observations from our review include the
following:

    (1) All but one of our autopsied children with
Reye's syndrome were well nourished in contradistinction
to those autopsied with other causes of death;

    (2) The age group autopsied with Reye's syndrome was
from 2 to 19 months;

    (3) Most of the children autopsied with Reye's syn-
drome were affected in spring and autumn months;

    (4) One of our cases of Reye's syndrome also had
meningitis, and we would stress the importance of not

ruling out the diagnosis of Reye's syndrome on the basis of a pleocytosis in the CSF.

(5) The precipitating factor in one of our patients appeared to be non-viral. This patient had an
acute attack of hereditary pancreatitis.

COMMENT

This paper emphasizes what we believe to be distinctive thymic changes in children dying with Reye's
Syndrome.

We suggest the thymic morphology be studied in the
various experimental models of Reye's Syndrome.

Many authors (4,5,6) have theorized the possibility
of a defect in cellular immunity in children with Reye
Syndrome. Whether the virus or viruses themselves may
cause defects in cellular immunity directly or a chemical toxin acting with a virus has this response, has
also been discussed in the literature.

Linneman et al (7) did a preliminary study of cellular immunity in this syndrome without positive results. However, they commented that a more extensive
study was necessary to be conclusive.

Millikin (8), Bourgeois (9) and Dvorackova (10)
mention an alteration in the lymphatic organs in Reye's
syndrome. This alteration consists of necrosis of the
follicular center at the sector B level. We have not
been able to identify these changes in our cases.

We do not know if these thymic changes of irregular
involution are cause or effect, nor do we know if they
are reversible or irreversible. To decide the significance of the changes observed, one should consider the
following:-

(1) The six children with irregular involution,
dying from illnesses other than Reye's syndrome, may
have gone on to develop Reye's syndrome had they survived;

(2) One of the six children with irregular involution dying from illnesses other than Reye's syndrome had chronic myeloid leukemia. Johnston (11) previously described a girl with chronic lymphatic leukemia who developed Reye's syndrome. This suggests transiently altered cellular immunity as a factor;

(3) The description of Reye's syndrome in families and of recurrent episodes in a single patient suggest familial and permanent defects in immunity;

(4) The fact that the peripheral lymphatic organs are not modified causes us to favour the theory of a transient alteration in immunity as a factor.

We feel it would be interesting to study the immune status of patients with Reye's syndrome, and of survivors of the acute illness. This would help identify functional alterations and the difference between those (actually patients and survivors), and would help clarify the permanent or transient nature of any observed alterations.

An additional question of importance is whether the thymic changes in Reye's syndrome are primary or secondary. We would be interested in the effects on thymic morphology in experimental animals after injections of exchange transfused blood from patients with Reye's syndrome.

As far as corticosteroids are concerned and the appearance of the irregular involution in Reye's syndrome, it seems that there is morphological evidence of a latent alteration.

ACKNOWLEDGEMENT
     I acknowledge all the people who have collaborated with this work in a personal way, or by sending their thymus cases: Dr.Gallardo from Argentina, Drs.Powell and Rosenberg from the U.S.A., Dr.Laxdall from Canada and, especially, Dr.Drut from La Platas Sor ludovica Hospital (Argentina) who contributed a great many cases.

I also acknowledge Dr. Natalio Guman, Chief of the
Pathology Service from Mariano Castex Hospital, where
this paper was written.

REFERENCES

1. Selye,H., and Horava,A. 1952. STRESS-Second
    Annual Report.*Acta Inc.,Med.Publishers,Montreal*.

2. Henry,L. 1967. Involution of the Human Thymus.
    Journ.Path. and Bact.93(2):661.

3. Henry,L. 1968. "Accidental' Involution of the
    Human Thymus.*Jöurn.Path.and Bact.96(2):337*.

4. Crocker,J.F.S.,Ozere,R.L.,Safe,S.H.,Digout,S.C.,
    Rozee,K.R.,Hutzinger,O. 1976. Lethal Interaction
    of Ubiquitous Insecticide Carriers with Virus.
    Science 192(1):331.

5. Stechenberger,B.W.,Keating,J.P.,Koslov,S.,
    Schecter,M.,Chang,M.,Haymond,M.W.,Feigin,R.D.,
    1975. Epidemiologic Investigation of Reye's
    Syndrome. *Journ. of Ped. 87(2):234*.

6. Tang,T.T.,Siegesmund,K.A.,Sedmah,G.V.,Casper,J.T.,
    Varma,R.R.,McCreadie,S.R. 1975. Reye's syndrome:
    a correlated electronmicroscopic, viral and bio-
    chemical observation.*J.A.M.A. 232(13):1339*.

7. Linneman,C.C.,Jr.,Shea,L.,Partin,J.C.,Schubert,
    W.K., Schiff,G.M. 1963-1974. Reye's Syndrome:
    Epidemiologic and Viral Studies.*Am.J.Epid.101(6):*
    517.

8. Millikin,P.D. 1977. Epitheloid Germinal Centres:
    An acquired immunologic deficit? *Am.J.Clin.Path.
    81:240*.

9. Bourgeois,C.H.,Shank,R.C.,Grossman,R.A.,Johnson,
    D.O.,Wooding,W.L. 1971. Acute Aflatoxin B,Toxici-
    ty in the Macaque and its similarities to Reye's
    Syndrome. *Lab. Invest. 24(3):206*.

10.   Dvorackova, I., Vortel, V.,Hroch,M. 1966. Enceph-
       alitic Syndrome with fatty degeneration of the
       viscera. *Arch. of Path. 81:* 240.

11.   Johnston, 1977. *Brit. Med.J. 22 Sept.,*640.

DISCUSSION

A.R. Colon (speaking in Spanish)- Was this an accelera-
     ted involution?

R.B. Cherjovsky   -   There was no gradiation.

A.R. Colon   -   Did you look for lymphoblastic
     transformation in these patients, accelerated
     transformation?

R.B. Cherjovsky   -   We had no facilities in which to
     look for transformation.

A.R. Colon   -   I gather, then, that you didn't
     look for specific T cells.

R.B. Cherjovsky   -   The facilities are lacking,and
     that is one of the reasons why I am here..in the
     hope of stimulating more research along these
     lines, to get people who can do lymphoblastic
     transformation and T cell rosette formation,work.

A.R. Colon   -   Did you study patients with hem-
     olytic uremic syndrome, mubucho fever or Argen-
     tinian hemorrhagic fever?

R.B. Cherjovsky   -   I have no hemorrhagic fever in
     my own cases. I have never seen hemorrhagic fever
     because it has been only in Surinam and surround-
     ing area.

A.R. Colon   -   I remember some studies that I
     have seen on hemorrhagic fevers, where thymuses
     were studied,and it was accelerated involution in

those cases.

R.B. Cherjovsky -   Oh,yes, but perhaps it hasn't
                       the irregular involution I've found in
                       Reye's syndrome.

A.R. Colon   -   The patients that did not have
                       Reye's syndrome; how long were they on
                       steroids?

R.B. Cherjovsky -   Of ten patients with Reye's
                       syndrome and with irregular involution,
                       only two have received corticosteroids,but
                       I don't know for how long.

THE ROLE OF CHEMICALS IN REYE's SYNDROME

S. Safe, Ph D., O. Hutzinger, Ph D., and
J.F.S. Crocker, M.D.

INTRODUCTION

Reye's syndrome (RS) is primarily a
children's disease which has been clinically
characterized as a non-specific encephalopathy associated with fatty degeneration of
the viscera (1). The disease occurs in children of all ages and both sexes with cases
being reported in diverse geographical locations. The etiology of RS has not yet been
elucidated, however, the most consistent
single factor appears to be an association
with a viral infection with viruses such as
influenza B, adenovirus type 3, Coxsackie A,
A9, B1 and B4, para influenza, measles, varicella, rubella, reovirus, polio type 1, Echo
8, influenza A, and herpes simplex (1,3). An
epidemiological survey in the United States
concluded that "two groups of cases of RS
emerge: those which occur in older children
(median age 11 years), cluster in time and
geographic region and are associated with
antecedent influenza B infection; and those
which occur sporadically throughout the year,
are isolated in occurrence, occur in younger
children (median age 6 years) and are associated with a wide variety of antecedent viral
illnesses" (2). A number of other reports
have suggested that a metabolic defect in the
urea cycle is also involved in RS. Reduced
levels of carbamyl phosphate synthetase and
ornithine transcarbamylase have been observed
in the liver of RS patients and this correlates with increased levels of ammonia and
decreased levels of citrulline in some patients (4). RS patients can also exhibit
other biochemical abnormalities which include
hypoglycemia elevated blood ammonia levels
(5), increased serum levels of free fatty
acids and diffuse serum triglycerides (6).

The latter two alterations are presumably associated with the fatty degeneration of the viscera and the metabolic alterations which accompany this disorder.

It has also been suggested that chemicals may play a significant role in RS (7,8) and this hypothesis has been supported by both human clinical studies and model animal studies.

HUMAN STUDIES - ROLE OF CHEMICALS

Aflatoxins. The aflatoxins are a group of fungal metabolites produced by the mold, Aspergillus Flavus. Aflatoxin B_1 is the most active compound in the series and is known to be one of the most potent animal hepatocarcinogens. In tropical and sub-tropical countries fungal infestation of stored crops (eg. peanuts and grains) has resulted in the introduction of this chemical into the food chain. Epidemiological studies have strongly suggested a relationship between this class of toxins and the high incidence of liver cancers in the susceptible geographical areas. Similarly, there is also clinical and analytical data which suggest a link between RS and aflatoxins in Thailand (9). The data indicated that the geographical and seasonal fluctuations in aflatoxins corresponded to the incidence of RS and, moreover, the toxin was identified in the autopsy specimens from the infected patients.

Salicylates. A number of reports have suggested a possible role of salicylates in RS (10, 11). It is well-known that salicylates and related drugs can induce a wide range of biological effects which include acute encephalopathy, uncoupling of oxidative phosphorylation, hepatic dysfunction, hypoglycemia and altered immune function. Since

many RS patients are likely to have used
this type of drug during the initial stages
of their illness an enhancement or potentiation of Reye's syndrome by the chemical is a
viable possibility.

__Other Xenobiotics.__ Pollack (8) has reviewed a number of other reports which have
suggested a possible involvement of diverse
chemicals in RS and these include warfarin
(12), isopropyl alcohol (13), lindane (14),
antihistamines, decongestants, unidentified
paints and pesticides (11).

ANIMAL MODEL STUDIES - ROLE OF CHEMICALS

__Fatty Acids.__ Some of the clinical,
pathological and biochemical aberrations
associated with RS involve fatty acids and
lipids and it has been suggested that these
compounds might also play a role in the observed mitochondrial damage in RS patients.
It is also known that the symptoms of Jamaican vomiting sickness and RS are similar
with a major difference between the two disorders being the prodromal viral illness
common to RS. Hypoglycin and its active metabolite, methylene-cyclopropyl acetic acid,
have been implicated as toxins in the Jamaican vomiting sickness and a related fatty
acid, 4-pentenoic acid, was used to determine
the effects on animals. The results supported a possible role of this type of chemical

$$CH_2=\overset{\overset{\displaystyle CH_2}{\diagup\diagdown}}{C}-CH-CH_2-\overset{\overset{\displaystyle NH_2}{|}}{CH}-COOH \qquad CH_2=\overset{\overset{\displaystyle CH_2}{\diagup\diagdown}}{C}-CH-CH_2-COOH$$

Hypoglycin   Methylene-cyclop-
                               ropyl acetic acid

in RS and Jamaican vomiting sickness. Administration of 4-pentenoic acid (15) to rodents
resulted in ureagenesis and hypoglycemia;

some brain edema was noted, medullary vacuolization was enhanced over control animals
and electron microscopy revealed fat droplets,
swollen mitochondria, cytoplasmic vacuole and
glycogen loss. In addition, prior exposure
to the mengo strain of the EMC virus and fasting,accelerated the effects of the chemical
in this animal model. Other chemicals such
as lindane, and the polychlorinated biphenyls
(PCB) had no visible effects and both aflatoxin and cuprizone did not potentiate the
viral infection (15).

Pesticides and Pollutants. A number of
groups have studied virus chemical interactions in insects, plants and tissue cell culture systems. Some of these reports have
indicated a synergistic effect in which the
combination of the two agents resulted in an
enhancement of diverse biological effects (11).
For example, it was shown that the larvae of
Bombyx Mori were more susceptible to the combination of chemical (fenitrothion) and virus
(polyhedrosis virus) than to either chemical
or virus alone (16). Friend and Trainer reported the first in vivo studies with chemicals and viruses using mallard ducks as the
animal model (17). Inoculation of the animals with duck hepatitis virus followed by
treatment with DDT resulted in a lessening
of the effects of the virus (18). The results
were interpreted in terms of a virus stimulation of microsomal enzyme activity and
the subsequent metabolic detoxication of the
chemical. DDT induces microsomal enzyme
activity although it is a very poor substrate
for this mixed function oxidase enzyme system.
More recent results in which the chemical was
administered followed by infection with the
virus showed that the chemical enhanced
viral mortality (19).

In 1974 and 1976, Crocker and co-workers

Table 1. The Composition of the Aromatic Solvent Aerotex 3470.

Chemical	Band	Relative %	Molecular Ion
1,3-Dimethyl-5-ethylbenzene	I	1.9	134
1,2-Dimethyl-4-ethylbenzene	I	4.4	134
1,2,3,5-Tetramethylbenzene	I	13.7	134
Short retention time alkylated benzenes (4 peaks)	I	1.4	120-134
Long retention-time alkylated benzenes (9 peaks)	I	24.8	148-162
Naphthalene	II	12.8[a]	128
1-Methylnaphthalene	II	17.5[a]	142
2-Methylnaphthalene	II	13.5[a]	142
2,6-Dimethylnaphthalene	II	3.4	156
2,3-Dimethylnaphthalene	II	4.1	156
1,5-Dimethylnaphthalene	II	.5	156
Long retention time alkylated naphthalenes	II	1.4	156-184
Alkylated biphenyls fluorenes and phenanthrenes (>30 peaks)	III	6.0	168-230
Alkylated bibenzyls (39 peaks)	IV	2.0	182-238

[a]major isomeric components.

(20, 21) developed a similar model using
young mice, mouse encephalomyocarditis (EMC)
virus and chemicals. DDT or commercial fenitrothion (FT) was topically painted on the
mice which were then exposed to a sublethal
dose of the virus. The two chemicals only
slightly enhanced viral lethality however, a
combination of the two insecticides resulted
in a 60% mortality. In addition fatty changes were noted in the liver and kidney. Subsequent work using commercial fenitrothion,
pure fenitrothion and the adjuncts present in
the commercial product pointed out the complexity of the problem. The commercial FT
product used was a mixture of anionic/non-
ionic surfactants (Atlox 3409 F, ICI Chemicals
Inc. or Toximul MP-8, Stephan Chemical Co.)
and an aromatic solvent (Aerotex 3470, Texaco
Canada Ltd.) all of which have been used in
an extensive forest spray program. The most
sensitive virus chemical combination was
obtained using the emulsifier/solvent combination (ie. 0.7% each of Toximul MP-8, Atlox
3409 and Aerotex 3470) in which 85% mortality
of the test animals was observed. Subsequent
studies using these commercial emulsifiers
and their purified components have also
shown their capability to enhance the infectivity of several single stranded RNA viruses
to mammalian cells in culture (22).

A striking feature of this latter work
is the fact that the chemicals which are the
most effective in the chemical-viral model
are widely used in food, shampoos and in a
myriad of other commercial applications. The
potential impact of any xenobiotic on mammalian systems depends on a number of factors
which include:

(a) the amount and frequency of exposure
(b) the biodegradability of the chemical
(c) the synergistic effects of chemical
     mixtures

(d)   the biological effects of individ-
      ual chemicals and chemical mixtures

These factors will be discussed in terms of
the specific chemicals used in the forest
spray program (and in the mouse virus-chemical
model studies) as well as other widely used
chemicals which are either persistent in
human tissue or are used frequently and are
more biodegradable. This latter class of
chemicals are usually the most environmentally
safe products since they do not accumulate
in the host animal and do not present a chronic toxicity problem. The results published
by Crocker and colleagues now challenge the
validity of this assumption since the emulsi-
fier/solvent carriers which they have studied
clearly potentiate viral lethality although
these chemicals are generally considered to
be non-toxic environmentally-acceptable products.

SOLVENTS AND SURFACTANTS

   Aerotex 3470. The commercial solvent,
Aerotex 3470 is marketed as a high boiling
petroleum distillate which is a by-product in
the fractionation of crude oil. The solvent
is aromatic in nature and several million
gallons of similar products are marketed as
industrial and commercial solvents. In
addition many more millions of gallons of
this material enter the environment annually
via crude oil spills. The analysis of Aerotex 3470 by gas chromatography (GC), mass
spectrometry (MS) and GC-MS indicated a complex mixture of over 100 components (23).
The analysis was simplified by prior separation of the mixture into 4 bands; bands 1 and
2 comprised over 91% by weight of the mixture
and contained an array of alkylated benzenes
and naphthalenes respectively (Table 1). 1,2,
3,5-Tetramethylbenzene and a series of isom-

eric C_5H_9-benzenes were the major components
of fraction 1, whereas naphthalene, 1 and 2-
methylnaphthalene,2,6 and 2, 3-dimethylnaph-
thalene were the major aromatics identified
in band 2. Previous studies have also shown
that alkylated naphthalenes and benzenes are
the most water soluble fraction (WSF) of
crude oil. Band 3 contained 6% by weight of
Aerotex and GC-MS analysis confirmed a highly
complex mixture of alkylated low molecular
weight polynuclear aromatics derived from
fluorene, biphenyl and phenanthrene. Band
4 (2% by weight of Aerotex) contained a complex series of alkylated bibenzyls which
have not hitherto been identified in aromatic
solvents (see Table 1).

The acute toxicities of these chemicals
vary considerably; the acute oral LD_{50} values
for naphthalene, phenanthrene, biphenyl and
bibenzyl are 2200, 700, 2180 and 1000mg/kg
respectively in rats (24); comparable in-
halation studies using mixed aromatic solvents confirmed the relatively low toxicity
of these chemicals to the test animals (cats,
dogs, rats) (25). These data are in contrast
to the highly toxic effects of the crude oil
WSF and related chemicals to aquatic organisms
The LC_{50} values of naphthalene, 1 and 2-meth-
ylnaphthalene and dimethylnaphthalenes to
<u>Cyprinodon</u> <u>variegatus</u>, <u>Paleamonetes</u> <u>pugio</u> and
<u>Penaeus</u> <u>aztecus</u> were in the ranges 2.0 - 5.1,
0.7 - 2.6 and 0.08 - 2.5 ppm (in water) respectively (26). Sub-acute toxicity studies
also indicated that these alkylated aromatics
also are inducers of microsomal enzyme activity (27).

Current experiments in our laboratory
are concerned with membrane perturbation of
these chemicals and their possible effects
on some aspect of lipid metabolism. The
physical toxicity of many chemicals has been

Table 2. Lysosomal Membrane Lysis by Aromatic Fractions and Specific Isomers[a]

Chemical Component	Concentration (M)		
	2×10^{-3}	2×10^{-4}	2×10^{-5}
Aerotex 3470	0.089±0.04	0.030±0.005	0.015±0.004
Band I	0.125±0.02	0.031±0.009	0.012±0.008
Band II	0.131±0.03	0.020±0.01	0.001±0.003
Band III	0.069±0.018	0.012±0.01	0.011±0.008
1,2,3,5-Tetramethylbenzene	0.070±0.030	0.007±0.006	0
Naphthalene	0.100±0.013	0.006±0.005	0
1-Methylnaphthalene	0.3065±0.050	0.020±0.010	0
2-Methylnaphthalene	0.230±0.040	0.021±0.007	0
Fluorene	0.015±0.003	0.016±0.006	0.008±0.002
Phenanthrene	0.054±0.014	0.021±0.015	0.011±0.002
Control[b]	0.005±0.010		

[a]Measured by the release of acid phosphatase enzyme release from lysosomes using β-glycerophosphate as substrate; each value is the mean of 4 incubations and the data represent the absorbance at 390 nm.

[b]The control values were obtained using the solvent, dimethylformamide.

related to their lipophilia, their uptake
into membranes and their ability to expand
membranes and impair their function. This
kind of physical toxicity has been well
correlated with anaethesia and narcosis (i.e.
physical toxicosis) however, membrane impairment can enhance an array of toxic effects
(29). The in vitro labilization of rat liver
lysosomes can be employed to measure the lytic
action of chemicals and this technique has
been used in the present study. The marker
enzyme measured was acid phosphates and the
results (table 2) suggest that the lytic
activity of Aerotex and related compounds
would be minimal for environmental exposures.

The impact of an environmental chemical
depends not only on contact but uptake and
persistence in biological systems. Anderson
and co-workers (26) have studied both the uptake and subsequent release of the alkylated
naphthalenes and naphthalene by the brown
shrimp Penaeus aztecus. The results indicated a rapid uptake of these chemicals by the
organism; transfer of the species to non-
polluted water resulted in the rapid release
of the chemicals with almost 100% depuration
within 10 hours. Comparable results were observed with the fish Cyprinodon variegatus
although the release time in a non-hydro-
carbon environment was extended to a few weeks
(26). A recent study in our laboratory
using the rat as a test animal has attempted
to evaluate the distribution and elimination
of Aerotex 3470 in this mammalian system.
The chemical was administered by intraperit-
oneal injection in corn oil (250 mg/kg in 2
ml corn oil) and the tissue and organs of
three test animals at each time point were
evaluated by GC analysis. The results are
summarized in Figures 1 and 2. The data
illustrate the pharmacokinetics of the three
major components of Aerotex 3470, namely

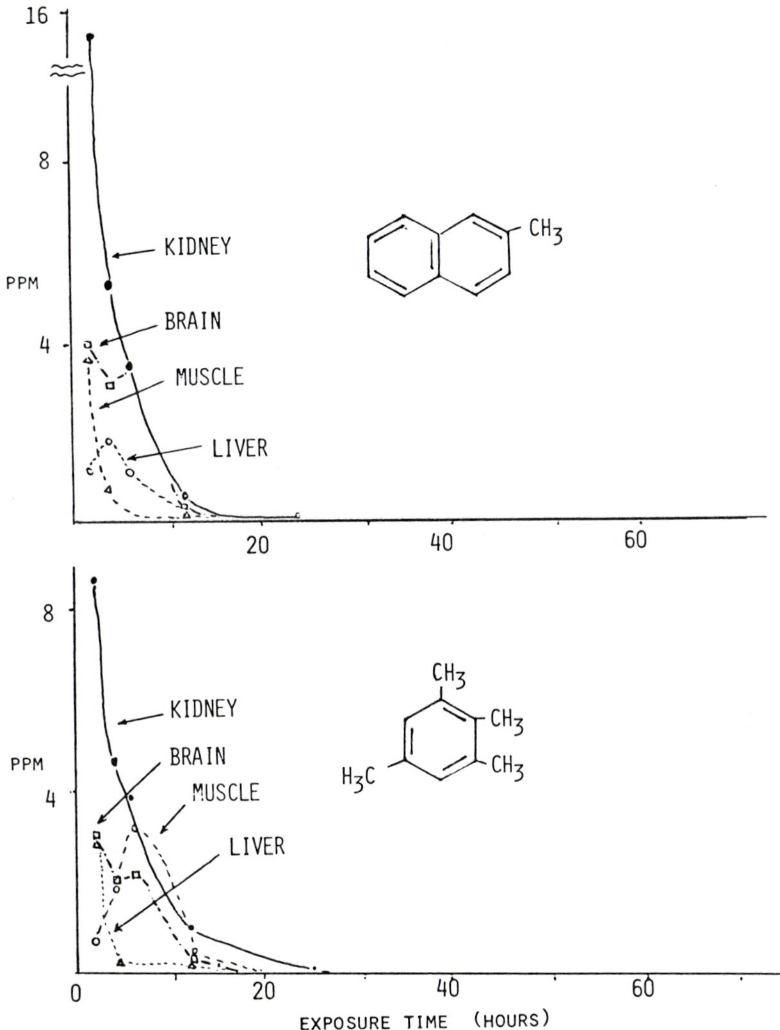

FIGURE I. PHARMACOKINETICS OF THE 2-METHYLNAPHTHALENE (TOP) AND 1,2,3,5,-TETRAMETHYLBENZENE (BOTTOM) COMPONENTS OF AEROTEX IN THE RAT.

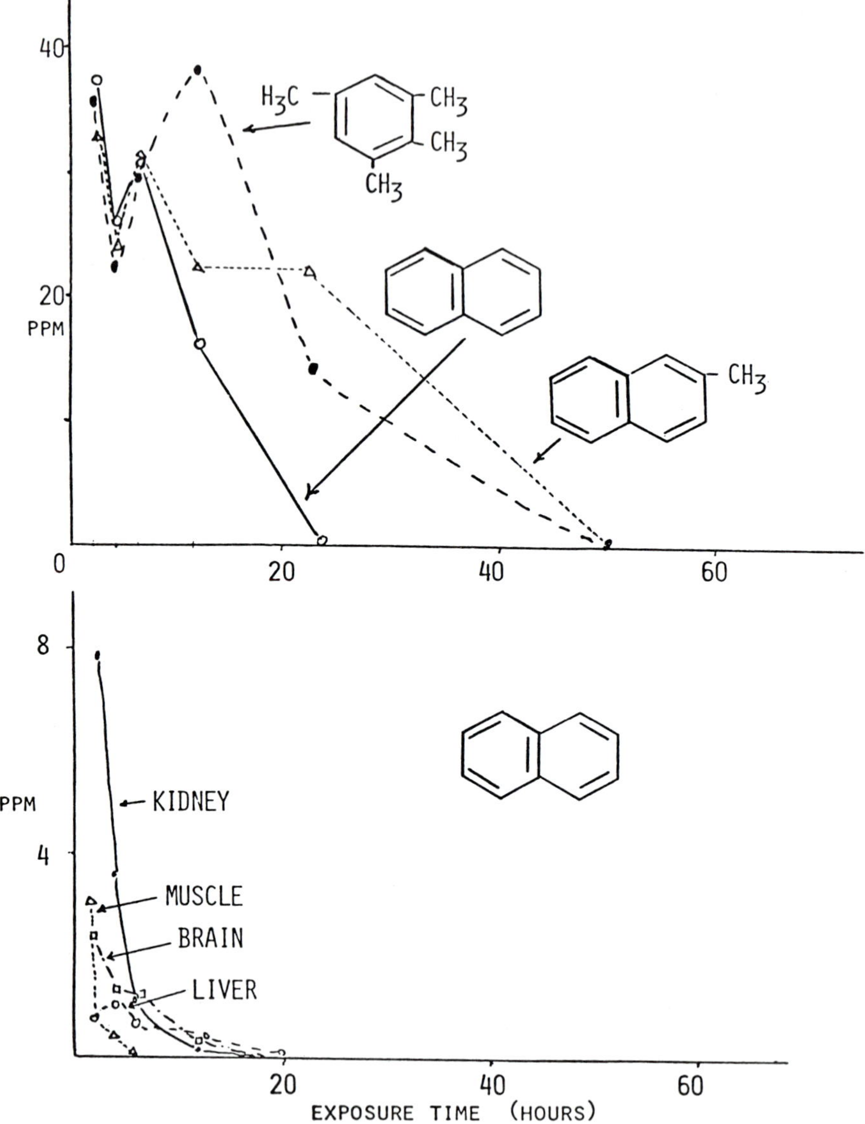

FIGURE 2   PHARMACOKINETICS OF THE MAJOR AEROTEX ISOMERS IN THE FAT (TOP) AND THE UPTAKE AND CLEARANCE OF NAPHTHALENE IN THE RAT (BOTTOM).

1,2,3,5-tetramethylbenzene, naphthalene and
2-methylnaphthalene. There is a rapid appearance of the aromatic hydrocarbons in the
tissue and organs followed by a complete removal of the chemical within 24 hours after
exposure from all samples with the exception
of the fat. The relatively rapid release of
the chemical complements the behaviour of
the major isomers in aquatic organisms. Not
surprisingly, the analysis of the tissue of
several RS patients from Eastern Canada failed to detect residues of the major isomeric
components of Aerotex 3470.

   Surfactants. The major nonionic and
anionic surfactant components of Toximul MP-8
and Atlox 3409F were described as calcium
dodecylbenzene sulfonate (anionic) and a
nonylphenol ethoxylate of polyethylene glycol.
These chemicals and related compounds are
widely used in detergents, cleansers, shampoos, foods and other industrial, consumer
and commercial products with several million
pounds produced annually (Table 3). The
linear alkylbenzene sulfonates (ABS) are particularly noteworthy since they are a major
component of detergents and vast quantities
of this chemical are introduced into the
environment, each year. The toxicity of the
ABS are species dependent with a number of
contrasting results. Several groups have
demonstrated the acute and chronic effects
of these chemicals in fish and invertebrates
with the larva stage in fish development
being the most susceptible to these surfactants (29). The mammalian LD_{50} values of ABS
are in the range of 500-3000 mg/kg indicating
a low acute toxicity (30), however, chronic
studies have suggested possible long term
health effects. ABS have been shown to cause
birth defects, teratogenic defects, and
fetal abnormalities in mice fed doses as low
as 2.75 mg/kg (31). Other studies with

Table 3. Present and Predicted Future Production of Surfactants[a]

| Millions of lb. | 1977 consumption | | | 1990 consumption total | Average annual growth rate 1977-90 |
	Total	Cleaning products	% of total		
Alkyl phenol ethoxylates	240	96	40%	184	-2.0%
Alcohol (C_{12}-C_{15}) surfactants	640	544	85	1206	5.0
Linear alkyl- benzene sulfon- ates	660	594	90	760	1.1
Soap	1180	944	80	1326	0.9
TOTAL	2720[a]	2178	80%	3476	2.0%

[a]from Chemical and Engineering News 1978. 56:12.

diverse mammalian systems have shown that
exposures to ABS which were up to several
thousand times the estimated human exposure
did not produce any significant deleterious
effects to the test animals (32). Itokawa
and co-workers (33) have shown that ABS
potentiated the hepatocellular damage induced
by polychlorinated biphenyls (PCB). This
synergism between a persistent pollutant
(i.e. PCB) and a "high-frequency" contact biodegradable chemical may be a key point in
considering the biological impact of chemicals.

Previous studies have shown that ABS
rapidly degraded in the environment (34) and
absorption distribution studies in rats showed that about 95% of the radiolabel was excreted within 72 hours. The relatively rapid
biodegradation of these chemicals mitigates
against their bioaccumulation. Studies in
our laboratory and others (34) have shown
that the most useful analytical technique
involves desulfonation and GC analysis of the
alkyl benzenes, i.e.

$$R\text{-}C_6H_4\text{-}SO_3^- \quad \xrightarrow[\text{acid, } 200^\circ\text{C.}]{\text{orthophosphoric}} \quad R\text{-}C_6H_5$$

Treatment of both Toximul MP-8 and Atlox 3409
with this reagent gave an alkylbenzene fraction. GC analysis of this product confirmed
the complexity of the mixture and it was not
possible to use this method to quantitate
ABS in tissue samples.

The polyethoxylate surfactants are widely used nonionic components of detergents,
cleansers, etc. as indicated in Table 3.

The polyethoxylates are readily manufac-
tured from the reaction of an alcohol with
ethylene oxide (EO) to yield a simple alcohol

ethoxylate $RO(CH_2-CH_2-O)_x H$ (x=1). Depending
on the reaction conditions and concentration
of EO one can prepare ethoxylates which vary
with respect to average EO content and which
in turn have varying chemical and surface
active characteristics. In practice the EO
number generally represents the average of a
wide spectrum of molecular species where x
is variable. Another factor which contributes
to the chemical complexity of the polyethoxylates is the diversity in the structure of
the lipophilic R component in the ether linkage. In many cases the ROH precursor is a
complex mixture of alcohols and this factor
contributes to the molecular complexity of
this class of surfactants. The acute toxicity
of this class of surfactants to mammals is
generally greater than 1000 mg/kg for most of
the mixtures studied (30). Recent subchronic
toxicity studies with alkylpolyethoxylates
correlated with the acute data with only
slightly increased liver/body weight ratios
and skin irritations observed in the test
animals (36, 37). Toxicological studies have
shown that these nonionic surfactants have
a relatively high acute toxicity to goldfish,
rainbow trout and Atlantic slamon using
concentrations of 1-10 mg/l (96 hour LC_{50})
(38, 39). A number of sub-lethal effects
were noted at these lower concentrations.

The interaction of surfactants and membranes has been well documented (43) and this
effect may play an important role in potent-
iating the toxicity of a number of chemical
carcinogens. The enhanced carcinogenicity
of N-methyl-N'-nitro-N-nitrosoguanidine and
20-methylcholanthrene in combination with
the nonionic surfactants Tween 80 (polyoxyethylene sorbitan monostearate) and Non-
ipol (nonylphenol polyethoxylate) has been
attributed to the interactions of the surfactants with the protective mucous barrier

of the stomach (40). Comparable results have also shown that surfactants enhance the carcinogenicity of benzo(a)pyrene, 4-nitro-3-guinoline-1-oxide and other chemicals in mammalian feeding studies (40-42).

The biodegradability of polyethoxylates in the environment is known to be rapid (34, 44, 45) with over 90% of the alkyl groups removed within 97 hours via mixed microbial degradation with secondary effluent.

$$RO(CH_2-CH_2-O)_x H \xrightarrow{\text{fast}} HO(CH_2-CH_2-O)_x H \xrightarrow{\text{slow}} (HO-CH_2-CHOH)_x$$

alkyl polyethoxylate   polyethyleneglycol

Recent data has also shown that the polyethylene glycol moiety is more long-lived with over 55% of the material remaining after 12 days (44, 45) and it is this partially degraded polymeric material which contributes to foaming in polluted water. Uptake studies with fish indicated that uptake through the gills reaches a steady state within 8 hours; when placed in pure water the surfactant is then rapidly eliminated partially.

The analysis of polyethoxylates has primarily centered around their breakdown and the widely used Wickbold procedure measures the hydrolysis of the hydrophobic moiety (46). Tobin and co-workers (44, 45) have shown the residual surfactant can be readily analysed using the following procedure which converts the alkyl polyethoxylate into an alkyl bromide and ethylene dibromide. Polyethylene

$$RO(CH_2-CH_2-O)_x H \xrightarrow{\text{HBr}} RBr + (Br-CH_2-CH_2-Br)_x$$

glycols can also be converted into the dibromide and the halogenated products can be

readily detected by GC using an electron
capture detector (ECD). This approach has
been used in our laboratory as a probe for
detecting residues of the surfactants in
tissue. Preliminary studies have used the
ethylene dibromide as an indicator of the
ethoxylate/polyethylene glycols and residues
could be detected in the low parts/trillion
range. However, control tissue treatment
with HBr also gave a significant quantity of
ethylene dibromide and this bio-analytical
approach was abandoned.

A second scheme has been devised in which
the polyethoxylates are isolated and the ether
linkages hydrolyzed using boron tribromide

$$RO(CH_2-CH_2-O)_x H \xrightarrow{BBr_3} ROH + (HOCH_2-CH_2OH)_x$$

The resulting hydrolyzate is reacted with
pentafluorobenzyl bromide (PFB) which forms
a PFB derivative that is sensitive to GC-ECD
analysis. The reaction of Igepal, a nonylphenol ethoxylate (Chemical Developments of
Canada Ltd.) followed by GC analysis of the
phenol and the PFB derivative resulted in
chromatograms which were similar to those
obtained for commercial nonylphenol. In all
cases the data resulting from Toximul MP-8
gave a more complex series of GC peaks (Figure 3) indicating the heterogeneity of the
alcohol used in this preparation. It should
also be noted, that the hydrolysis/derivat-
ization procedure is limited to the detection
of the alcohol moiety present in the parent
ethoxylates or present in tissues as the free
alcohol.

Examination of tissue from Reye's synd-
rom patients did not give any detectable
PFB-nonylphenol residues.

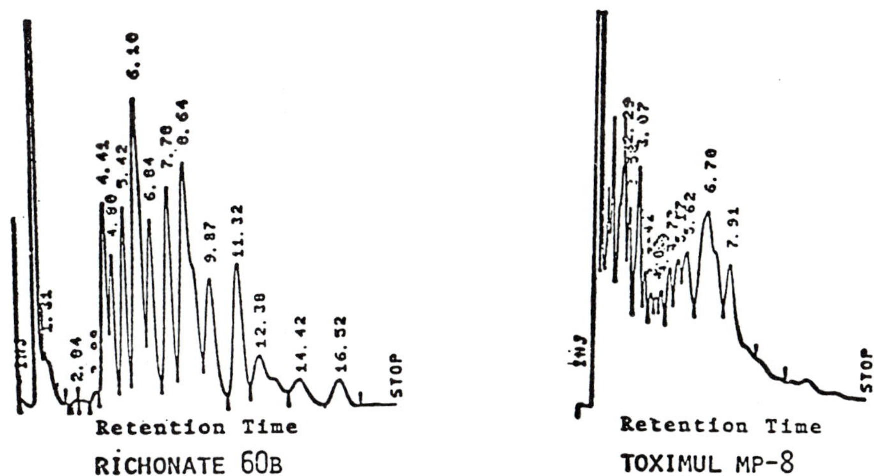

FIGURE 3. DESULFONATION OF ABS (TOP) AND THE GC ANALYSIS OF RICHONATE 60B (A DODECYLBENZENE SULPHONATE) AND TOXIMUL MP-8.

Chemicals Which are Potential Human Health
Hazards.

It is clear that the role of chemicals
in diseases is a complex multifactorial
problem and it is difficult to single out
individual chemicals as causal agents. There
are exceptions to this statement particularly
with respect to industrial chemical hazards
(ie. vinyl chloride, asbestos, benzidine,
lead etc). This also applies to some environmental chemicals which become major problems
in specific areas. Polychlorinated biphenyl
(PCB) pollution in southwestern Japan, poly-
brominated biphenyls (PBB) in Michigan and
mercury in Minamata, Japan are examples of
environmental pollutants which contribute
to health problems. These occurrences usually
result from specific point pollution problems
which then magnifies the health impact of the
chemical.

The chemicals which are an obvious potential long term health hazard are those
which have been identified as residues in
humans and which are known to possess some
toxic properties. These chemicals are
primarily the persistent aromatic pesticides
and pollutants and include; DDT and its related metabolites and degredation products
(p,p'-DDT, o,p'-DDT, p,p'-DDE, o,p'-DDE,
p,p'-DDD and o,p'-DDD), hexachlorocyclohexanes
(ie. including lindane and related stereois-
omers), aldrin, dieldrin, heptachlor, heptachlor epoxide, endrin, mirex, oxychlordane,
trans-nonachlor, PCB and hexachlorobenzene.
Most of these chemicals along with toxaphene,
methoxychlor, phthalic acid esters and kepone
are included in the persistent toxic substances list #1 proposed by the International
Joint Commission (47). A second toxic substances list includes a number of other chemicals which also pose a threat to human and

animal health. These chemicals include volatile halohydrocarbons commonly found in drinking water (chloroform, bromoform, tetrachloroethylene and carbon tetrachloride), aromatic hydrocarbons (benzene, toluene and alkylated naphthalenes), halogenated aromatic industrial chemicals (chlorinated phenols, chlorinated benzenes, chlorinated styrenes, chlorinated naphthalenes, chlorinated terphenyls, brominated biphenyls and pentabromotoluene) and the ubiquitous polynuclear aromatic hydrocarbons. In addition a number of toxic inorganic substances including arsenic, cadmium, mercury, lead, selenium, zinc, nickel, copper, iron and chromium are also contained in the toxic substances list. This rather extensive compilation of toxic chemicals by no means covers the diversity of compounds which are a potential human health hazard. A recent report by the United States Environmental Protection agency lists no less than 1259 different chemicals which have been identified in water.

As noted previously in this paper the synergistic effects of chemicals in combination may be an important contributing factor in human health in general and Reye's syndrome in particular. The constant exposure of the population to chemical pollutants and the uptake and retention of the more persistent lipophilic chemical species serves as a relatively permanent body reservoir of toxic substances. It has been illustrated that "multiple exposure" chemicals such as the surfactants which are not persistent in the environment and are readily biodegradable can enhance viral lethality and the toxicity of other chemicals. This viral-chemical and chemical-chemical synergism may play a major role in Reye's syndrome and other chemically related diseases.

ACKNOWLEDGEMENT

The authors gratefully acknowledge the
financial assistance of the National Research
Council of Canada and the Department of Natural Resources, Province of New Brunswick.

<u>REFERENCES</u>

1. Reye, R.D.K., Morgan, G. and Baral, J.
    1963. Encephalopathy and fatty degenerat-
    ion of the viscera - a disease entity in
    childhood, Lancet 2: 749.
2. Corey, L., Rubin, R.J., Hattwick, M.A.W.,
    Noble, G.R. and Cassidy, E. 1976. A
    nationwide outbreak of Reye's syndrome.
    Amer. J. Med. 61: 615.
3. Corey, L., Rubin, R.J., Thompson, T.R.,
    Noble, G.R., Cassidy, E., Hattwick, M.A.W.
    Gregg, M.B. and Eddins, D. 1977. Influ-
    enza B- associated Reye's syndrome: in-
    cidence in Michigan and potential for
    prevention. J. Infect. Dis. 135: 398.
4. Brown, T., Hug, G., Lansky, L., Bove, K.
    E., Ryan, M., Brown, H., Schubert, W.K.,
    Partin, J.C. and Lloyd-Still, J. 1976.
    Transiently reduced activity of carbamyl
    phosphate synthetase and ornithine trans-
    carbamylase in liver of children with
    Reye's syndrome. N. Engl. J. Med. 294:861
5. Haller, J.S. 1975. Clinical experience
    with Reye's syndrome, p.1. In Reye's
    Syndrome. J.D. Pollack (ed.), Grune and
    Stratton, New York.
6. Pollack, J.D., Cramblett, H.G., Flynn, D.
    and Clark, D. 1975, p.227. Serum and
    tissue lipids in Reye's syndrome. In
    Reye's Syndrome, J.D. Pollack (ed.),
    Grune and Stratton, New York.
7. Mullen, P.W. 1978. Immunopharmacological
    considerations in Reye's syndrome: a poss-
    ible xenobiotic initiated disorder. Bio-
    chem Pharmacol. 27:145
8. Pollack, J.D., Burech, D. and Hamparian,
    V.V. 1977. The role of chemicals in pot-
    entiating viral infections and Reye's
    syndrome, p.519. In Fenitrothion: The
    Long-Term Effects of its Use in Forest
    Systems. J.R. Roberts, R. Greenhalgh and
    W.K. Marshall (ed.). National Research
    Council of Canada, No. 16073. Ottawa.

9.   Bourgeois, C.H. 1975. Encephalopathy
     and fatty viscera: a possible response
     to acute aflatoxin poisoning, p.131. In
     Reye's Syndrome, J.D. Pollack (ed.).
     Grune and Stratton, New York.
10. Hilty, M.D. 1975. Etiology of Reye's
     Syndrome, p.383. In Reye's Syndrome, J.D.
     Pollack (ed.). Grune and Stratton, New
     York.
11. Linneman, C.C. Jr., Shea, L., Kauffman,
     C.A., Schiff, G.M., Partin, J.C. and
     Schubert, W.K. 1974. Association of
     Reye's syndrome with viral infection.
     Lancet 2: 179.
12. Mogilner, B., Freeman, J., Blashar, Y.
     and Pincus, F. 1974. Reye's syndrome in
     three Israeli children. Possible relation-
     ship to warfarin toxicity. Isr. J. Med.
     Sci. 10:1117.
13. Glasgow, A. M.,and Ferris, J.A. 1968.
     Encephalopathy and visceral fatty in-
     filtration of probable toxic aetiology.
     Lancet 1: 451.
14. Black, J.T. Luchtan, A. and Radomski,J.L.
     1972. Reye's syndrome due to pesticide
     intoxication: treated with exchange trans-
     fusion p.132. In Neuro-opthalmology:
     symposium of the University of Miami and
     the Bascom Palmer Eye Institute J.L.
     Smith (ed.). C.V. Mosby Co. St. Louis,Mo.
15. Colon, A.R., Pardo, V. and Sandberg, D.H.
     1975. Experimental Reye's syndrome ind-
     uced by viral potentiation of chemical
     toxin, p.199. In Reye's Syndrome, J.D.
     Pollack (ed.). Grune and Stratton, New
     York.
16. Watanabe, H. 1971. Polyhedrosis-virus
     infection in the silkworm, Bombyx mori,
     applied topically with sablethal doses
     of insecticides, J. Sericulf Sci. Japan
     40: 350.
17. Friend, M. and Trainer, D.O. 1970. Poly-
     chlorinated biphenyl: interaction with

duck hepatitis virus. Science 170:1314

18. Ragland, W.L., Friend, M., Trainer, D.O. and Sladik, N.E. 1971. Interaction between duck hepatitis virus and DDT in ducks. Res. Commun. Chem. Pathol. Pharmacol 2: 236.

19. Friend, M. and Trainer, D.O. 1974. Experimental DDT-duck hepatitis virus interaction studies. J. Widl. Manage. 38:887

20. Crocker, J.F.S., Rozee, K.R., Ozere, R.L. Digout, S.C. and Hutzinger, O. 1974. Insecticide and viral interaction as a cause of fatty visceral changes and encephalopathy in the mouse. Lancet 2: 22.

21. Crocker, J.F.S., Ozere, R.L., Safe, S.H., Digout, S.C., Rozee, K.R. and Hutzinger, O. 1976. Lethal interaction of ubiquitous insecticide carrier with virus. Science 192: 1351.

22. Rozee, K.R., Lee, S.H.S., Crocker, J.F.S. and Safe, S. 1978. Enhanced virus replication in mammalian cells exposed to commercial emulsifiers. Appl. Environ. Microbiol. 35: 297.

23. Safe, S. Plugge, H..and Crocker, J.F.S. 1977. Analysis of an aromatic solvent used in a forest spray program. Chemos. 6: 641.

24. U.S. Dept. of Health Education and Welfare 1974. NIEHS Toxic Substances List.

25. Carpenter, C.P., Geary, D.L. Jr., Meyers, R.C., Nackreiner, D.S.,Sullivan,L.J. and King, J.B. 1977. Petroleum hydrocarbon toxicity studies. XIV. Animal and human responses to vapours of "high aromatic solvent. Toxicol. Appl. Pharmacol. 41:235.

26. Anderson, J.W., Neff, J.M., Cox, B.A., Tatem, H.E. and Hightower, G.M. 1974. The effects of oil on estuarine animals: toxicity uptake, depuration, respiration, p. 285. In Pollution and Physiology of Marine Organisms, J.F. Vernberg and W.B. Vernberg (eds.) Academic Press, New York.

27.   Fabacher, D.L. and Hodgson, E. 1977.
       Hepatic mixed function oxidase activity
       in mice treated with methylated benzenes
       and methylated naphthalenes. J. Toxicol.
       Environ. Health, 2: 1143.
28.   Lysosomes in Biology and Pathology, 1969,
       J.T. Dingle and H.B. Fell, eds. Volume
       2. North Holland, Amsterdam
29.   McKim, J.M., Arthur, J.W. and Thorslund,
       T.W. 1975. Toxicity of a linear alkyl
       sulfonate detergent to larvae of four
       species of freshwater fish. Bull Environ.
       Contam. Toxicol. 14:1.
30.   Swisher, R.D. 1975. Exposure levels and
       oral toxicity of surfactants. Arch.
       Environ. Health 17:232.
31.   Mikami, Y., Sakae, Y. and Miyamoto, I.
       1973. Anomalies induced by ABS applied
       to the skin. Teratol. 8: 98.
32.   Nolen, G.A., Klusman, L.W., Patrick, L.F.,
       and Geil, R.G. 1975. Teratology studies
       of a mixture of tallow alcohol ethoxylate
       and linear alkylbenzene sulfonate in rats
       and rabbits. Toxicol. 4: 231
33.   Itokawa, Y., Kamohara, K. and Fujiwara,
       K. 1973. Toxicity of polychlorinated Bip-
       henyls increased with simultaneous ing-
       estion of alkylbenzene sulfonic acid salt.
       Exper. 29:822.
34.   Swisher, R.D. 1970. Surfactant Biodegrad-
       ation. Marcel Dekker Inc., New York.
35.   Otvos, I., Bartha, B., Balthazar, Z. and
       Palyi, G. 1974. Petrochemical analytical
       problems. IV. Gas-liquid chromatographic
       mass spectrometric investigation of the
       desulfonation of dodecylbenzene sulfonic
       acids. J. Chem. 94:330.
36.   Benke, G.M., Brown, N.M., Walsh, M.J. and
       Drotman, R.B. 1977. Safety testing of
       alkyl polyethoxylate nonionic surfactants.
       I. Acute effects. Food Cosmet. Toxicol.
       15: 319.
37.   Brown, N.M. and Benke, G.M. 1977. Safety

testing of alkyl polyethoxylate nonionic
surfactants. II. Subchronic studies. Fd.
Cosmet. Toxicol. 15: 319.

38. Wildish, D.J. 1974. Lethal response by
Atlantic salmon parr to some polyethoxy-
lated cationic and nonionic surfactants.
Water Res. 8: 433.

39. Wildish, D.J. 1972. Acute toxicity of
polyoxyethylene esters and polyoxyethylene
ethers to S. salar and G. oceanicus,
Water Res. 6: 759.

40. Fukushimo, S. 1973. The combined effects
of N-methyl-N'-nitro-N-nitrosoguanidine
and 20-methylcholanthrene associated with
surfactants on the induction of cancer
of the glandular stomach in rats. Nagoya
Med. J. 18: 143.

41. Ekwall, P., Ermallo, P., Setala, K. and
Sjoblom, P. 1951. Gastric absorption of
3,4-benzpyrene II. Significance of the
solvent for the penetration of 3,4-benz-
pyrene into the stomach wall. Cancer Res.
11: 758.

42. Takuhashi, M. and Sato, H. 1969. Effect
of 4-nitroquinoline-1-oxide with alkylbenzene sulfonate in gastric carcinogenesis. In Exp. Carcinoma Glandular
Stomach U.S. - Japan Symp. p. 241.

43. Shelton, K.R. 1976. Selective effects of
nonionic detergent and salt solution in
dissolving nuclear envelope protein.
Biochim. Biophys. Acta 455: 937.

44. Tobin,R.S., Onuska, F.I., Anthony, D.H.J.
and Comba, M.E. 1974. Biodegradation
test methods do not detect persistent
polyglycol products. Ambio 5:30.

45. Tobin, R.S. Onuska, F.I., Brownlee, B.G.,
Anthony, D.II.J. and Comba, M.E. 1976.
The application of ether cleavage technique to a study of the biodegradation
of a linear alcohol ethoxylate nonionic
surfactant. Water Res. 10: 529.

46. Wickbold, R. 1972. Zur bestimmung nicht-
     ionischer tenside in flussund abwasser.
     Tenside Deterg. 9:173.
47. Great Lakes Water Quality - Appendix E.
     Status Report on the Persistent Toxic
     Pollutants in the Lake Ontario Basin 1977.
     Great Lakes Water Quality Board, Inter-
     national Joint Commission.

DISCUSSION

M.D. Hilty -   I wonder if you had the opportunity to look for PCB's or DDT or some
of the other organochlorines in either
blood or fat specimens of patients with
Reye's syndrome and, especially, have you
had a chance to look sequentially to see
if there is any evidence of mobilization
of these compounds from fat stores?

S.Safe   -   No, we haven't. The first work
really that we have done on the PCB's is
we have identified them at fairly low levels in the brain, but we haven't analysed fat as yet.

M.D. Hilty -   Now in Ohio some of the water
towers in some of the small towns are
periodically lined with what looks like
grease. Are you familiar with this compound? It has to be repeated every 3 or
4 years. What I have been able to determine is it is a by-product of the petroleum industry. It has Stoddard solvent in
it and a few other things, and I know
that this one family that I mentioned this
morning live at the dead end of a water
line and their water tower in that particular town had been treated the summer
before they moved to this community, and
in that winter when the children developed
their chicken pox, all three developed

Reye's syndrome.

S.Safe   -   I'm not sure what the liner would
     be. Certainly, Stoddard solvent is not that dis-
     similar to Aerotex 3470 and the water soluble
     fraction of crude oil.

Unidentified -   Does anybody know how DDT or simi-
     lar compounds ever become eliminated from the
     body?

S.Safe   -   I think presumably it's a slow me-
     tabolic process. I mean DDT is metabolized, and
     PCB's are metabolized; it is slow and presumably
     when they are mobilized and circulating there is
     some metabolism, probably redeposition - that's
     the reason why they are persistent.

Same Speaker-   Under normal circumstances, it
     might take a century to get rid of any signifi-
     cant amount?

S.Safe   -   DDT and most of these others are
     pretty good microsomal enzyme inducers so it is a
     protective thing;but,although they are good mi-
     crosomal enzyme inducers, DDT is still a lousy
     substrate for the microsomes. It is still only
     very slowly metabolized, although much better
     than a non-induced system.

B.C. Reiner-   The Environmental Protection Agen-
     cy for many years were collecting fat obtained at
     autopsy, and we at the Children's Hospital were
     contributing tissue for analysis of such lipid -
     deposited materials. I don't know of any correla-
     tion of these findings with Reye's syndrome, and
     I was wondering if you had any?

S. Safe   -   I don't know of any data that cor-
     relates the two. I think that this was an area
     that the Halifax group was initially interested in
     and our interest went down, primarily because of
     the animal model studies. Now that our interest
     in the possible correlation between these chemi-
     cals and Reye's is re-kindled,we'll look again.

FURTHER EVIDENCE FOR ABNORMALITIES IN LYSINE
CATABOLISM IN REYE'S SYNDROME PATIENTS

Judith W. Rittenhouse, Ph.D.,
Merle Mason, Ph.D., and Joseph V. Baublis, M.D.

Many Reye's syndrome (RS) patients have been reported to have elevated serum levels of amino acids,
with especially high levels of lysine, alanine, glutamine, and α-amino-N-butyrate (1,2). A brief undocumen-
ted report suggested that a lysine catabolite, saccharopine is also present in serum (2). A second lysine
metabolite, α-aminoadipate, was briefly reported to
occur in the urine of Reye's patients (3). We have
been interested in the incidence of these abnormalities
of lysine metabolism in RS and why they occur.

Figure 1 shows the major pathway of lysine catabolism. Hydroxylysine and tryptophan catabolites share
part of the pathway. The major pathway as shown occurs
primarily in liver mitochondria. Saccharopine and
α-aminoadipate are early metabolites of the pathway.

In preliminary studies of lysine catabolism in RS
we have analyzed the sera of seven RS patients with a
Beckman Model 120C amino acid analyzer using sodium
citrate buffers in a two-column system. Urines from
two of the patients were also analyzed. Identification
of lysine intermediates was based on cochromatography
with authentic standards both on the analyzer and with
two dimensional thin-layer chromatography. All patients were hospitalized at Mott Children's Hospital,
The University of Michigan, between 1974 and 1978. RS
was diagnosed by histobiochemistry. Samples were taken
within two days of admission and stored frozen.

THE MAJOR LYSINE CATABOLIC PATHWAY

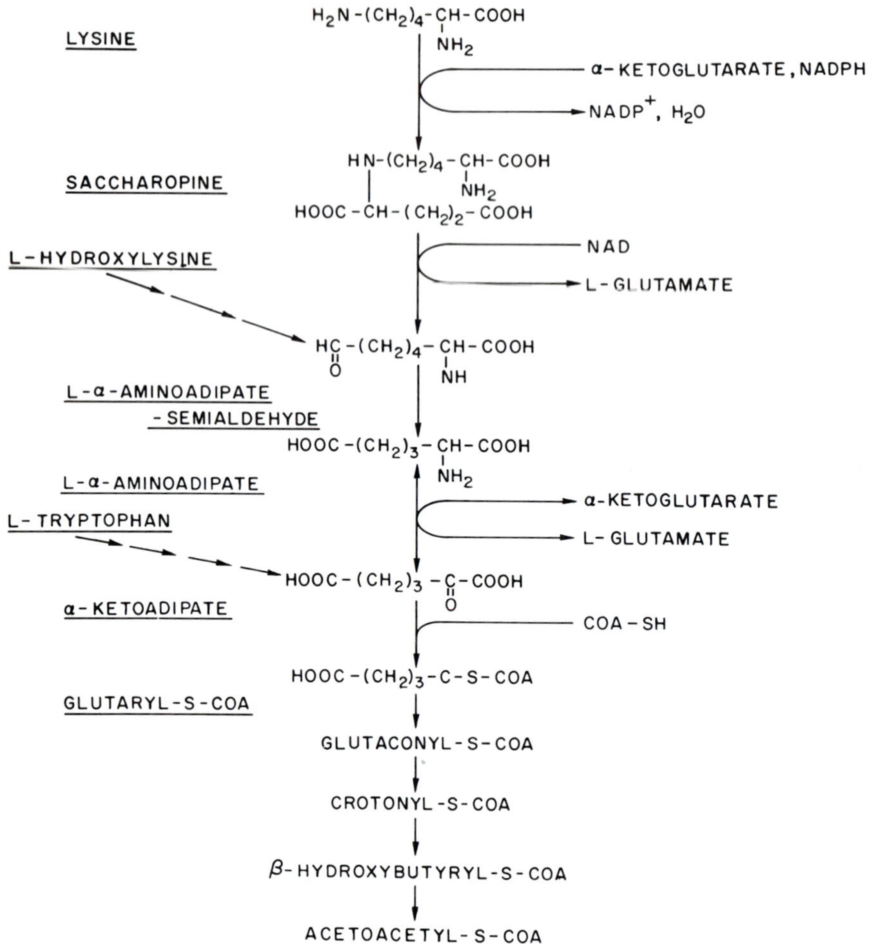

Figure 1.   The major pathway of lysine catabolism.

Figure 2 illustrates cochromatography in the analyzer.   The lower tracing is a segment of the elution profile of the urine of one patient, and the upper one is of the same urine to which authentic saccharopine and α-aminoadipate were added.   With standard conditions cystine tends to cochromatograph with saccharopine.   To avoid this interference in our system cystine was made to cochromatograph with valine instead by adjusting the pH of the eluting buffer.

Homocitrulline, which tends to comigrate with saccharopine, is another lysine catabolite, apparently formed by substitution of lysine for ornithine in the urea cycle. It is interesting that it was detected in the urine of patient number 7 according to thin-layer chromatography. However it is sometimes present in the urine of normal children. The amounts were small enough to cause only a slight error in the quantitative measurement of saccharopine.

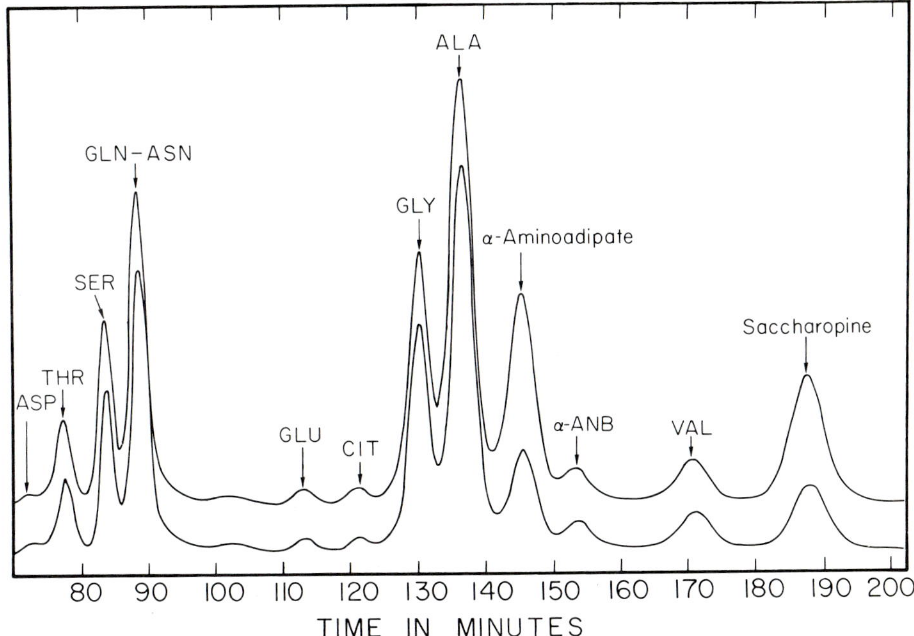

Figure 2.   Amino acid analysis of the urine of a Reye's syndrome patient, before and after the addition of authentic saccharopine and α-aminoadipate. Both tracings (with baselines displaced to facilitate comparison) represent absorbance at 570 nm.

Table 1 shows the levels of lysine and of the two catabolites in the sera of seven RS patients and in the urine of 2 of the 7. Control values from the literature are also shown and data from the recent study by

TABLE 1

URINARY AND SERUM LEVELS OF LYSINE AND ITS
CATABOLITES IN REYE'S SYNDROME PATIENTS

| | | URINE (mg/g CREATININE) | | |
| | | RS Patients | | Glutaric |
	Normal*	2	7	Aciduria**
Lysine	16-172	1128	58	110.1
Saccharopine	0	358	242	617.7
α-Aminoadipate	0-5.5	240	430	682.3
Outcome	--	died	S	--

| | Serum (μMoles/100 ml) | | | |
Patient	Lysine	Saccha-ropine	α-Amino adipate	Outcome
Normal[1]	11-27	0	0	--
RS 1	85	trace	trace	died
RS 2	83	0	2	died
RS 3	12	trace	trace	died
RS 4	162	trace	5	died
RS 5	54	0	0	S
RS 6	17	0	0	S
RS 7	53	0	trace	S

*Reference 4

**Reference 1

Goodman et al (4) of a patient with glutaricaciduria
type 1 is also presented.

     Moderate to severe hyperaminoacidemia was seen in
sera of 4 of the 7 patients, the degree apparently
correlating with survival. Lysine was elevated in the
sera of 5 of the 7 patients, and in one case was almost
10 times the normal level. α-Aminoadipate, which is
not detectable in normal serum by standard amino acid
analysis, was found in trace to moderate concentrations
in the sera of 5 of the 7 patients. Sera from 3 of the
5 also contained traces of saccharopine.

     Urine levels of lysine and its catabolites from
patients number 2 and 7 are also shown in Table 1 and
compared with those of the glutaricaciduria patient.

     Although it is not shown here, we also analyzed
the amino acids of cerebrospinal fluid of patients 4
and 5. These did not contain detectable levels of
either aminoadipate or saccharopine. Glutamine was
greatly elevated as reported by others for RS patients
(5,6).

     This report is preliminary. Further work is
underway to determine more exactly the incidence of
these abnormalities, their duration, relationship to
other metabolic changes, and to patient treatment. We
also plan to look for the presence of some of the other
lysine catabolites that would not have been detected
with the analyzer.

     The reason for accumulation of lysine and its
intermediate catabolites is not clear but several factors that may possibly be involved may be mentioned.
Lysine is an essential amino acid, so its accumulation
and that of its catabolites are dependent on increased
supply, as by increased protein breakdown, and/or on
decreased catabolism, as by blockage or absence of a
catabolic enzyme. The glutaricaciduria patient cited
in Table 1 may exhibit such blockage, apparently at
the glutaryl-CoA dehydrogenase stage (4). The striking
similarity of the symptoms and laboratory observations
of that patient with those of Reye's patients suggests

a similar underlying disease mechanism, as noted by the
authors (4). They also suggest that the proposed
enzymatic defect may cause or render more likely the
development of the syndrome. In this regard, it is
noteworthy that the symptoms and hyperaminoacidemia
were episodic whereas the enzymatic defect is assumed
to be continuous, suggesting that factors other than
the enzymatic defect were involved. In spite of the
similarities, the absence of glutaricaciduria reported
in Reye's patients (7,8) suggests that glutaryl-CoA
dehydrogenase deficiency per se is not a factor in RS.

Elevated serum lysine levels commonly accompany
hyperammonemia from various causes, and hyperammonemia
is a well-known feature of RS. However the excretion
of lysine catabolites has not been routinely found in
these disorders although amino acid levels have been
studied extensively, in some cases with a specific
attempt to detect lysine catabolites. Thus, although
ammonia might theoretically donate amino groups to
cause accumulation of certain amino acids, its elevation appears not to adequately explain the abnormalities of amino acid excretion in RS.

Reactions of the lysine pathway may be directly
inhibited by the fatty acids known to accumulate in
tissues of such patients (9). Adipate and various
mono- and dicarboxylic fatty acids of moderate chain
length that are elevated in such patients strongly
inhibit α-aminoadipate (kynurenine) aminotransferase in
animals (10,11). The elevated saccharopine and lysine
levels cannot be rationalized by such inhibitions,
although the effects of these agents or of blockage
of aminoadipate aminotransferase on saccharopine
synthesis and degradation have apparently not been
reported.

Other workers have suggested (12) that alterations
in mitochondrial membranes, possibly of viral origin,
may cause the multiple metabolic disorders seen in the
syndrome. Such alterations, presumably associated
with failure of fundamental transport and compartment-
ation functions of the inner membrane, might permit
the escape of saccharopine and aminoadipate from the

mitochondrial matrix. Since the lysine catabolic enzymes are probably largely restricted to the liver mitochondria, judging from animal models, further breakdown of lysine catabolites in other tissues would not occur, and they would therefore accumulate relative to other amino acids whose catabolic enzymes are more widely distributed. Failure of the lysine catabolic pathway in liver mitochondria might also occur as a result of decreased enzyme activities of unknown origin,such as those seen with all other liver mitochondrial enzymes so far examined in Reye's patients.

Clearly these possible relationships of the observations to other expressions of the disease can only be tested by additional experiments.

ACKNOWLEDGEMENTS

This work was supported by U.S.P.H.S. Grant AM186-47.3.

REFERENCES

1.   Hilty,M.D.,Romshe,C.A. and Delamater,P.V. 1974. Reye's syndrome and hyperaminoacidemia.*J.Ped.84*:362.

2.   Kang,E.S. and Gerald,P.S. 1972. Hyperammonemia and Reye's syndrome.*New Engl.J. Med.286*:1216.

3.   Shih,V.E.,Glick,T.N. and Bercu,B.B. 1974. Lysine Metabolism in Reye's Syndrome.*Lancet II*:163.

4.   Goodman,S.I.,Norenberg,M.D.,Shikes,R.H.,Breslich, D.J. and Moe,P.G. 1977. Glutaric aciduria:Biochemical and morphologic considerations·*J.Pediatr.90*:746.

5.   Zacarias,J.,Harum,A.,and Brinck,P. 1971.Glutamine values in cerebrospinal fluid of children:some observations on clinical application.*J.Pediatr.78*: 318.

6.   Glasgow,A.M. and Dhiensiri,K. 1974. Improved Assay for Spinal Fluid Glutamine and Values for Children with Reye's syndrome.*Clin.Chem. 20*:642.

7. Tanaka,K.,Kean,E.A. and Johnson,B. 1976. Jamaican
    Vomiting Sickness:Biochemical Investigation of Two
    Cases.*New Engl.J. Med. 295:461.*

8. Harrington,W.,Liu,A.,Lonsdale,D. and Igow,D. 1977.
    Urinary Organic Acid Profiles of Reye's Syndrome
    Patients. *Clin.Chem.Acta. 74:247.*

9. Bourgeois,C.,Olson,L.,Comer,D.,Evans,H.,Keschamaras,
    N.,Cotton,R.,Grossman,R.,and Smith,T. 1971. Enceph-
    alopathy and Fatty Degeneration of the Viscera: A
    Clinicopathologic Analysis of 40 Cases. *Am.J.Clin.
    Pathol. 56:558.*

10. Tobes,M.C. and Mason,M. 1977. L-Aminoadipate Amino-
    transferase and Kynurenine aminotransferase.*J.Biol.
    Chem. 252:4591.*

11. Mason,M., 1959. Kynurenine Transaminase: A study of
    Inhibitors and their Relationship to the Active
    Site. *J.Biol.Chem. 234:2770.*

12. DeVivo,D.C., 1978. Reye Syndrome: A metabolic re-
    sponse to an acute mitochondrial insult. *Neurology
    28:105.*

REYE'S SYNDROME IN THE NEWBORN

I. Dvorackova,M.D., C. Proks, M.D.

The occurence of Reye's syndrome in the neonatal
period is quite unusual. In the world literature, only
two cases have been published. The first case of a 4-
day-old infant with the clinical and morphological
picture of Reye's syndrome was described by Papageour-
giou in 1972 (1). The second neonatal case fulfilled
the clinical, non-histologic criteria for this syndrome; the infant survived and was reported by Harris
(2) in 1976.

Our report is concerned with the observations of
six newborns with the morphological changes characteristic of Reye's syndrome.

Case 1: K.J., a premature boy (1550g), the product
of a third uncomplicated pregnancy, who had two healthy brothers. The mother worked in a co-operative
farm. The infant was well after delivery. Several
hours after birth, he developed apneic spells and hy-
potonia. The child died within 32 hours with the clinical diagnosis of Respiratory Distress syndrome (RDS).
Autopsy showed atelectases of the lungs and a fatty
liver.

Case 2: V.M., a premature girl (2150g), the product of an uneventful pregnancy. The child's mother is
a clerk and the family lives in a city. Shortly after
delivery,respiratory distress and acidosis were noted.
Intensive alcalic therapy was utilized without any effect. The child died 67 hours after birth with a
clinical diagnosis of immaturity and RDS. Autopsy findings showed a subdural haematoma, haematocephalus,and
atelectases of the lungs.

Case 3: V., a premature male (1300g), the product of a
first pregnancy. The child's mother is a worker in a
factory and the family lived in the country. The infant
was well and normally active until 20 hours of age when
tachypnea,acidosis and respiratory distress were noted.
The intensive alcalic therapy was without any effect.
Immediately before death, the infant vomited blood and
died at 75 hours of age, with the clinical diagnosis of
immaturity and Respiratory Distress syndrome. Autopsy
findings showed haematocephalus and a yellow liver.

Case 4: V.M., a premature male (1330g), second of twins
(twin B) from a first pregnancy. The mother was a laboratory technician on a co-operative farm. The family
lived in the country. Respiratory distress,acidosis and
tachypnea were noted several hours after birth. The infant died within 70 hours with the clinical diagnosis
of pneumonia. Autopsy findings showed a subdural haematoma, haematocephalus, and atelectases of the lungs. A
five-year-old boy (twin A) and the other three siblings
(2 boys, 1 girl) are healthy.

Case 5: V.K., was born at 40 weeks' gestation, weighing
3200 g., and was the product of a third pregnancy. Two
boys from the first and second pregnancy are healthy.
The mother works on a co-operative farm and the family
lives in the country. The child was well and active.The
second day, two hours after breast feeding,the infant
became pallid and had frequent apneic spells. The infant died 45 hours after delivery,with the clinical diagnosis of Sudden Infant Death syndrome. Autopsy findings revealed a yellow liver and a yellow tinge to the
cortex of kidneys and heart.

Case 6: V.O.,full-term male (3400g) from the fifth normal pregnancy (a brother of the Case 5). The infant
apparently did well until 48 hours after birth when pallor,temperature instability and a heart disorder were
noted. The infant died at 72 hours, with the clinical
diagnosis of Sudden Infant Death syndrome and suspected
heart disease. Autopsy findings showed a yellow liver,
brain edema, a yellow tinge to the cortex of the kidneys,heart and striated muscle.A boy from the mother's

fourth pregnancy is healthy. (Familial and clinical
data are summarized in Tables 1 and 2).

TABLE 1

| FAMILIAL DATA | | | | | |
CASE	SEX	AGE	YEAR OF DEATH	COUNTRY	CITY
1. K.J.	m	32 hrs.	1972	*	
2. V.M.	f	71 hrs.	1972		*
3. V.	m	72 hrs.	1972	*	
4. V.M.	m	70 hrs.	1972	*	
5. V.K.+	f	45 hrs.	1972	*	
6. V.O.+	m	72 hrs.	1976	*	

	EMPLOYMENT OF MOTHER	PREGNANCY	BROTHERS AND SISTERS
1. K.J.	co-op.farm worker	III	2
2. V.M.	clerk	I	
3. V.	co-op.farm worker	I	
4. V.M.	co-op.farm technician	I	4
5. V.K.+	co-op.farm clerk	III	3
6. V.O.+	co-op.farm clerk	V	3

+(Case 5 and 6: brother and sister)

TABLE 2.

CLINICAL DATA

CASE	SEX	BIRTH WEIGHT AND LENGTH	CLIN. SYMPTOMS
1. K.J.	m	1520/40	hypotonia acidosis
2. V.M.	f	2060/42	tachypnoe acidosis
3. V.	m	1250/37	hypotonia acidosis
4. V.M.	m	1330/41	hypotonia acidosis
5. V.K.	f	3200/50	
6.	m	3140/48	EKG-changes

	CLIN. DIAGNOSIS	DEATH AFTER BIRTH
1. K.J.	Immaturity RD Syndrome	32 hrs
2. V.M.	Immaturity RD Syndrome	71 hrs
3. V.	Immaturity RD Syndrome	72 hrs
4. V.M.	Immaturity Gemellus B RD Syndrome	70 hrs
5. V.K.	Sudden death	45 hrs
6. V.O.	Sudden death	72 hrs

Histopathological study of all 6 cases showed
generalized fatty infiltration of the liver, kidney,
heart and striated muscles (diaphragm, and psoas muscle)

and brain oedema (Figure 1-5). The findings differed
only in the intensity of fatty degeneration in various
organs. (The difference is shown in Table 3). In three
cases (3,5,6) granular decomposition of muscle fibres
resembling Zenker's degeneration was found (Fig.6,7).

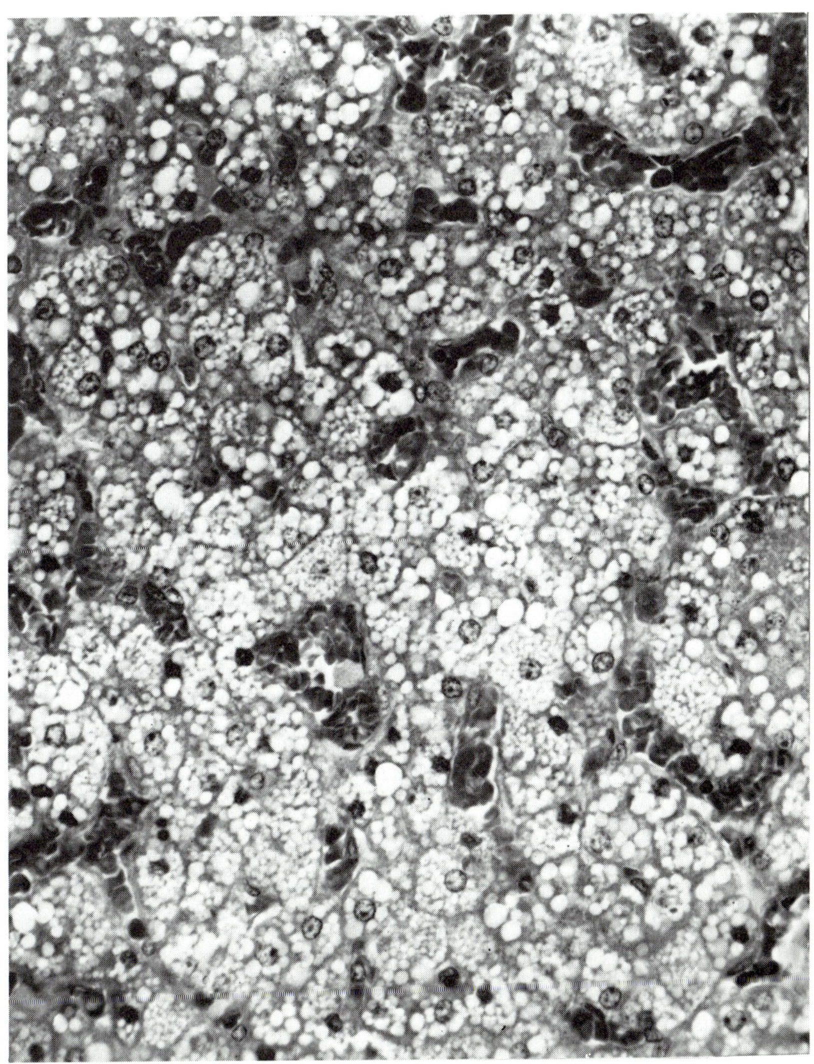

Figure 1. Diffuse fatty degeneration of the liver
           (Case 3).

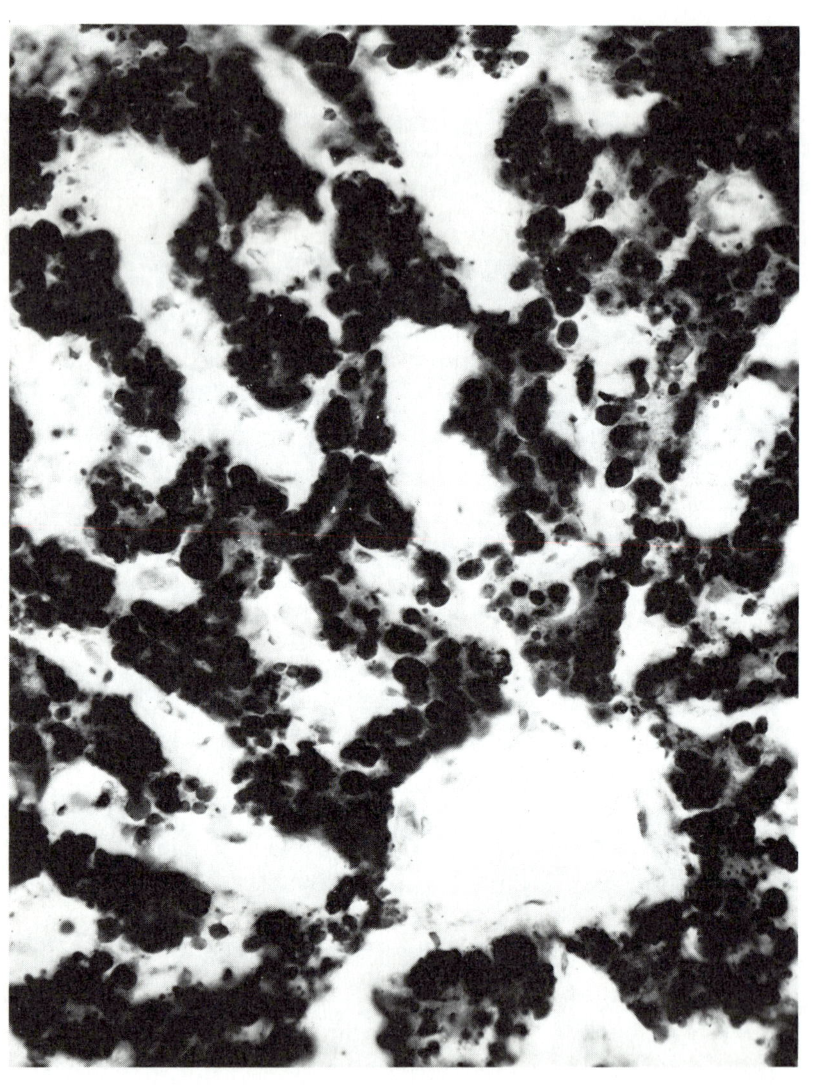

Figure 2. Section of the same liver (Sudan III stain).

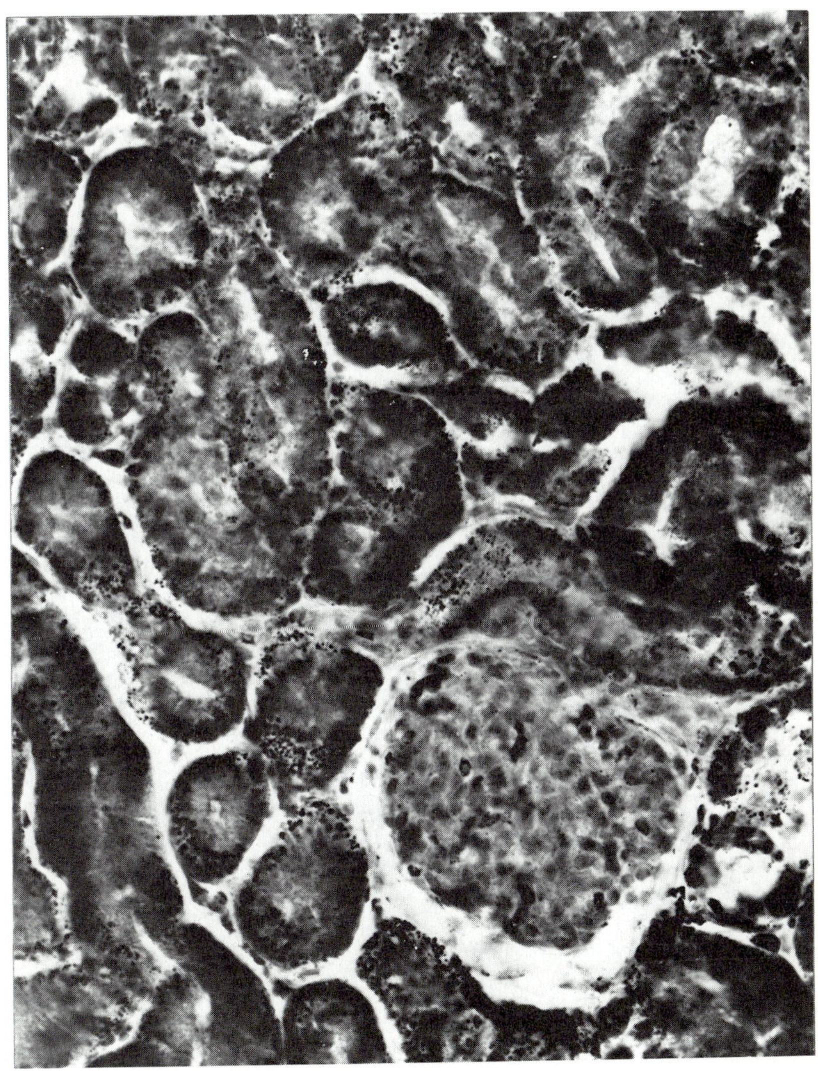

Figure 3. Fatty degeneration of proximal
tubules of the kidney (case 6)
(Sudan III stain).

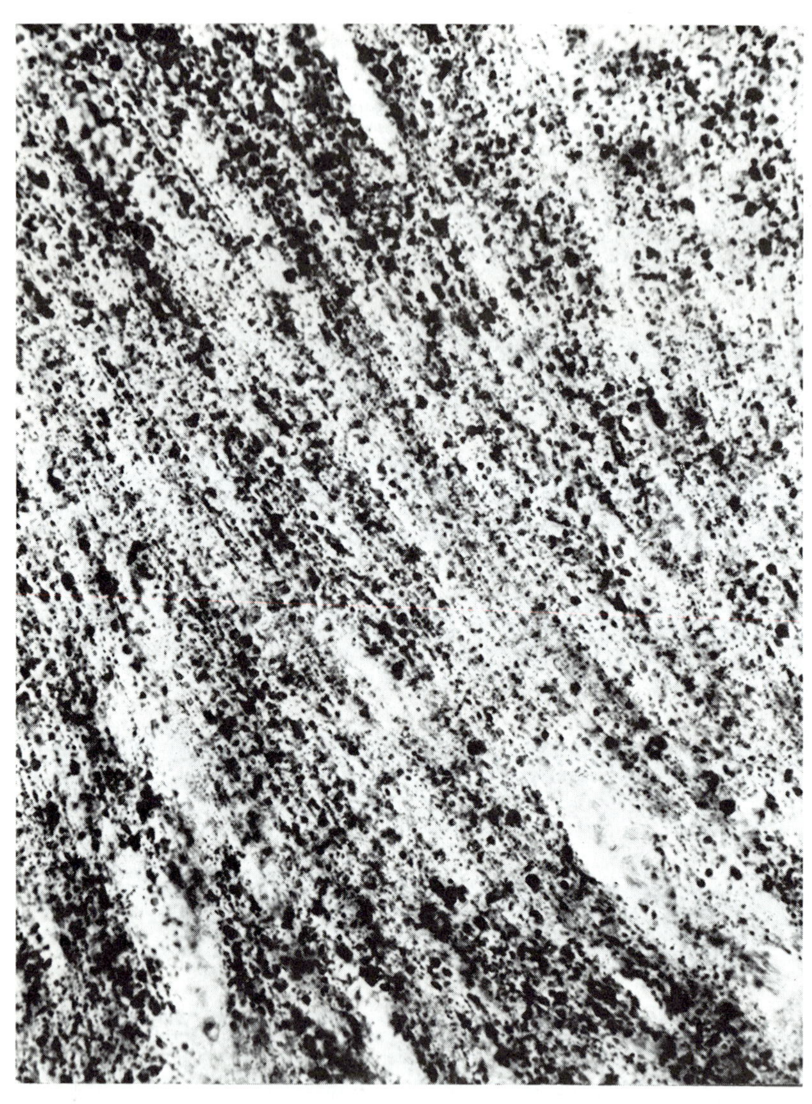

Figure 4.   Fatty degeneration of the myocardium
(case 5) (Sudan III stain)

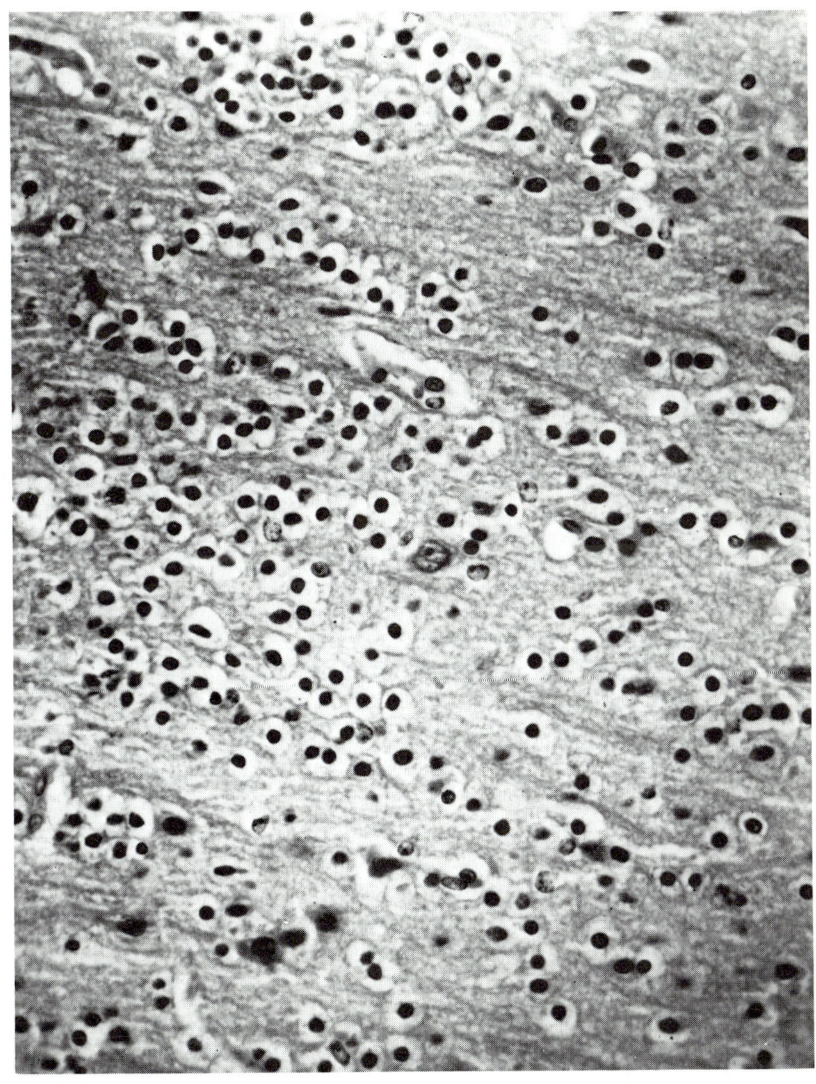

Figure 5. Pericellular brain oedema (case 6).

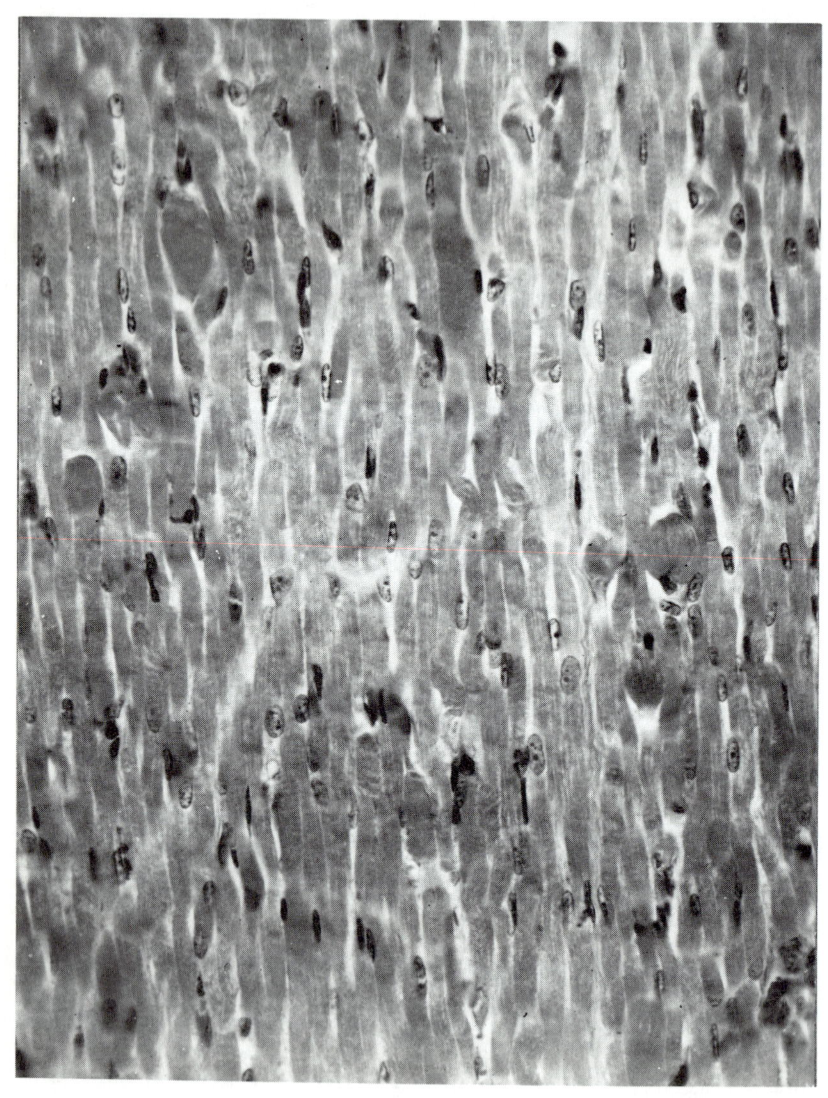

Figure 6. Granular disruption of muscle
fibres of diaphragm (case 6).

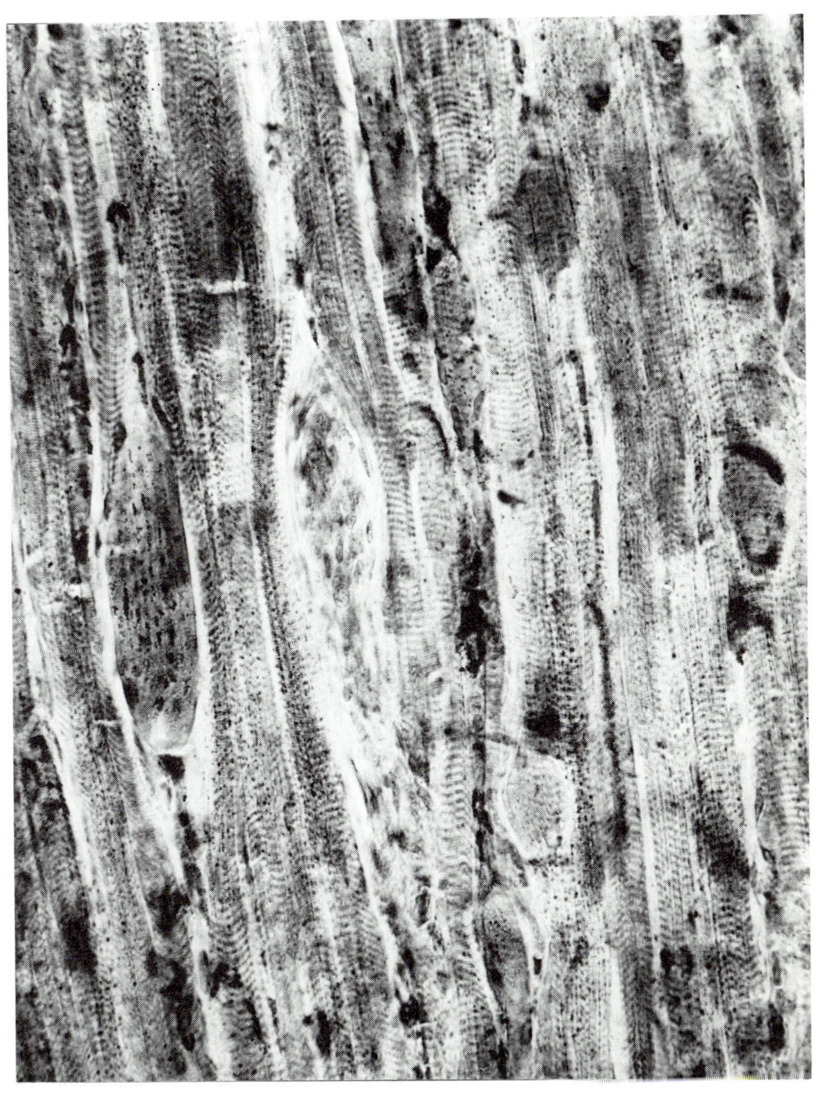

Figure 7.   Fatty degeneration of altered
            muscle fibres (Sudan III stain).

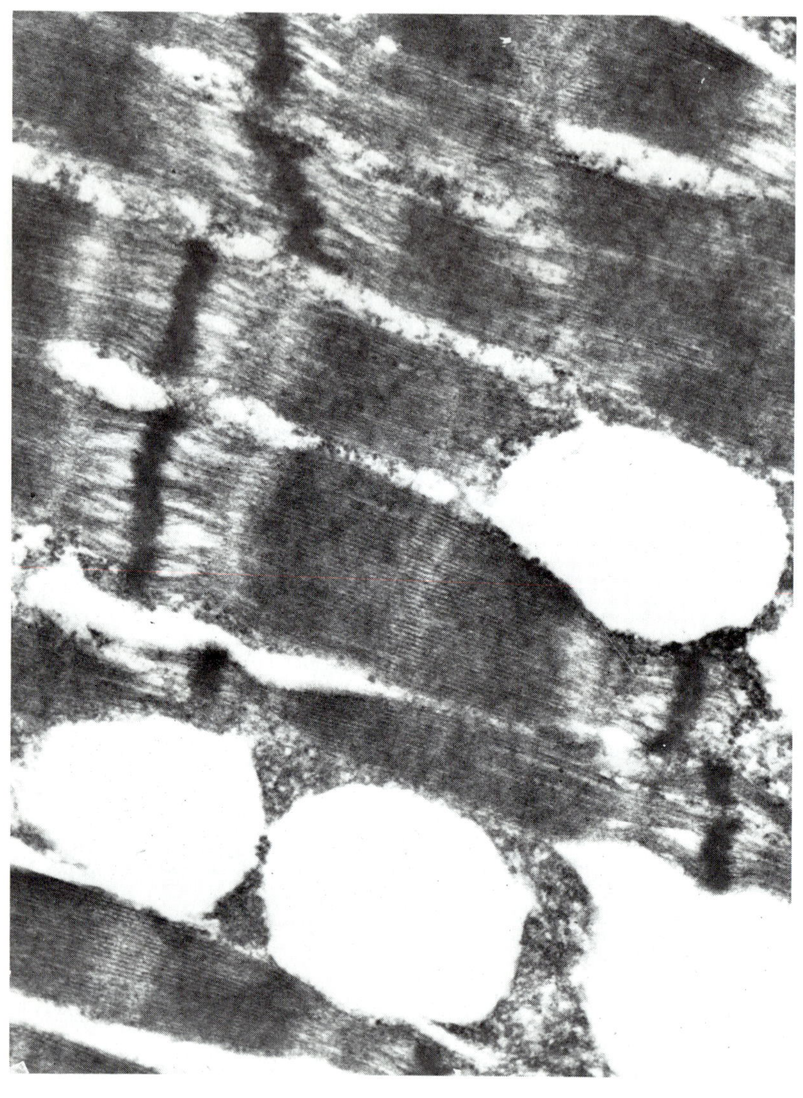

Figure 8: Electron micrograph of Case 6.
Psoas muscle; loss of cross banding;
Empty membrane-free vacuoles between
myofibrils.

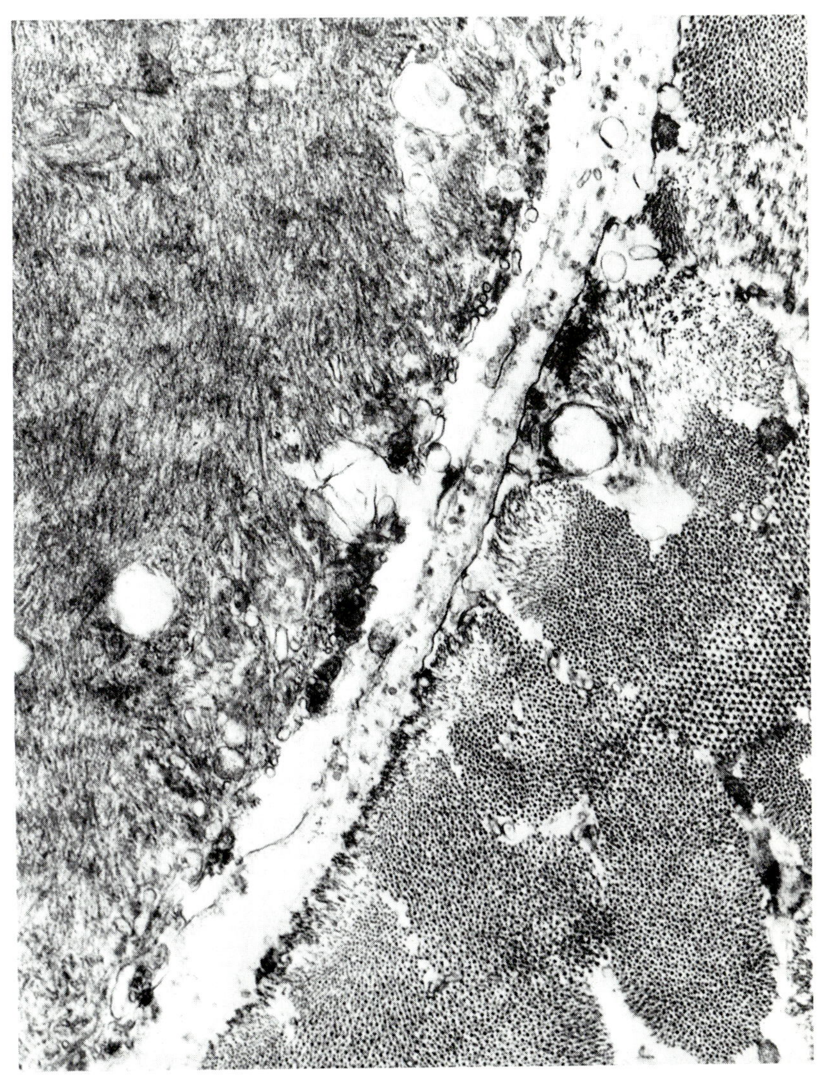

Figure 9. Electron micrograph of Case 3.
Psoas muscle; homogenization of
muscle fibre. Border between normal
and altered muscle fibre.

TABLE 3

DEGREE OF STEATOSIS

CASE	SEX	AGE	LIVER	KIDNEY	HEART	STRIATED MUSCLE
1. K.J.	m	32 hrs.	+++	+++	++	++
2. V.M.	f	71 hrs.	+++	++	++	+
3. V.	m	72 hrs.	+++	+++	+++	++
4. V.M.	m	70 hrs.	+++	++	+++	+
5. V.K.	f	45 hrs.	+++	+++	+++	++
6. V.O.	m	72 hrs	+++	+++	+++	+++

+++ massive
 ++ middle
  + mild

Samples of psoas muscle and of the diaphragm fixed in 10% formalin (case 3) and paraffin blocked (case 6) were additionally processed for electron microscopy. Two kinds of changes were present: the first one, which corresponded with the granular disruption of muscle fibres on light microscopy,was the loss of the cross banding of the sarcomeres. Empty, membrane-free vacuoles (probably dissolved lipids) were present between the myofibrils. The second change observed was homogenization of muscle fibres due to the disintegration of A- and I-bands (Figure 8 and 9).

Virological investigation (case 5,6) of myocardium gave negative results. Liver samples of 3 cases (3, 4, 6) were investigated for the presence of aflatoxin.

Chemical Analysis

In case 3, the presence of aflatoxin was studied by chromatography. Aflatoxin B_1 obtained from Calbiochem (California) was used as a standard. The homogenized tissue sample, 50g by weight, was subjected to lyophilization. The sample was extracted with chloroform, purified on a silica-gel column, and subjected to thin layer chromatography (TLC) on silica-gel (Silufol 365 UV, Kavalier,Czechoslovakia). Solvent system (I) petroleum ether: chloroform: ethyl ether (40:10:50) and (II) chloroform:acetone:ethyl ether (30:10:60) were employed; the first was used for washing of the material spotted on the TLC plates at the origin. Spots were detected under a 365 nm UV light.

The results of TLC were as follows: the liver sample extract showed spots with blue fluorescence,like that of aflatoxin B_1 in 365 nm UV light; also, the same color change as B_1 was found when treated with 50% H_2SO_4 and R_F values identical to that of the commercial product of aflatoxin B_1.

Chemical investigation of the liver sample from case 4 gave a negative result.

Case 6': The liver sample was studied by chromatography and spectrophotometry. Aflatoxin B_1 and M_1 obtained from IEM,CSAV (Prague) were used as standards. Homogenized liver tissue(110g) was subjected to lyophilization. The sample was extracted three times with chloroform. The pooled extract was taken to dryness and the residue dissolved in methanol-acetone mixture.10 ml of 20% aqueous solution of lead acetic acid was added to the suspension,and within five minutes another 10 ml of saturated aqueous solution of sodium sulphate was added. The precipitate obtained was separated by centrifugation and the clear solution was poured into a separatory funnel. The solution was extracted five times by 50 ml n-hexane. The aqueous layer was extracted three times with chloroform. Extracts were pooled and filtered through anhydrous sodium sulphate and chloroform and removed in a rotary vacuum evaporator. The residue was dissolved in a small known amount of chloroform,and this small portion tested by TLC with aflatoxin standard on the Kieselgel G (Type 60) eluting systems as follows:-

1. chloroform: acetone: isopropanol   (85:10:5)
2. chloroform: n-hexane:pyridine   (75:20:5)
3. chloroform: acetone   (90:10)

Results: The liver sample extract showed spots with blue fluorescence like that of commercial aflatoxin B_1 and M_1 in 365 nm UV light, also the same color change when treated with 40% H_2SO_4 and R_F values which are shown in Figure 10.

For the spectrophotometric measurements, a substantial portion of the evaporated residue was put on the chromatographic column of a Kieselgel H (Type 60) and the aflatoxin was eluted with the chloroform:acetone (90:10) system. The solvent was removed from the fraction containing aflatoxin by evaporation and the residue having been dissolved in methanol was measured spectrophotometrically. (The spectra were measured with the SP8000 Unicam Spectrophotometer).

<u>Results:</u>
Spectral maxima of aflatoxin B_1 max 262nm, max 362 nm

aflatoxin M_1 max 265nm, max 357 nm

metabolites X1,X2 max 263 nm, max 364 nm
Quantitative analysis showed a concentration of 1015 µg/
kg aflatoxin B_1, 9 µg/kg aflatoxin M_1, and two undefined
metabolites X1,X2 450 µg/kg in the liver.

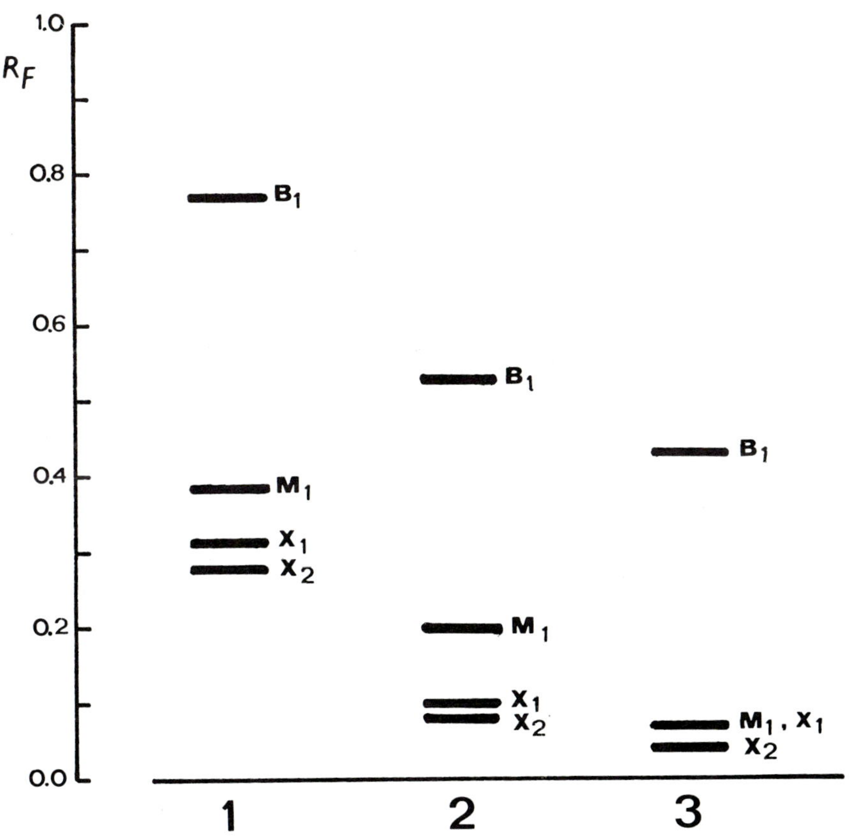

Fig.10. R_F values of aflatoxin B_1, M_1 and two
metabolites X1, X2.

Discussion: The diagnosis of Reye's syndrome is usually
based on the clinical course,biochemical findings and
morphological changes characterized by fatty degeneration of the viscera.

Unlike the clinical picture in older children, in our cases there **was no prodromal** respiratory infection, followed by the onset of vomiting and neurological symptoms.

The clinical course in the first 4 premature newborns did not differ in the symptoms from other common cases of prematurity in which respiratory distress is the initial abnormality noted. The death of the sibs (case 5,6) was sudden and unexpected. The diagnosis in all 6 cases was suspected on the basis of histological investigation. The morphological changes found in the organs fulfilled the criteria for Reye's syndrome. Degenerative changes of striated muscles in the 3 cases (3,5,6) was not an exceptional finding, and was observed and described by us in 1966 in older children with this syndrome (3). The character of the muscle changes is similar to that of Zenker's degeneration in which excessive accumulation of lactic acid is the proposed pathogenic mechanism (4). We propose a hypothesis that a similar pathogenic mechanism could lead to changes in the striated muscle in this syndrome, in which the Kreb's cycle metabolic pathway is impaired.

The etiology of Reye's syndrome seems to be most likely multifactorial. Viral infection, inborn metabolic disorders, toxins or the combination of these factors are presumed. The attempt at virus isolation in our two cases was negative. The possibility of a genetic metabolic disorder cannot be excluded in one of our familial cases. Analogous cases of familial fatal steatosis in newborn infants with some striking pathological resemblance to our patients have been previously reported by Peremans (5) and Satran (6). The authors assumed that it was a disorder genetically transmitted.

We suggest that the aflatoxin demonstrated in the liver samples in two of our three cases could be an important factor in the etiology of this syndrome. It is known that this mycotoxin produces Reye's-like morphological changes in experimental animals (7,8)and has also been demonstrated in the organs of children with Reye's syndrome (9,10,11,12,13).

Hypothetically, there are two possibilities of intoxication in the noenatal period: through the gastro-intestinal tract during the breast feeding of mothers' contaminated milk, or transplacentally; the latter has been seen in animals (14). Our hypothesis concerning the etiologic role of aflatoxin in our cases is demonstrated by:

1. All the cases except for one were observed in one geographic region in the year 1972.

2. Except for one case, all the children came from the families living in the country.

3. The mothers of most of our newborn worked on co-operative farms where the contact with aflatoxin (contaminated agriculture products) is more probably than in the city.

Although it seems that Reye's syndrome in the neonate is quite exceptional, it is likely that similar cases exist but escape our attention.

Acknowledgement

Appreciation is expressed to Dr. F. Brodsky, State Veterinary Institute, Hradec Kralove, and to Ing. D. Vesely, IEM, CSAV, Prague, for the chemical investigation. Thanks are due to Dr. J. Spacek for his help in electron microscopy.

REFERENCES

1. Papageorgiou,A.,Wigglesworth,F.W.,Schiff,D.,Stern, L. 1973. Reye's syndrome in a newborn infant. *Can. Med.Assoc.J. 109* :717-720.
2. Harris,H.B.,Vogler,L.B.,Cassady,C. 1976. Reye's syndrome in a neonate.*South.Med.Journ.69* :1511-1512.
3. Dvorackova,I.,Vortel,V.,Hroch,M. 1966. Encephalitic syndrome with fatty degeneration of viscera. *Arch. Path. 81:*240-246.
4. Anderson,W.A.D. 1971. Zenker's degeneration. *Pathology I, Ed.6,* p.79,C.V. Mosby Comp., St. Louis.

5.   Peremans,J.,DeGraef,P.J.,Strubbe,G.,DeBlock,G.
      1966. Familial metabolic disorder with fatty
      metamorphosis of the viscera.*J.Pediatr.69:*1108-
      1112.

6.   Satran,L.,Sharp,H.L.,Schenker,J.R.,Krivit,N.1969.
      Fatal neonatal hepatic steatosis:a new familial
      disorder.*Journ.Pediatr. 75:*39-46.

7.   Bourgeois,C.H.,Shank,R.C.,Grossman,R.A.,Johnson,
      D.O.,Wooding,P.,Chandavimol,P. 1971. Acute afla-
      toxin B_1 toxicity in the Macaque,and its similar-
      ities to Reye's syndrome. *Lab.Investig.24:*206-
      216.

8.   Shank,R.C.,Johnson,D.O.,Tanticharvenyos,P.1971.
      Acute toxicity of aflatoxin B_1 in the macaque
      monkey. *Toxicol.Appl.Pharmacol. 20:*227-231.

9.   Becroft,D.M.O.,Webster,D.R. 1972. Aflatoxins and
      Reye's disease.*Brit. Med.Journal 4:*117.

10.   Chaves-Carballo,E.,Ellefson,P.D.,Gomez,M.R.1976.
      An aflatoxin in the liver of a patient with Reye-
      Johnson syndrome. *Mayo Clin.Proc. 51:* 48-50.

11.   Dvorackova,I.,Zilkova,J.,Brodsky,F. 1972. Afla-
      toxin and liver damage with encephalopathy. *Sb.
      Ved.Pr.Lek.Fak.Karlovy Univ. 15:*521-524.

12.   Dvorackova,I.,Kusak,V.,Vesely,D.,Vesela,J. 1977.
      Aflatoxin and encephalopathy with fatty degener-
      ation of viscera (Reye). *Ann.Nutr.Aliment.31:*977-
      990.

13.   Shank,R.C.,Bourgeois,C.H.,Keschamras,N. 1971.
      Aflatoxins in autopsy specimens from Thai chil-
      dren with an acute disease of unknown etiology.
      *Food.Cosmet.Toxicol. 9:*501-507.

14.   Butler,W.H.,Wiglesworth,J.S. 1966. Effects of af-
      latoxin B_1 on the pregnant rat. *Brit.J.Exp.Path.
      47:*242-247.

SECTION IV

EXPERIMENTAL MODELS AND PATHOGENESIS

MODELS OF CHEMICAL AND VIRUS INTER-
ACTION AND THEIR RELATION TO A
MULTIPLE ETIOLOGY OF REYE'S SYNDROME

J. D. Pollack, Ph. D.

The interaction of viruses and chemicals has been
suggested as a possible etiology for Reye's syndrome.
Although such synergism has not been proven in humans
there are data, somewhat unappreciated, I believe,which
do show that in other biological systems combinations
of viruses and chemicals result in greater pathology
than when either is administered alone (1).

I would like to review these findings and relate
these data to two speculative schemes for the pathogenesis of Reye's syndrome.

Some workers have used insects, cells in culture,
rodents and ducks as indicators of the enhanced pathology of virus-chemical combinations. Unfortunately in
some cases, the purity of the experimental chemicals,
often of commercial grade, was not determined and, in
others, the chemicals were known to be impure. In most
of the work, the presence or toxicity of these carriers
or other impurities was not considered.

Though the number of reported synergisms of non-
lethal concentrations of insecticides and viruses is
relatively small, the findings suggest that such synergisms exist. In Table 1 are listed, apparently far
afield from Reye's syndrome, researches showing potentiation of insect mortality by insecticides after viral
exposure. As an example, Schnyder and Benz (2)
reported that combination of the insecticide DDD and
the granulosis virus of the moth Zeiraphera diniana in

TABLE 1

Potentiation of Insect Mortality by Insecticides After Viral Exposure

VIRUS	INSECTICIDE	HOST	REFERENCE
Polyhedrosis	TEPP	*T. ni*	McEwen and Hervey, 1958 (3)
Polyhedrosis	Toxaphene	*T. ni*	Genung, 1960 (4)
Polyhedrosis	Parathion	*T. ni*	Getzin, 1962 (5)
Polyhedrosis	Endrin	*T. ni*	Wolfenbarger, 1965 (6)
Polyhedrosis	Endrin Trichlofon, Endosulfan	*T. ni*	Girardeau and Mitchell, 1968 (7)
Granulosis	DDD	*Z. diniana*	Schnyder and Benz, cited in Benz, 1971 (2)
Polyhedrosis	DDT	*I. seriata*	Schnyder and Benz, cited in Benz, 1971 (2)
Polyhedrosis, Entomopox	Fenitrothion	*C. fumiferana*	Morris *et al.*, 1974; Morris, 1977 (8,9)
Nuclear polyhe-drosis	Rotenone	*G. mellonella*	Hsieh *et al.*, 1974 (10)
Granulosis	Malathion	*P. interpunctella*	Hunter, *et al*, 1975 (11)

Z. diniana larvae would increase mortality. In the
same report these workers also noted the synergistic
effect of oral DDT on the mortality of larvae of
the looper Idaea seriata with the polyhedrosis virus of
I. seriata.

There are other examples of chemical and virus potentiation of insect mortality listed in this table.
Of particular note are the findings of Morris and co-
workers (8,9). Their data is of especial interest
because of the use in Canada of the insecticide
fenitrothion in effective combination with either nuclear polyhedrosis or entomopox viruses against the
spruce budworm Choristoneura fumiferana. These workers
found in the population of insects surviving the entomo-
pox-fenitrothion combination that the number of males
outnumbered the females two to one.

These reports indicated that there is a synergism
between insecticides and virus. The mechanism of this
synergism is not known, but in its simplest form if the
insecticide follows virus exposure, that is, when the
insecticide is the synergist of the virus, there may be
stimulation of virus production, or the toxin may stress
the insect, making it more susceptible to the viral infection. As suggested by Telenga (2) the latter
situation could occur by reducing the number of protective hemocytes through the insecticide-mediated
release of physiologic stressors, such as neurohormones.
This synergism results in a fatal infection. It is also
possible that the virus is the synergist of the insecticide. In this case, an infection subsequent to toxin
exposure alters the host's ability to detoxify or elimi-
nate already present insecticide or its degradation
products. This synergism results in a fatal intoxication.

Other investigators have examined virus-chemical
interactions in tissue culture systems (Table 2). Gabliks and coworkers (12,13,14) for example, examined
the replication of poliovirus in HeLa cells and
vaccinia virus in rabbit kidney and Chang liver cells
which had been exposed first to insecticides. They

TABLE 2

Potentiation of Cellular Pathology by Combinations of Virus and Insecticide or Emulsifier

VIRUS	INSECTICIDE	HOST CELL	REFERENCE
Poliovirus	Karathane	HeLa	Gabliks, 1965 (12)
Vaccinia	DDT	Rabbit Kidney	Bantug-Jurilla and Gabliks, 1966 (16)
Poliovirus	DDT, Dicofol	HeLa	Gabliks, 1967 (13)
Foot-and-Mouth	Dimethoate	Swine	Puga and Rodrigues, 1974 (17)
Vesicular Stomatitis	Fenitrothion, Toximul MP8, etc.	L-929, HeLa	Rozee *et al.*, 1978 (15)

found that HeLa cells treated with karathane, a dinitrophenol insecticide, and poliovirus, resulted in a virus
yield per cell about 18 times more than from HeLa cells
not treated with insecticide. Rozee and coworkers
(15), using the pesticide fenitrothion, recently demonstrated a significant enhancing effect on the replication of vesicular stomatitis virus in L-929 cells.

The works noted in this table indicate that pre-
treatment of host cells with some insecticides, such as
karathane or fenitrothion, significantly increase viral
yields and host cell mortality. The increased mortality
may also be relatable to an increase in host cell susceptibility or to a stimulation of viral synthesis.

The effect of emulsifiers in enhancing viral infections in tissue culture was also reported by Rozee and
coworkers. Out of 17 emulsifiers tested, 9 were found
to enhance viral replication. Viruses having single-
stranded RNA responded to enhancing emulsifiers but
double-stranded viruses showed no significant increase
in viral yields over controls. Non-ionic polymers of
polyoxyethylene had the most activity, while mixtures of
ionic surfactants and/or polyoxyethylene alcohols displayed reduced or no activity. Optimum emulsifier concentrations for enhancement were at subtoxic doses.
Enhancement was not demonstrated if the emulsifier was
added simultaneously with virus. The investigators concluded that certain metabolic events were necessary for
enhancement and that enhancement was reversible.

A possible explanation for the effects seen with
insecticide solvents or emulsifiers may be attributed to
the activity of microsomal mixed-function oxidase systems. Brattsten and Wilkinson (18) have reported that
a mixed function oxidase system can be induced by insecticide solvents. Induction may have a marked effect on
susceptibility. In fact, susceptibility may even be decreased. Thus, carriers used for pesticides cannot be
regarded as inert agents with little or no biological
activity.

Among the first animal interaction studies of viruses and pesticides, such as DDT, were those conducted by Friend and Trainer (19) with mallards (Table 3). DDT followed by duck hepatitis virus resulted in increased duck mortality. Presumably the DDT altered the host defenses rendering mallards more susceptible to the virus. It was also suggested that the host immune response was impaired by DDT exposure. These and other investigators noted that the duck and mouse hepatitis viruses were morphologically associated with the endoplasmic reticulum where the microsomal mixed-function oxidases that probably detoxify DDT are localized, an observation I feel of much import.

Crocker and coworkers (23) indicated that insecticide preparations have a "priming" effect in increasing the viral susceptibility of the young mouse. They demonstrated fatty changes in the livers of animals treated with insecticides and then virus. They suggested that the disease produced by the interaction of the virus and toxin may be quite different from the pathology resulting from the action of either alone.

Colon and associates (24) explored the hypothesis that viral infection with toxin potentiated the development of encephalopathy with fatty changes of the viscera. They tested, in rats, the effects of a number of compounds administered simultaneously with an infective dose of the mengo strain of EMC virus, and found that the most significant histologic and biologic changes occurred when 4-pentenoic acid was used. The biochemical alterations noted were hepatic triglyceride steatosis and lowered glycogen levels. Colon and his associates hypothesized that the disease was caused by a hepatic mitochondrial toxin which is activated or potentiated by viral infection. Subsequent abnormalities in mitochondrial metabolism contributed to the cerebral edema and hepatic steatosis.

Crocker and coworkers (25) showed that painting young mice with presumably non-toxic petroleum by-products as emulsifiers or impurities increased the lethality of subsequent infection with EMC virus. In their

TABLE 3

Effect of Combinations of Virus and Insecticide or Emulsifiers on Animals.

VIRUS	CHEMICAL	ANIMAL	EFFECT	REFERENCES
Duck hepatitis	DDT	Mallard	Protection	Friend and Trainer, 1970 (19)
Duck hepatitis	DDT	Mallard	Protection	Ragland *et al.*, 1971 (20)
Duck hepatitis	Dieldrin	Mallard	Protection	Friend and Trainer, 1972 (21)
Duck hepatitis	DDT, Dieldrin	Mallard	Potentiation	Friend and Trainer, 1974 (22)
EMC*	DDT, Fenitrothion	Mouse	Potentiation	Crocker *et al.*, 1974 (23)
EMC*	4-pentenoic acid	Rat	Potentiation	Colon *et al.*, 1974 (24)
EMC*	Petroleum by-products	Mouse	Potentiation	Crocker *et al.*, 1976 (25)

* Encephalomyocarditis virus

experiments the maximum mortality of 85% was observed
in groups of animals that had been exposed to both virus and emulsifier-solvent. The mortality was lower in
groups of animals exposed to virus and insecticide.
They also observed fatty liver changes in some animals.
They suggested that there could be some direct interaction or combination of virus and toxin,or that the
viral infection allowed either release of stored toxin
or effected increased viral replication and spread.
These products,as noted by Dr. Safe in this Symposium,
are in widespread use as pesticide dispersal agents and
emulsifiers and their role in human disease has received very little attention.

The accumulated data indicates that there exists
an apparently subtle experimental association of virus
and certain chemicals resulting in increased morbidity
and mortality in animals,insects and cell cultures. As
this pathologic association can occur in a variety of
cells, it may also occur in humans.

Peter Mullen (26) evaluated the recent laboratory,
clinical and epidemiological data relevant to Reye's
syndrome from a biochemical and immunopharmacological
perspective.He considered that environmental exposure
to various potentially toxic,foreign compounds or
their biotransformation products, called xenobiotics,
may be responsible for the early pathogenesis.Mullen
proposed,as briefly shown in Figure 1,that subsequent
to initiating xenobiotic factor or factors there resulted biochemical and functional anomalies of the
liver and,in turn, impairment of normal immune defenses
against subsequent viral infections. The prodromal illness leads to further biochemical and immunologic abnormalities, possibly exacerbated by toxic residuum or
still abnormal cellular function,progressing to the extensive liver degeneration and encephalopathy of Reye's
syndrome.

Central to this proposal for the pathogenesis of
Reye's syndrome were the xenobiotic initiating factors
and the secondary impaired immune defenses.One possible
xenobiotic initiating factor is aflatoxin.
With Drs.Dennis Burech and Charles Reiner of
Children's Hospital in Columbus,we have examined Reyes

*Figure 1. Abbreviated Outline of Xenobiotic Initiated
Pathogenic Mechanisms in Reye's Syndrome, adapted from
Mullen (1978).*   (26)

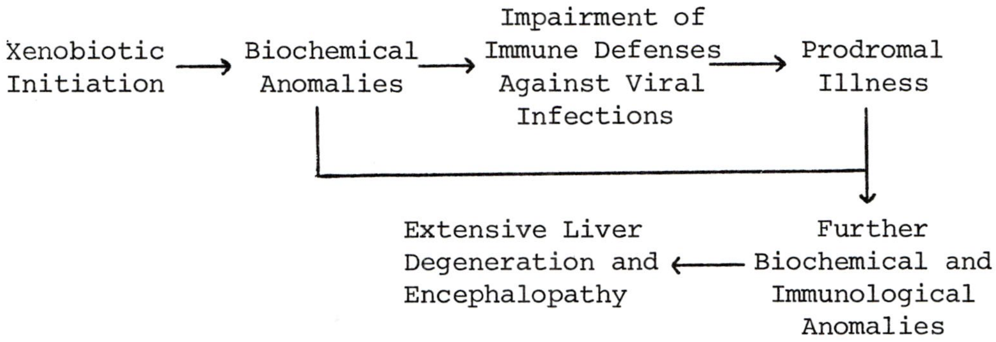

Xenobiotic Initiation → Biochemical Anomalies → Impairment of Immune Defenses Against Viral Infections → Prodromal Illness → Further Biochemical and Immunological Anomalies → Extensive Liver Degeneration and Encephalopathy

Syndrome tissues from nine patients for aflatoxins. We
found no aflatoxin in the liver, kidney, fat, or brain
tissues from these patients. We are capable of detecting 5.2 μg of aflatoxin B_1, or 25.5 μg of aflatoxin B_2,
in a kilogram of wet liver. Including the study of
Chaves-Carballo et al (27) with our data, the analysis for aflatoxin in hepatic tissue from 18 cases of
Reye's syndrome in the U.S. has been reported. No aflatoxin has been found in 17; an aflatoxin-like substance
was found in one but positive identification could not
be made. Recently, Hogan and associates (28) have reported low levels of aflatoxin in the blood of two
patients during the acute phase of Reye's syndrome.
Re-examining three of our liver specimens by their
techniques, we still did not detect any aflatoxin.
Although we feel it unlikely that aflatoxicosis is important in the pathogenesis of Reye's syndrome in the
U.S., we do not exclude the possibility that it could
be one of many xenobiotic initiating factors.

The most difficult problem we have had in attempting to develop a working hypothesis for the pathogenesis of Reye's Syndrome is to decide which data or
theory to emphasize.

Most reports associate a virus with the etiology
of Reye's syndrome. The evidence has been reviewed in
a number of papers by Corey (29) and Noble (30) and
their coworkers. The most convincing data associate
varicella and influenza B with the onset of Reye's syndrome. Partin and associates (31) hypothesized that
Reye's syndrome, like influenza pneumonia, may be an
epiphenomenon occurring about 7 days after the first
clinical evidence of influenza. Corey's analysis revealed a geographic clustering and a rural distribution
of cases, which suggested a contributory factor in addition to antecedent viral infections. An extrinsic or
an environmental agent is postulated as playing a possible important role in the pathogenesis of Reye's
syndrome.

In some cases of Reye's syndrome there is evidence
of genetic abnormalities or defects (32,33,34). The
possibility that Reye's syndrome may involve a double

viral infection (31) or an impaired immunologic
system (35,26) has been reported. The role of a
"serum factor", the urea cycle, toxic levels of ammonia,
free fatty acids, the involvement of cyclic AMP or
orotic acid endogenously liberated, have been considered,
and are discussed in this Symposium.

As I have noted, Crocker and Colon and their co-
workers (23,24) were apparently the first groups to
examine virus-toxin interactions in some relationship
to Reye's syndrome or encephalopathy with fatty degeneration of the viscera. The possibility that the syndrome has a multiple etiology or is affected by the relationship of two or more agents such as viruses, chemicals or both working simultaneously or with some temporal separation we find plausible. However, in few
cases have there been any evidence of unusual levels of
drugs or toxins in serum or tissue of Reye's syndrome
patients. Of course, exposures to low non-toxic levels
of chemicals might still be sufficient to interact or
"prime" the host or modify the virus as I have already
inferred.

As an experimental working hypothesis, we consider,
as shown in Figure 2, that the evidence suggests a multiple etiology for Reye's syndrome. Our speculation
considers that there are possibly three initiators of
Reye's syndrome: a virus, an exogenous toxin or a virus-
chemical interaction. First, in the case of an apparent
viral etiology: as noted by others, under stress, lipolysis of depot fat is associated with an abnormal lipid
metabolism responsible for the release of high levels
of toxic free fatty acids (36) or other innocuously
accumulated toxic chemicals compartmentalized in
adipose. These secondary incitants may lead to structural and further biochemical abnormalities. Endogenous toxins originating from tissues other than fat,
such as tyramine, noted by Dr. Faraj in this Symposium,
may also lead to structural and biochemical abnormalities.

Second, such exogenous toxins as aflatoxins, herbicides, insecticides, or surfactants are also consid-

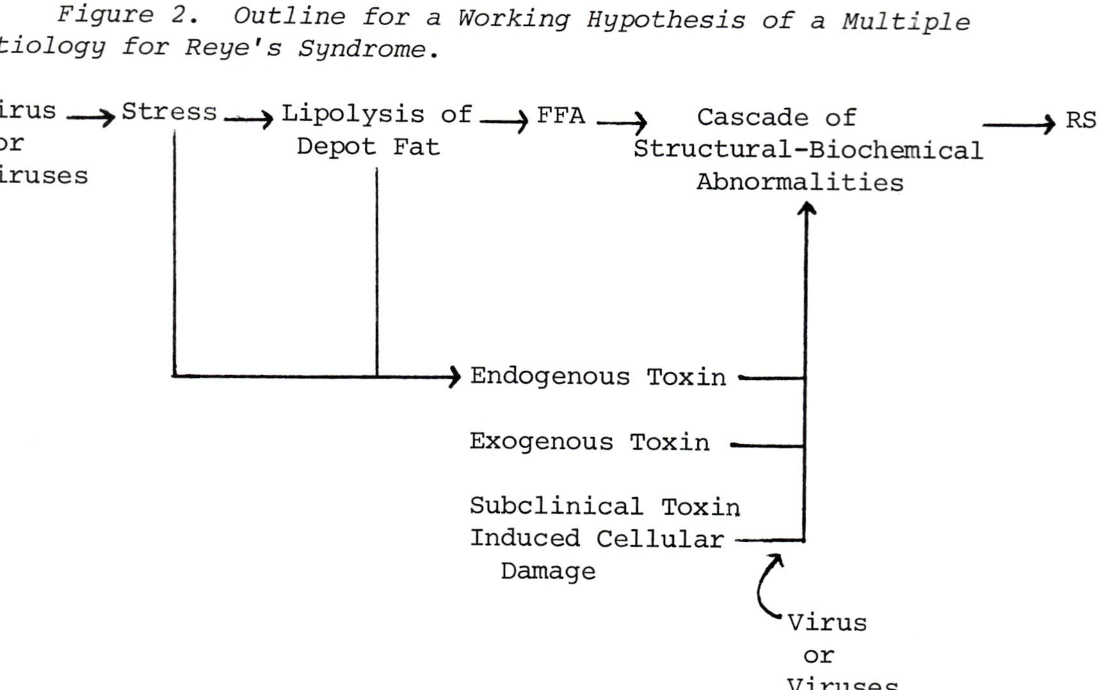

Figure 2. Outline for a Working Hypothesis of a Multiple Etiology for Reye's Syndrome.

ered to be able to directly affect the normal structure
and metabolism of cellular organelles leading to Reye's
syndrome or a Reye's syndrome-like disease. Finally,
the synergistic action of prior toxin damaged cells and
virus has already been emphasized.

Our speculations include that primary or secondary
effectors act either directly or indirectly at a common cellular locus, perhaps the fat cell, mitochondrion
or at the smooth endoplasmic reticulum-Golgi complex
membrane.

We observed by electron microscopy, marked proli-
feration of hepatic smooth endoplasmic reticulum in
four of five non-comatose patients examined. The concentric whorls of hyperplastic smooth endoplasmic reticulum reported by Schubert and associates (37) were
not observed. We associate the hepatic steatosis, decrease in circulating lipoprotein, increase in lipopoly-
sis, circulating free fatty acids and cholesteryl esters
of Reye's syndrome with changes in the Golgi apparatus
and SER. We further speculate that these Golgi-SER
changes follow or are concomitant with fat cell changes
and may precede mitochondrial pathology and possibly
the encephalopathy of Reye's syndrome.

In summary, there is evidence of increased morbidity and mortality in various insects, tissue cultures,
rodents, and mallards when they are exposed to both
chemicals and viruses.

Reye's syndrome or encephalopathy with fatty degeneration of the viscera are diseases that have been
etiologically associated with viruses or environmental
toxins. The association of Reye's syndrome with viruses is presently more certain. There is little evidence
for the association of Reye's syndrome with extraordin-
ary levels of environmental toxins. In the largest pertinent series, Bourgeois and colleagues (38) found
aflatoxin in Thailand children but not significant antecedent viral infection. In the United States, of the
18 Reye's syndrome hepatic specimens that have been
examined, in only one case was a substance found that

resembled an aflatoxin. The role of aflatoxin in the
pathogenesis of Reye's Syndrome has not been generally
and convincingly demonstrated.

It is presently difficult to involve, except co-
incidentally, other environmental toxins in the pathogenesis of Reye's Syndrome. Hardly any reports present
data for the presence of these substances in cases of
Reye's Syndrome. Until general evidence is offered
that these substances are present in patients, their
role in the pathogenesis of Reye's syndrome, though
suspected, can be questioned. In addition, it will be
important to determine both the levels of these substances in the patients and their environment and the
ability of these substances to interact in cell culture
and animals with viruses associated with Reye's syndrome.

REFERENCES

1. Pollack, J.D., Hughes, J.H., Hamparian, V.V. and
    Burech, D. 1978. The interaction of Chemicals
    and Viruses and their Role in Reye's Syndrome.
    Chemosphere 7:7 551-563.
2. Benz, G. 1971. Synergism of micro-organisms and
    chemical insecticides. In Microbial control of
    insects and mites. Edited by H.D. Burges and
    N. N. Hussey. Academic Press, New York. 327-355.
3. McEwen, F.L. and Hervey, G.E.R. 1958. Control of
    cabbage looper with a virus disease. *J. Insect
    Pathol. 51:626-631.*
4. Genung, W.G. 1960. Comparison of insecticides,
    insect pathogens and insecticide-pathogen combin-
    ations for control of cabbage looper Trichoplusia
    ni (Hbn.). *Fla. Entomol. 43:* 65-68.
5. Getzin, L.W. 1962. The effectiveness of the polyhe-
    drosis virus for control of the cabbage looper,
    Trichoplusia ni. *J. Econ. Entomol. 55:* 442-445.
6. Wolfenbarger, D.A. 1965. Polyhedrosis-virus
    surfactant and insecticide combinations, and Bacil-
    lus thuringiensis surfactant combinations for
    cabbage looper control. *J. Invertebr. Pathol.
    7:* 33-38.

7. Girardeau, Jr., J.H. and Mitchell, E.R. 1968.
    The influence of a subacute infection of polyhed-
    rosis virus in the cabbage looper on susceptibil-
    ity to chemical insecticides. *J. Econ. Entomol.*
    61: 312-313.

8. Morris, O.N., Armstrong, J.A., Howse, G.M. and
    Cunningham, J.C. 1974. A 2-year study of virus-
    chemical insecticide combination in the integrated
    control of the sprude budworm, Choristoneura fumi-
    ferana (Tortricidae:Lepidoptera). *Can. Entomol.*
    106: 813-824.

9. Morris, O.N. 1977. Long-term effects of aerial
    applications of virus-fenitrothion combinations
    against the spruce budworm, Chorisoneura fumiferana
    (Lepidoptera:Torticidae). *Can. Entomol. 109:*9-14.

10. Hsieh, M.L., Collins, W.J. and Stairs, G.R. 1974.
    Interaction of nuclear-polyhedrosis virus, DDT,
    rotenone and peanut oil in Galleria mellonella
    larvae. *Environ. Entomol. 3:*567-569.

11. Hunter, D.K., Collier, S.J. and Hoffman, D.F. 1975.
    Compatibility of malathion and the granulosis virus
    of the Indian meal moth. *J. Invertebr. Pathol.*
    25: 389-390.

12. Gabliks, J. 1965. Responses of cell cultures to
    insecticides. III. Altered susceptibility to
    polio virus and diphtheria toxin. *Proc. Soc. Exp.*
    Biol. Med. 120: 172-175.

13. Gabliks, J. 1967. Insecticidal compounds. Effects
    on replication of vaccinia and polio viruses in
    human Chang-strain liver cells. *Arch. Environ.*
    Health 14: 698-702.

14. Gabliks, J. and Friedman, L. 1969. Effects of
    insecticides on mammalian cells and virus infect-
    ions. *Proc. N.Y. Acad. Sci. 160:* 254-271.

15. Rozee, K.R., Lee, S.H.S., Crocker, J.F.S. and
    Safe, S. 1978. Enhanced virus replication in
    mammalian cells exposed to commerical emulsifiers.
    Appl. Environ. Microbiol. 35: 297-300.

16. Bantug-Jurilla, M. and Gabliks, J. 1966. Responses
    of cell cultures to insecticides. *Fed. Proc. 25:*
    447.

17.   Puga, F.R. and Rodrigues, M.A.I.R. 1974. Efeito
      de insecticidas sobre o metabolismo e a susceptib-
      ilidade de celulas IB-RS-2 ao virus da febre aftosa.
      Arq. Inst. Biol., Sao Paulo 41: 141-145.
18.   Brattsten, L.B. and Wilkinson, C.F. 1977. Insect-
      icide solvents: interference with insecticidal
      action. *Science 196:* 1211-1213.
19.   Friend, M. and Trainer, D.O. 1970. Polychlorinated
      biphenyl: interaction with duck hepatitis virus.
      Science 170: 1314-1316.
20.   Ragland, W.L., Friend, M., Trainer, D.O. and
      Sladek, N.E. 1971. Interaction between duck hepa-
      titis virus and DDT in ducks. *Res. Commun. Chem.
      Pathol. Pharmacol.* 2:236-244.
21.   Friend, M. and Trainer, D.O. 1972. Duck hepatitis
      interactions with DDT and dieldrin in adult mallards.
      Bull. Environ. Contam. Toxicol. 7:202-206.
22.   Friend, M. and Trainer, D.O. 1974. Experimental DDT-
      duck hepatitis virus interaction studies. *J.
      Wildl. Manage. 38:* 887-895.
23.   Crocker, J.F.S., Rozee, K.R., Ozere, R.L.,
      Digout, S.C. and Hutzinger, O. 1974. Insecticide
      and viral interaction as a cause of fatty visceral
      changes and encephalopathy in the mouse. *Lancet
      2:* 22-24.
24.   Colon, A.R., Ledesma, F., Pardo, V. and Sandberg,
      D.H. 1974. Viral potentiation of chemical toxins
      in the experimental syndrome of hypoglycemia,
      encephalopathy, and visceral fatty degeneration.
      Am. J. Digest Dis. 19: 1091-1101.
25.   Crocker, J.F.S., Ozere, R.L., Safe, S.H., Digout,
      S.C., Rozee, K.R. and Hutzinger, O. 1976. Lethal
      interaction of ubiquitous insecticide carriers with
      virus. *Science 192:* 1351-1353.
26.   Mullen, P.W. 1978. Immunopharmacological consider-
      ations in Reye's Syndrome: A possible xenobiotic
      initiated disorder? *Biochem. Pharmacol. 27:* 145-
      149.
27.   Chaves-Carballo, E., Ellefson, R.D. and Gomez, M.R.
      1976. An aflatoxin in the liver of a patient with
      Reye-Johnson Syndrome. *Mayo Clin. Proc.* 51:48-50.

28. Hogan, G.R., Ryan, N.J. and Hayes, A.W. 1978. Aflatoxin B and Reye's Syndrome. *Lancet 1*:561.

29. Corey, L., Rubin, R.J., Thompson, T.R., Noble, G.R. Cassidy, E., Hattwick, M.A.W., Gregg, M.B., and Eddins, D. 1977. Influenza B-associated Reye's Syndrome: incidence in Michigan and potential for prevention. *J. Infec. Dis. 135:* 398-407.

30. Noble, G.R., Corey, L. and Rubin, R.J. 1975. Virologic components of Reye's Syndrome. In Reye's Syndrome. Edited by J.D. Pollack. Grune and Stratton, New York. pp. 189-197.

31. Partin, J.C., Schubert, W.K., Partin, J.S., Jacobs R. and Saalfeld, K. 1976. Isolation of influenza virus from liver and muscle biopsy specimens from a surviving case of Reye's Syndrome. *Lancet 2:* 599-602.

32. Abraham, J.L. 1971. Dermatoglyphics and Reye's Syndrome. *Lancet 1:* 969-970.

33. Thaler, M.M., Hoogenraad, N.J. and Boswell, M. 1974. Reye's Syndrome due to a novel protein-tolerant variant of ornithine-transcarbamylase deficiency. *Lancet 2:* 438-440.

34. Brown, T., Brown, H., Lansky, L. and Hug, G. 1974. Carbamyl phosphate synthetase and ornithine trans-carbamylase in liver of Reye's Syndrome. *N. Engl. J. Med. 291:* 797.

35. Linnemann, Jr., C.C., Shea, L., Kauffman, C.A., Schiff, G.M., Partin, J.C. and Schubert, W.K. 1974. Association of Reye's Syndrome with viral infection. *Lancet 2:* 179-182.

36. Pollack, J.D., Cramblett, H.G., Flynn, D. and Clark, D. 1975. Serum and tissue lipids in Reye's Syndrome. In Reye's Syndrome. Edited by J.D. Pollack. Grune and Stratton, New York. pp. 227-243.

37. Schubert, W.K., Partin, J.C. and Partin, J.S. 1972. Encephalopathy and fatty liver (Reye's Syndrome). In Progress in liver diseases, vol. 4. Edited by H. Popper and F. Schaffner. Grune and Stratton, New York. pp. 489-510.

38. Bourgeois, C., Olson, L., Comer, D., Evans, H. Keschamras, N., Cotton, R., Grossman, R. and Smith, T. 1971. Encephalopathy and fatty degeneration of the viscera: A clinicopathologic analysis of 40 cases. *Am. J. Clin. Path. 56:* 558-571.

DISCUSSION

K.Dhiensiri   -   Doctor Pollack, we were told yesterday
        that organic chemicals may not be found in the
        liver after a few hours, because of high degra-
        dation rates. I don't know if this is true of
        the aflatoxin, and wonder whether the aflatox-
        ins used in experimental models with mice or
        mallard ducks exhibited a potentiating effect
        on the virus?

J.D. Pollack -   There is evidence with Rhesus monkeys
        that some aflatoxins shortly after administra-
        tion are almost undetectable; they may be rap-
        idly excreted. There have been some experiments
        with the mouse model, using viruses and afla-
        toxins reported by Dr.Colon and his colleagues.

A.R. Colon   -   No; I have had no luck with potentia-
        ting the effect of aflatoxins. I don't want to
        dismiss the aflatoxin - that's why I'm here. I,
        too, have looked for aflatoxin in patients with
        Reye's syndrome and I have not found any; but I
        find it hard to overlook the incredible evidence
        that Bourgeois and his colleagues from Thailand
        put together. Aflatoxin,I think, is a remarka-
        ble agent. If you take it in very tiny doses
        over a period of a year, speculation is that it
        produces cirrhosis, the prime example is child-
        hood cirrhosis which is now thought to be re-
        lated to chronic aflatoxin intoxication. If you
        take it in little larger doses over a period of
        six months, the association is that of adult
        hepatoma. If you take aflatoxin in moderate do-
        ses over a period of six weeks, you get hepati-
        tis. Admittedly,most of the hepatitis has been
        reported out of Central Africa, Western Africa;
        nonetheless, there is a human-associated afla-
        toxin hepatitis.   If you take aflatoxin in
        large doses as Bourgeois and his colleagues sug-
        gested over a short period of time (7-10 days)
        you end up with a Reye's syndrome. This brings

to mind the question that, perhaps in Thailand
there is a group of genetically predisposed
cases who, when they come in contact with aflatoxin, will develop the Reye's syndrome.Might
it not be worthwhile to, at the very least, do
some tissue typing - HLA typing on some of
these kids in Thailand, to see if anyone has a
group of children who in any way were homogenous genetically?

J.D. Pollack -   Yes; I think it would be a very good
        idea. Dr. Glasgow, who is in the audience, has
        addressed some of the things you've brought up
        both publicly and privately, and may wish to
        comment. We are quite concerned when working
        with aflatoxin B, as it is one of the most po-
        tent hepatocarcinogens known; it's about 100
        times more hepatocarcinogenic than butter yel-
        low, and it has a marked propensity to stick to
        glass. I was disappointed that Dr. Dhiensiri
        didn't have the opportunity to check the chil-
        dren in Thailand for aflatoxin, because I would
        like to put that Thailand story to rest, if
        possible, and I am also sorry that Dr. Dvorack-
        ova is not here. You will note in her paper that
        she finds aflatoxin in some patients. She has
        observed and reported this before. My view is
        that aflatoxin may be a possible xenobiotic-
        initiating factor,but apparently not in this
        country.

E.S. Kang   -   The vast majority of children have
        been exposed to presumably the viral stress of
        influenza or varicella and have not developed
        Reye's syndrome. Varicella itself is character-
        istically a very mild disorder, and there is no
        evidence clinically reported that the viral in-
        fection, which preceded the episode of Reye's
        syndrome, was of unusual severity. Therefore, I
        wonder what is the role of the particular virus.

        Earlier at this meeting, other inves-
        tigators very pertinently brought up the fact

that these viruses are enveloped. The envelope
may have some unique role to play in this interaction.

J.D. Pollack   - Yes; I agree. Also, there may be
other pertinent differences in the affecting
viruses; for example, the nature of their nu-
cleoprotein.

L.D.O. Schneiderman - We're doing HLA typing in Detroit. We have done thirty families and our
preliminary results, which are not significant
right now, tend toward BW7, B6. This July and
August we are going to record 30 more families.
Institutions who might want to participate
would be welcome.

A PATHOGENIC ROLE FOR A SERUM FACTOR
IN REYE'S SYNDROME

June R. Aprille, Ph. D., and
Gregory K. Asimakis, Jr., Ph. D.

INTRODUCTION

Even though Reye's syndrome has been recognized
since 1963 (1), its etiology and pathogenic mechanisms
remain a puzzle. In 1971, a key observation by Dr.
Partin and his colleagues showed that liver mitochondrial injury is associated with Reye's syndrome (2).
Since then morphological changes in mitochondria of
other organs have been described (3,4,5,6,7). Numerous
metabolic features of the illness suggest that an insult
to mitochondrial function in several tissues underlies
the clinical presentation (8,9,10,11). The idea that a
toxic substance may be causing mitochondrial damage has
been considered (2). The substance could be thought of
as an accumulating intrinsic metabolite or an exogen-
ously acquired toxin. In either case, one might expect
to find the harmful substance in the serum of afflicted
children. We therefore decided to look for a substance
in serum which might have an effect on mitochondria.

Isolated rat liver mitochondria were evaluated for
classical parameters of respiratory function _in vitro_
in the presence or absence of Reye's syndrome serum. In
this way, it was shown that serum from Reye's syndrome
patients has unusual effects on both the structure and
function of isolated mitochondria (8,9). The findings
suggest that the substance responsible for these effects _in vitro_ may be relevant to the pathophysiology
of Reye's syndrome. However many important questions
are yet to be answered before that hypothesis can be
verified. The object of this paper is to report

recent progress toward defining the mechanism of action
of the supposed serum factor, its molecular characteristics, and the circumstances of its occurrence.

METHODS

Preparation of Serum. Serum or plasma samples
were graciously provided by colleagues from several
hospitals at widely separated locations (see Acknowledgements). Some samples had been stored frozen for
several years, others were from recent admissions. All
samples were routinely lyophilized to dryness. An
amount of water equal to one-fifth the original volume
was added to reconstitute the sample. For some
experiments, serum was passed through an ultrafil-
tration membrane (type XM50, Amicon Corp.) under
nitrogen pressure to remove large proteins ($>$50,000 MW)
before lyophilization and reconstitution. Ultrafil-
trates have been shown to be as potent as whole serum
in the bioassay for the Reye's syndrome serum factor
(see Results). In a typical experiment, 10 ul of the
approximately five-fold concentrated whole serum or
filtrate was tested for an effect on mitochondrial
function in the 1 ml assay system described below.
Unless otherwise stated, the Reye's syndrome sera used
in all the experiments discussed here were obtained
from patients at admission in Stage III or IV coma,
Lovejoy classification (12).

Mitochondrial Respiration. For most of the
experiments, mitochondria were isolated from rat liver
by the usual method of differential centrifugation (9).
Respiratory activity was assayed polarographically in a
1 ml chamber at 30°C. The incubation medium described
earlier (9) was used in some experiments. In more
recent experiments, a mixture consisting of 0.225 M
sucrose, 10 mM Tris-HCL, 10 mM KCl, 1 mM EDTA, 5 mM
$MgCl_2$, 10 mM $K-PO_4$ buffer, pH 7.4 was employed. About
0.7 - 1 mg mitochondrial protein was used in each
assay. The substrate was 5 mM glutamate + 5 mM malate;
90 - 120 umoles ADP was used to initiate state 3
respiration. Deviations from these procedures which
were a necessary part of certain experiments are
described in the text.

RESULTS AND DISCUSSION

Effects of serum on mitochondria in vitro.

<u>Respiration.</u> Reye's syndrome serum caused a marked increase in state 4 respiration in isolated mitochondria. This effect was observed most directly if serum was added after a normal state 4 rate was established (Fig. 1). A similar addition of control serum had only a slight effect (Fig. 1). The effect of Reye's serum on state 4 was also seen if serum was added during state 3 or even before the addition of ADP and substrate (Fig. 1). The magnitude of the effect of Reye's

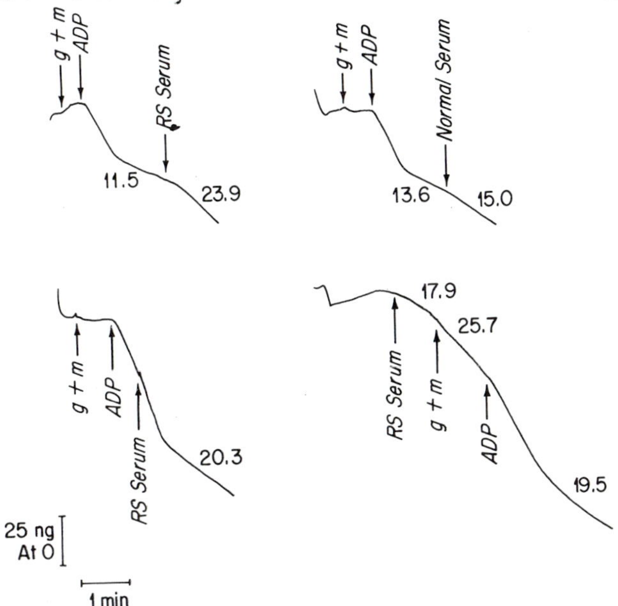

<u>Figure 1.</u> Recordings of the polarographic assay of mitochondrial respiration show the increase in state 4 respiratory rate caused by the addition of Reye's syndrome (RS) serum. In the upper left panel RS serum was added during state 4 at the time indicated by the arrow. For comparison, a similar addition of normal serum is shown in the upper right panel. The effects of adding RS serum during state 3 (lower left) or before the addition of substrate (lower right) are also shown. Numbers refer to rates of oxygen consumption in units of nanogram atoms O/min. Details of the assay are given in Methods. Abbreviations: g+m, glutamate + malate; ADP, adenosine-5'-diphosphate.

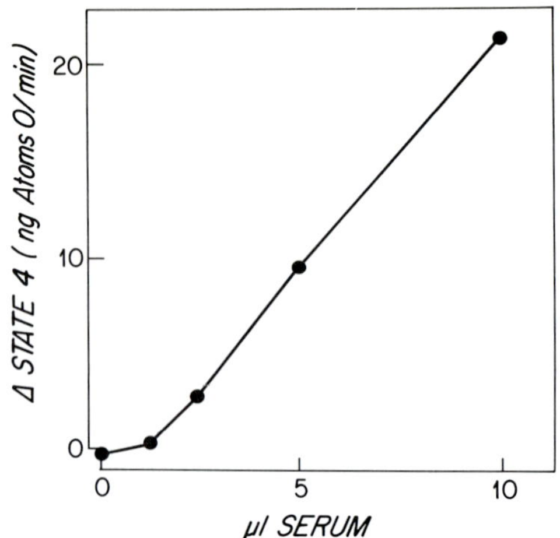

Figure 2. The magnitude of the increase in state 4
respiratory rate (Δngatoms O/min) was directly related
to the amount (ul) of Reye's syndrome serum added to
the assay during state 4 respiration. The assay was
performed as described in Methods and Figure 1.

syndrome serum was dependent on the amount of serum
added (Fig. 2).
     A number of substances, including ions, respiratory
substrates, ADP, and uncouplers (e.g. free fatty acids),
could be expected to stimulate respiration as did RS
serum (13). It is possible to distinguish among these
potential mechanisms by using their specific inhibitors.
We previously reported (9) that inhibitors of mitochondrial ATPase, or Ca^{++} transport did not antagonize the
effect of Reye's syndrome serum on liver mitochondria.
Furthermore, the site-specific electron transport chain
inhibitors rotenone (phosphorylation site I) and antimycin A (phosphorylation site II) did not block stimulation of oxygen consumption by Reye's syndrome serum.
Of the inhibitors tested only KCN (phosphorylation
site III) completely abolished all respiratory activity
in the presence of Reye's syndrome serum. More recently,
we have also found that H_2S, another blocker of electron
transport which acts at the terminal phosphorylation site,
will block the effect of Reye's syndrome serum (Fig. 3).
     These results suggest that in the presence of
antimycin A, a serum factor is able to stimulate oxygen
consumption by interacting directly or indirectly with

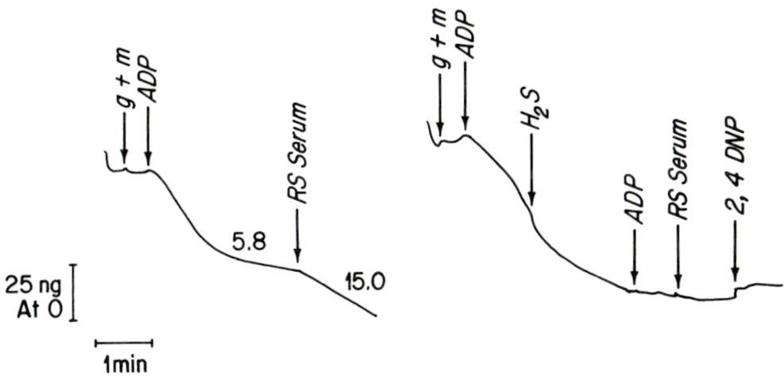

Figure 3. Hydrogen sulfide (H_2S) was shown to block
the effect of Reye's syndrome (RS) serum on mitochondrial respiratory rate. On the left, an addition of RS
serum done during state 4 respiration caused the usual
increase in oxygen consumption. On the right, H_2S (f.c.
~ 20 uM) was added to block electron transport.
Another addition of ADP demonstrated that the H_2S was
effective. The subsequent addition of RS serum caused
no change in oxygen consumption. A final addition of
2,4 dinitrophenol (2,4 DNP, f.c. 40 uM) verified that
electron transport was still inhibited. Other details
and abbreviations same as Figure 1.

the electron transport chain of liver mitochondria at
a point beyond phosphorylation site II (Fig. 4). (This
does not obviate the possibility that in the absence of
any inhibitors, the serum factor may interact at other
sites in the cytochrome chain as well). If the factor
is able to cause a reduction of cytochromes cc_1 or aa_3
in a way that does not depend on electron transport
from the first part of the respiratory chain, it is
possible that electron flow from normal substrates
could be impaired.
     Because the effect is insensitive to antimycin A,
it cannot be attributed to a classic uncoupling mechanism which depends upon the normal flow of electrons
from an NADH- or FADH-linked substrate. This would seem
to rule out substances such as salicylates, bile acids
or free fatty acids, all of which are known uncouplers
which might be suspected to be in excess in Reye's syndrome serum. Further evidence that the effect of Reye's
syndrome serum is not due to free fatty acids nor to
bilirubin is derived from the observation that it cannot

be antagonized by excess bovine serum albumin (Fig. 5).
Albumin has been shown to reverse the uncoupling effect
of free fatty acids and bilirubin when added to respiring
mitochondria _in vitro_ (14, 15). Because of the special
attention that the short-chain acid, pent-4-enoate, has
received as an agent which produces Reye's syndrome-
like features in animals (16), we tested this compound
directly in our assay system. At a concentration of
1 mM, no change in state 4 respiration was observed.

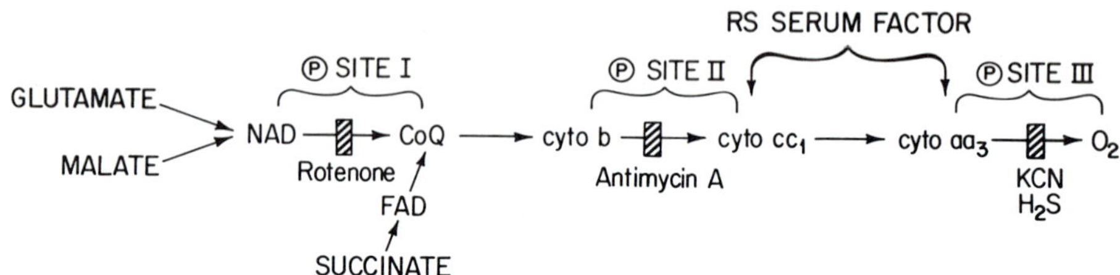

Figure 4. A diagrammatic representation of the known
sites of action of specific electron transport chain
inhibitors as these relate to the probable site of
action of a Reye's syndrome (RS) serum factor. The
inhibitors rotenone, antimycin A and KCN interfere with
electron transport at phosphorylation sites I, II, and
III respectively. H_2S also inhibits at site III. Since
the effect of RS serum on O_2 consumption was not blocked
by rotenone or antimycin A, but was blocked by KCN and
H_2S, the RS serum factor is probably able to interact
with the terminal region of the chain, between sites II
and III as indicated by the bracketed arrows.

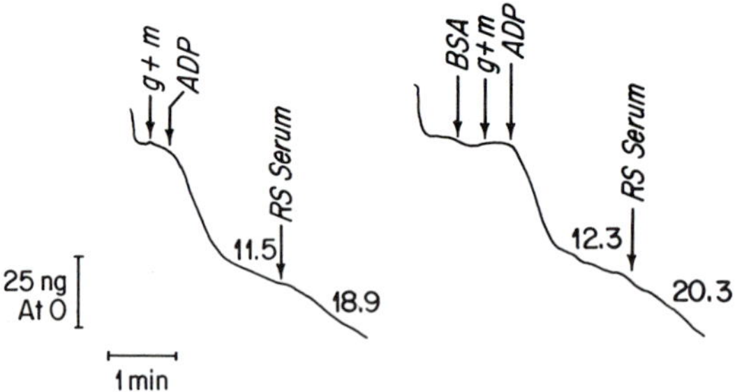

Figure 5. The effect of Reye's syndrome serum was not
blocked by the prior addition of bovine serum albumin
(BSA, f.c. 3.0 mg/ml) to the mitochondrial assay. Assay
details are the same as Figure 1.

We have also tested NH_4Cl directly at concentrations which mimic the extraordinarily high ammonia levels often seen in Reye's syndrome serum (8). No effect of NH_4Cl was apparent. If Reye's syndrome serum was deaminated (by repeated additions of NaOH and degassing to neutral pH), the effect of serum on state 4 respiration was not diminished.

<u>Structure</u>. We have previously shown by electron microscopy that Reye's syndrome serum causes morphological changes in isolated rat liver mitochondria that qualitatively resemble mitochondrial changes seen in liver biopsies from Reye's syndrome patients. The matrix appeared swollen and cristae were disorganized (8).

Mitochondrial swelling can be followed in a more quantitative fashion spectrophotometrically. Increases in swelling are measured as decreases in light-scattering, or more properly, as decreases in non-specific absorbance. For the experiment shown in Figure 6-A, the difference in optical density at 520 nm between a reference and sample cuvette was continuously recorded using an Aminco DW 2a spectrophotometer in the split-beam mode. The first recording in Figure 6-A shows the effect of adding normal serum filtrate to the sample cuvette. A slow rate of limited swelling (3.25×10^{-3} O.D. units/min) was observed. If serum filtrate from a Reye's syndrome patient was added to the sample cuvette instead of normal serum, continuous rapid swelling (8.75×10^{-3} O.D./min) occurred as shown by the second recording in Figure 6-A. Figure 6-B is included to show that the control and Reye's sera used in this particular experiment had the usual disparate effects on state 4 respiration which mirrored their respective effects on mitochondrial swelling.

The significance of mitochondrial swelling is a complicated topic (17, 18) and will not be discussed in detail here. However it should be noted that swelling can occur in an energy-linked respiration-dependent mode. The degree of swelling is dependent upon the particular electron donor available and is greater for substrates which support bi-directional electron transport. It is thus possible that the change in respiratory activity caused by Reye's

Syndrome serum is directly related to the concomitant
swelling. It is also possible that the swelling caused
by Reye's syndrome "serum factor" may be osmotic,
perhaps due to a change in the otherwise selective permeability of the inner mitochondrial membrane.
Therefore, at this stage of the investigation, both
swelling and respiratory changes can be attributed
to Reye's syndrome serum, but the cause-effect
relationship of these two phenomena is not clear.

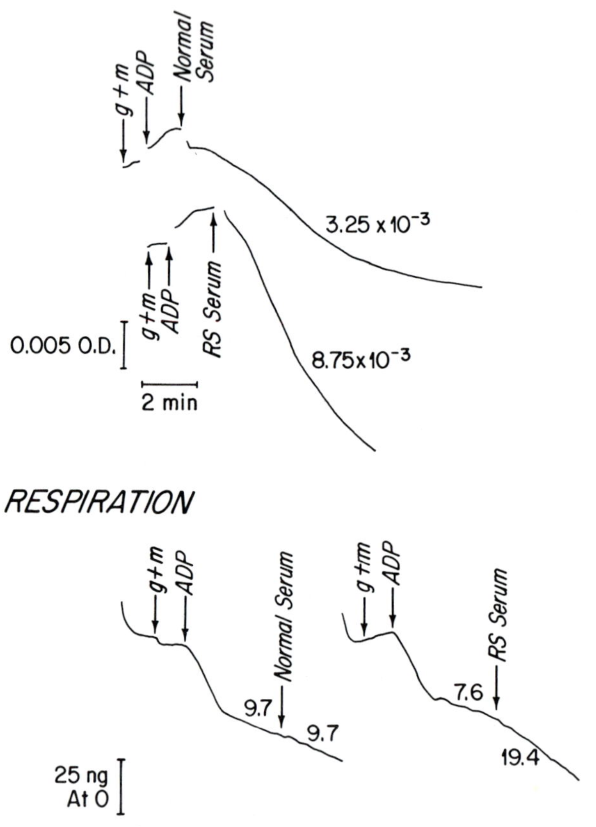

Figure 6. The effects of normal serum and Reye's syndrome serum on mitochondrial swelling (A), compared
with the effects of these same sera on respiratory rate
(B). In A, non-specific absorbance was recorded as a
function of time. The polarographic assays in B were
performed as described in previous figures. In A, rates
are in units of O.D./min; in B, units are ngatoms O/min.

Molecular characterization

     Serum was passed through filters having defined
pore sizes in an attempt to estimate molecular weight.
The series of filters used (Amicon, Lexington, MA) had
nominal molecular cut-offs of approximately 50,000 MW,
1000 MW and 500 MW. After every filtration step, the
material retained on the filter as well as the filtrate
were tested in the bioassay for the expected effect on
rat-liver mitochondria. The filtrate was positive in
each case (Table 1). The retained fractions were negative. There was occasionally a small amount of activity
detected in the fraction retained by the 500 MW filter.
However, this was barely significant compared to the
500 MW filtrate which was strongly positive in the
bioassay. On the basis of these experiments, we guessed
the molecular weight of the active substance to be less
than approximately 500 daltons.

Table 1. Molecular weight characterization of Reye's
syndrome serum factor by filtration under N_2 pressure
through Amicon filters of defined pore size.

AMICON FILTER	MW CUT-OFF	ACTIVITY (ΔngAt O/MIN) RETENTATE	FILTRATE
XM 50	50,000	0	17.0
UM 2	1,000	0	16.0
UM 05	500	1.9	10.3

     In another experiment, an ultrafiltrate of Reye's
syndrome serum was fractionated by gel chromatography
in Bio-gel P-2 which has a range of 200-2000 daltons.
Each of the eluted fractions was tested in the bioassay
for an effect on rat liver mitochondria. As shown in
Figure 7, all the positive activity was found in fractions eluting in a region associated with a molecular
weight of no more than about 450 daltons. This rough
estimate agrees with the results obtained by ultra-
filtration.

Because the "serum factor" eluted at the lower limit of the fractionation range for Bio-gel P-2, the possibility that it might be a simple ion has been considered. We have ruled out Ca^{++}, NH_4^+, Cl^-, and Na^+ by direct tests in the bioassay (8,9). $PO_4^=$, K^+, and Mg^{++} are already present in excess in the bioassay medium. No ions other than some of those considered here have been reported to be in unusually high concentrations in Reye's syndrome. Furthermore, it would be difficult to relate the observed effects on respiratory activity to any other common ions.

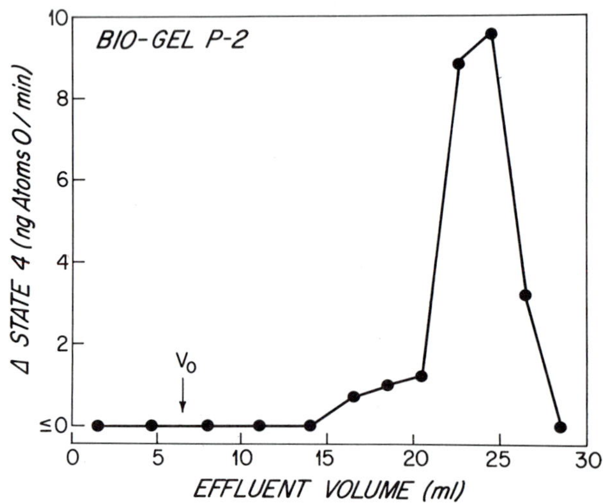

Figure 7. Molecular weight characterization of Reye's syndrome serum factor by column chromatography. 0.5 ml of a 20-fold concentrate of an ultrafiltrate (UM 2 filter) of RS serum was layered onto a Bio-gel P-2 column and was eluted with distilled water. Fractions of approximately 3 ml were collected through the first 15 ml of effluent; 2 ml fractions were collected thereafter. All fractions were lyophilized and reconstituted to one-tenth volume with distilled water. Each was tested for an effect on state 4 respiratory activity as described in the text and in Figure 1. The value obtained (Δngatoms O/min) for each fraction was plotted as a function of the midpoint of the fraction volume. The column dimensions were 1.5 X 11.5 cm. The void volume (V_o) was determined to be 6.5 ml using dextran blue.

Since the putative factor appears to be of small molecular weight, it is reasonable to suppose that it might cross the cell membrane _in vivo_, but at present this remains speculative. The molecular weight of ≤ 450 certainly precludes the possibility of a large protein. This conjecture is further supported by the observation that the effect of Reye's syndrome serum is stable to 5 minutes of boiling and to repeated freeze-thawing.

Occurrence

Data from tests using sera from 9 Reye's patients in Stage III-IV coma, and a number of control patients (including those in hepatic coma with liver cirrhosis, chronic active liver disease, or salicylate poisoning) were compared in an earlier report (8). Since that time, other additional sera have been tested. Of a total of 23 Reye's patient sera tested since we began the study three years ago only one has failed to cause any change in state 4 respiratory activity. Results from a recent series are summarized in Table 2.

Table 2. The effect of sera from several groups of donors on state 4 respiratory rate.

DONOR	n	Δ RATE (ngAt O/min) $\bar{x}$	S.E.M.	RANGE
NORMAL	4	2.1	1.0	-0.7-5.5
PARENTS, SIBLINGS	6	2.4	0.6	0-3.6
CHRON. ACT. HEPATITIS	3	3.3	1.5	0.4-5.2
ENCEPHALITIS	2	4.8	-	4.7-4.8
RS STAGE III or IV	8	9.7	2.3	1.5-19.0

The average change in state 4 respiration was higher for sera from Reye's syndrome patients as compared to sera from normal donors, siblings and parents of Reye's

syndrome patients, or patients with encephalitis or
chronic active hepatitis. The distribution of individual values is depicted in Figure 8. Using a simple
paired Student's test we determined that the Reye's
syndrome group shown in Figure 8 was different from
both the normal group and parent-sibling group at a
confidence level of p<.06 and p<.02 respectively. The
small number of individuals in the other control groups
did not justify a statistical comparison, but the mean
increase in state 4 respiration in the Reye's group
was at least twice the average of any of the other
groups.

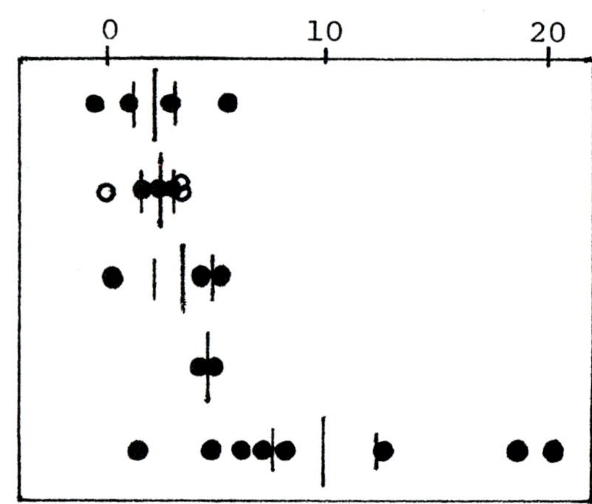

Figure 8. Sera from Reye's syndrome (RS) patients,
or from those in the several normal and disease control groups listed here were tested for an effect on
state 4 respiratory rate as described in Methods and
Figure 1.   The value obtained (Δnanogram-atoms
O/min) for each individual serum sample is displayed
here to show the group distributions.

One might ask whether the positive effect of
Reye's syndrome serum is due to the presence of a
unique substance, or due to the absence of the normally occurring inhibitor of a deleterious substance.
The latter possibility does not appear to be correct,
because the addition of excess normal serum prior to
the addition of Reye's syndrome serum in the bioassay
did not prevent the expected stimulation of state 4
respiration (Fig. 9).

We have noted that some normal sera do have a
slight stimulatory effect on state 4 respiration.
When it occurs, this small effect shows sensitivity
to several inhibitors that is identical to that seen
with the larger effect of Reye's syndrome serum. This
suggests that the active substance may be present at
very low concentrations in normal individuals. It is
conceivable that the pathogenic mechanism in Reye's
involves an abnormal accumulation of an intrinsic
substance which at high concentrations is deleterious
to mitochondria.

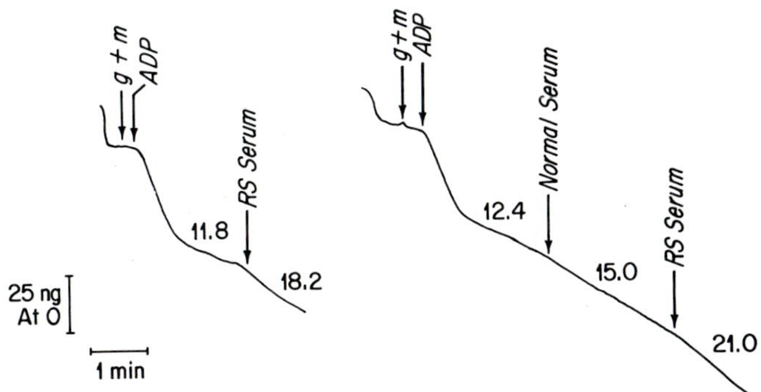

Figure 9. The effect of Reye's syndrome (RS) serum
on state 4 respiratory rate is not prevented by the
prior addition of excess normal serum. On the left,
the change in state 4 respiration caused by the
addition of 5 ul RS serum (5-fold concentrated) is
shown. On the right, 10 ul normal serum (also 5-
fold concentrated) preceded the addition of 5 ul RS
serum. Other details and abbreviations given in
Figure 1.

SUMMARY AND SPECULATION

We have described an unusual effect of Reye's syndrome serum on mitochondria. The specific molecule which mediates the alteration in mitochondrial structure and function has not yet been identified, but progress has been made toward that end. We do know that it must have a molecular weight of less than 500 daltons and that it is heat-stable. It is not likely to be a free fatty acid nor any of the following ions: NH_4^+, K^+, Mg^{++}, $PO_4^=$, Cl^-, Na^+, Ca^{++}. We also have gained some insights into the _in vitro_ mechanism of action of the putative serum factor. In liver mitochondria, the factor does not appear to behave as a true uncoupler of oxidative phosphorylation. The factor is able to interact at the terminal region of the cytochrome chain in a way that suggests electron transport in that region is stimulated. In some ways, the factor behaves as though it were an electron donor itself. Since oxygen consumption continues in the presence of the factor, the substance cannot be viewed as an absolute respiratory blocker.

The relationship of these observations to the compromised state of energy metabolism in Reye's syndrome remains to be clarified. In spite of the obvious pitfalls of extrapolating from mitochondria _in vitro_ to an _in situ_ mechanism, we will (for the sake of discussion) allow the speculation that the factor may have a role in the pathophysiology of Reye's syndrome. At present, a hypothetical mechanism is envisioned in which the steady state redox potential of the cytochromes may be changed sufficiently to alter the kinetics of oxidative phosphorylation via NADH and FADH-linked electron donors.

The serum factor we have described is not likely to be the primary etiologic agent in Reye's syndrome, since preliminary evidence suggests that it may be present at very low levels in normal serum. Instead it probably arises as an overproduction (or decreased clearance) of an intrinsic metabolite, as a consequence of the response of certain cells to a critical combination of etiologic circumstances (see Fig. 10). It is most certain that Reye's syndrome is related to an antecedent viral illness; synergistic effects of

enviromental toxins and/or genetic factors may further predispose the victim to develop the clinical
features finally identified as Reye's syndrome. We
can even suppose that several different combinations
of etiological circumstances may find a common final
metabolic pathway that is altered to result in the
accumulation of the deleterious factor ("x" in Figure
10). This substance "x" then may interfere with
mitochondrial function in several tissues, resulting
in an interdependent cascading sequence of metabolic
changes. For example, the function of mitochondria
in neurons may be directly affected by the substance.

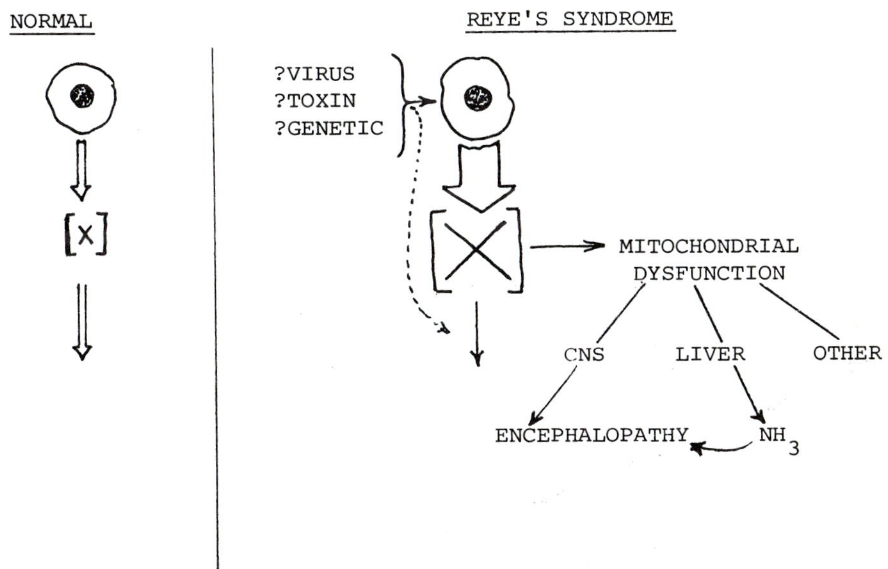

Figure 10. Hypothetical scheme depicting a possible
role for an endogenously produced serum factor in
Reye's Syndrome. The factor ("x") may be present at
low levels in normal individuals as shown on the left,
where production balances clearance. In Reye's syndrome, (right side of diagram) several etiologic circumstances may combine to trigger an accumulation of
"x" by increasing production (large arrow) or
impairing clearance (small arrow). At high concentrations "x" is deleterious to mitochondria. See
text for additional explanation.

If CNS endothelium were also affected, ion transport
(an ATP dependent process) would be impaired so that
cerebral edema would contribute further to the encephalopathy. In some cases, aerobic metabolism may be
further compromised by increasing ammonia concentrations; ammonia concentrations may be increased due to
the effect of the substance "x" on liver mitochondrial
functions, which include critical steps in ammonia detoxification. The possible relationship of mitochondrial injury to other clinical symptoms in Reye's
syndrome has been discussed in further detail elsewhere
(8,9) and recently reviewed (10).

Does the serum factor have a pathogenic role in
Reye's syndrome? Further investigation of the serum
factor's mechanism of action at the cellular and biochemical level will provide the information necessary
to decide whether the ideas presented here are correct.
This approach holds a great deal of promise as a step
toward understanding an extremely complicated illness.

ACKNOWLEDGEMENTS

We gratefully acknowledge the generous and gracious
cooperation of the following individuals who have provided the serum samples necessary for the progress of
this work.

G. Carpenter	L. Lansky	J.S. Partin
D. DeVivo	I. Lotte	D. Shannon
J. Fisher	F. Lovejoy	A. Silverman
H. Green	R. Mathis	J. Sones
J. Haller	S. Palfrey	W.A. Walker
A. Lake	J.C. Partin	

The study was supported in part by a grant from the
Charles H. Hood Foundation. We thank Peter Tullson and
Mark Buseck for assistance in some of the laboratory
work.

REFERENCES

1. Reye, R.D.K., Morgan, G. and Baral, J. 1963.
    Encephalopathy and fatty degeneration of the vis-
    cera: A disease entity in childhood. Lancet 2:749.

2. Partin, J.C., Schubert, W.K. and Partin, J.S. 1971.
    Mitochondrial ultrastructure in Reye's syndrome
    (encephalopathy and fatty degeneration of the vis-
    cera). N. Engl. J. Med. 285:1339.

3. Chang, L.W., Gilbert, E.F., Tanner, W. and Moffat,
    H.L. 1973. Reye syndrome. Light and electron
    microscopic studies. Arch. Pathol. 96:127.

4. Partin, J.C., Partin, J.S. and Schubert, W.K. 1977.
    Muscle ultrastructure in Reye's syndrome. Pediatr.
    Res. 11:564.

5. Partin, J.C., Partin, J.S., Schubert, W.K., and
    McLauren, R.L. 1975. Brain ultrastructure in
    Reye's syndrome (encephalopathy and fatty altera-
    tion of the viscera). J. Neuropathol. Exp. Neurol.
    34:425.

6. Collins, D.N. 1974. Ultrastructural study of
    intranuclear inclusions in the endocrine pancreas
    in Reye's syndrome. Lab. Invest. 30:333.

7. Morales, A.R., Bourgeois, C.H. and Chulacharit, E.
    1971. Pathology of the heart in Reye's syndrome.
    Am. J. Cardiol. 27:314.

8. Aprille, J.R. 1977. Reye's syndrome: patient serum
    alters mitochondrial function and morphology _in_
    vitro. Science 197:908.

9. Aprille, J.R. and Asimakis, G.K. 1977. Reye's
    syndrome: the effect of patient serum on mito-
    chondrial respiration _in vitro_. Biochem. Biophys.
    Res. Comm. 79:1122.

10. DeVivo, D.C. 1978. Reye syndrome: A metabolic
    response to an acute mitochondrial insult? Neurol.
    28:105.

11. Haymond, M.W., Karl, I.E., Keating, J.P. and DeVivo,
    D.C. 1978. Metabolic response to hypertonic
    glucose administration in Reye syndrome. Ann.
    Neurol. 3:207.

12. Lovejoy, F.H., Smith, A.L., and Bresnan, M.J. 1974.
    Clinical staging in Reye syndrome. Am. J. Dis.
    Child. 128:36.

13. Kessler, R.J., Tyson, C.A. and Green, D.E. 1976.
    Mechanism of uncoupling in mitochondria: Uncoup-
    lers as ionophores for cycling cations and protons.
    Proc. Natl. Acad. Sci. (U.S.A.) 73:2141.

14. Weinbach, E.C. and Garbus, J. 1966. Restoration by
    albumin of oxidative phosphorylation and related
    reactions. J. Biol. Chem. 241:169.

15. Bjorntorp, P., Ells, H.A. and Bradford, R.H. 1964.
    Albumin antagonism of fatty acid effects on
    oxidation and phosphorylation reactions in rat
    liver mitochondria. J. Biol. Chem. 239:339.

16. Glasgow, A. and Chase, H.P. 1975. Production of
    the features of Reye's syndrome in rats with 4-pen-
    tenoic acid. Pediatr. Res. 9:133.

17. Packer, L. 1967. Energy-linked low amplitude
    mitochondrial swelling. In Methods in Enzy-
    mology X, M.E. Pullman, Ed. pp. 685-689.
    Academic Press, New York, N.Y.

18. Hunter, F.E. and Smith, E.E. 1967. Measurement of
    mitochondrial swelling and shrinking-High amplitude.
    In Methods in Enzymology X, M.E. Pullman, Ed. pp.
    689-696. Academic Press, New York, N.Y.

DISCUSSION

C. Solomons -   Did you have an opportunity to do
             any PO ratios on your mitochondria?

J.R.Aprille   -   In these studies,we were adding ser-
             um to the assay during state 4 respiration.
             In order to do PO ratios, serum would have
             to be added at the beginning of state 3.That
             was done in some of my earlier work,and
             there was an apparent increase in the PO,as

though oxygen consumption was unproductive-
ly stimulated, but the statistics were marginally significant. I might add also that
in this system we are looking at changes in
the mitochondria within a few minutes of
the addition of serum, whereas in vivo the
situation is very different, because there
is a chronic exposure to this factor over a
long period of time.

G.D. Gall   -   I wonder if you've looked at pyruvate
or lactic acid in your experimental system,
to see if there is any effect on respiration?

J.R. Aprille-   Pyruvic acid or lactic acid have not
specifically been looked at. Either of
these might serve as a substrate for oxada-
tive phosphorylation, so they might be expected to change the rate of respiration.
But such an effect would certainly be
blocked by antimycin A. You will recall
that the effect of serum factor is NOT
blocked by antimycin A.

S.H. Lee   -   Can you tell me if anybody looked for
the serum factor in urine, in light of its
low molecular weight?

J.R. Aprille-   That has occurred to us. I have one
Reye's patient urine sample recently obtained from Dr. Haller, but I have not yet
tested it. I have one other urine that had
been stored since 1974 which was negative,
even though the serum for that patient was
very positive. However, I dug the urine
sample out of somebody's freezer and I
don't know the storage history, so I can't
draw a general conclusion.

S.H. Lee   -   Are these specifically for liver mitochondria?

J.R. Aprille-   We have tested mitochondria from a
                  number of other tissues. There is an ef-
                  fect of Reye's serum on mitochondria iso-
                  lated from brain but the mechanism appears
                  different from that in liver. The serum
                  appears to be acting more like an un-
                  coupler in brain, because the effect is
                  blocked by antimycin A, but not by oligo-
                  mycin. Interestingly, we have not been
                  able to show a consistent effect on mus-
                  cle mitochondria. This is due to one of
                  two reasons: either there is something
                  different about muscle mitochondria which
                  predisposes them differently to the fac-
                  tor, or we haven't quite got the condi-
                  tions right in the assay to see an effect.
                  In any case, I remember yesterday Doctor
                  Partin showed electron micrographs of bi-
                  opsied muscle mitochondria that were very
                  different than those seen in liver, sug-
                  gesting that the muscle mitochondria are
                  not affected to the same extent. This a-
                  grees very well with what we have seen in
                  vitro.

M.R. Hurley -   Do the survivors have this serum
                  factor?

J.R. Aprille -   Do you mean after they have recover-
                  ed, as opposed to the critical stages of
                  illness?

M.R. Hurley -   Yes.

J.R. Aprille -   No,they don't. They're back to nor-
                  mal, but I can't remember offhand the num-
                  ber of patients that we've tested in that
                  category.

M.R. Hurley -   But,those that you did do, do they
                  still retain the factor?

J.R. Aprille -   No,they don't. I might add that we
                  tested one patient who died, who had a

very large titre of this factor, the most positive we've ever seen at the early stage of the
illness. She died within 72 hours of admission.
A premortem blood sample was negative; which is
interesting because it appears as though the
factor had come and gone by the time that she
expired.

J.C. Partin   - In your Britton Chance - type mitochondrial swelling studies, do you think that
there was actually an increase in volume of the
mitochondria to account for the change in optical density, or was there a change in matrix
conformation first?

J.R. Aprille   - I think there is change in matrix
composition first,followed by a change in volume.
Let me simplify that a bit. The electron micrograph published in an earlier report showed a
clearing of the matrix which would account for
a decrease in optical density. That was after
a 10-minute exposure to serum. We had also a
30-minute exposure to serum, which I am not prepared to show as yet because we'd like to do a
much more careful time sequence of the change,
but at 30 minutes the mitochondria were completely blown apart.

J.C. Partin   - So, you initially see low amplitude
swelling in the old terminology?

J.R. Aprille - Yes; I would say so. But it is hard to
distinguish because the low amplitude swelling
probably progresses quickly to high amplitude
swelling in the first few minutes. Therefore, I
really don't want to distinguish between the two
on the basis of that experiment.

Unidentified   - What about storage of activity,either
in the whole serum or after it has been concentrated? Do you know anything about stability of
the activity?

J.R. Aprille   -   We have tested positive samples
            that have been in people's freezers since
            1974. We obviously didn't test them in 1974
            so we don't know if activity has diminished
            since then, but we have repeatedly freeze-
            thawed all of our samples and a couple of
            times they have accidentally been left on the
            table, with no loss of activity. The activity
            is also stable to boiling.

Unidentified   -   I can't remember from your writing
            whether you have looked at the total serum
            osmolarity or osmotic strength before you
            start concentrating it.

J.R. Aprille   -   No; we have not but we are only
            adding 10 microlitres of the concentrated
            serum to a 1 ml. assay, so osmotic effects on
            the mitochondria probably are not the over-
            whelming factor in any case. We were worried
            about that possibility and did test super-
            concentrated salt solutions in 10 micro-
            litre quantities directly added to the as-
            says, but we saw nothing like what we see
            with the serum.

B.A. Faraj   -   Have you simply tried to take your
            serum, precipitate your protein out, and
            check the supernatant, to see whether it has
            any effect or not?

J.R. Aprille   -   No; but we have effectively done
            that in another way, using the filtration
            techniques. The serum was filtered through
            filters,cutting everything off above molecu-
            lar weight 500, which certainly removes any-
            thing that would be precipitated in an acid
            precipitation. The activity remains in the
            low molecular weight fraction, and we are
            not faced with the problem of getting rid of
            the acid. Because we have small quantities of
            serum,we have avoided multistep procedures.

B.A. Faraj   -   And also, if you have enough serum
                you can extract your protein free fraction
                under different pH medium and check the acti-
                vity under acidic extraction or basic extrac-
                tion. You can get a fairly good idea what
                you're looking at as to whether the compound
                is an amine or is an acidic compound, or
                whether it is an aromatic.

J.R. Aprille   -   Yes; we have some experiments plan-
                ned like that, but we are trying to concen-
                trate on micro techniques in the interest of
                making the most use of what serum we have. I
                would also like to try, for example, a DEAE
                column which should tell us what the charge
                is, and some electrophoresis which should
                give us new information.

D.B. Tower   -   The molecular weight puts it in
                the class most likely of amino acids or pur-
                ine, pyrimidine nucleotides or something of
                that sort. These can be looked at rather easi-
                ly in a gross fashion. The nucleotides can be
                looked at fluorometrically and, since we know
                certain amino acids are elevated in Reye's
                serum, these could be looked at unofficially,
                so to speak. Have you checked any of those
                possibilities?

J.R. Aprille   -   No; this is a matter of philosophy,
                I think, because if you think about what we
                have with the semi-purified fraction, which
                is everything under 500 molecular weight,
                there must be a huge number of substances(in-
                cluding those you mentioned) that are still
                present. We could hypothesize about what's
                there and start testing a number of those
                different things. We have tested some obvious
                substances,like the 4-pentenoic, and we will
                now test tyramine and some other things that
                we hear about from time to time. But I think
                we are going to put most of our efforts into
                continuing purification, in order to limit
                the possibilities that we have to test.

RECENT DEVELOPMENTS AND CONTRIBUTIONS FROM
EXPERIMENTAL MODELS OF REYE'S SYNDROME

Frederick L. Ruben, M.D.

INTRODUCTION

Reye's syndrome (RS) may well be a disease of
diverse etiology. The wide range of animal models
studied to date, many of which show fatty involvement
of organs and biochemical derangements, lend support to
the notion of multiple causation for RS. This paper
addresses the role of influenza virus infection in producing the picture of RS in animals. Surprisingly,
there are very few studies to cite despite the fifteen-
year-long association between influenza virus and RS
(1). It is true, however, that the great bulk of
data associating RS and influenza has come within the
past five years with the RS epidemic of 1973-74 associated with influenza B virus (2) and the recent
report of Partin et al showing recovery of influenza A
from liver, muscle, cerebrospinal fluid and respiratory
secretions of a male with RS (3).

I would first like to report on studies in Pitts-
burgh in collaboration with Dr. Harvey Mendelow of
Montefiore Hospital and Dr. R. E. Brown of Huntingdon,
PA.

Stimulated by our finding of large clusters of RS
cases in association with epidemic influenza, particularly type B but also with type A (4), and the
peculiar geographic distribution of RS cases, all from
suburban or rural areas outside the city of Pittsburgh
(5), we were encouraged by the reports of Crocker and

colleagues that viral-toxin interactions might precipitate RS in susceptible children (6). We studied
in a baby hamster model, the biochemical and
histologic effects of selected chemicals with and without influenza infection.

MATERIALS AND METHODS

     We used three week old Syrian hamsters of mixed
sexes. The toxins studied are shown in Table I.

TABLE I.   Toxins for Exposing Animals

Category	Toxins
1. Brush killer	Esteron, Amdon 101, Daconate 6
2. Insecticide	Sevin 4 oil, Dylox 4, Malathion
3. Solvent	Xylene, SC-100, 654 solvent (HAN)
4. Emulsifier	Atlox 3406-F, Atlox 3409-F, Toximul R, Toximul S

They fall into four general categories. Categories 1
and 2 are the active ingredients for many commercial
and government spray operations, while categories 3
and 4 are widely used vehicles for spraying insecticides and herbicides. We found that undiluted toxins
in most cases were fatal to animals; therefore, toxins
were diluted 1:100 in corn oil and were brush painted
to the animals' backsides daily for ten days. Egg
grown influenza A/Eng/74 or influenza B/HK/74 virus
(isolates came from patients with proven RS) was then
administered via syringe intranasally. Animals were
sacrificed using ether anesthetic two weeks following
infection. They were bled by cardiac puncture and
tissues were removed, fixed in formalin and representative portions were processed for standard hematoxylin
and eosin (H and E) staining. In some cases oil red O
staining for lipid was performed on formalin-fixed
frozen sections. Sera were tested for glucose, alka-

line phosphatase, SGOT, and SGPT, triglycerides, and cholinesterase. Hemagglutination inhibiting (HAI) antibodies against influenza were measured pre and post infection in all animals. Control animals received either corn oil alone, influenza alone, or toxin alone. There were 10 - 20 animals per corn oil or virus alone group and 3 - 4 animals per toxin or toxin-virus group.

RESULTS

The toxins diluted 1:100 in corn oil produced some apparent listlessness in a few animals but were not fatal. Influenza A or B, alone or following toxins, never perceptibly affected any animals. All animals had homologous virus antibody titer rises. There were no cross infections, and non-infected animals remained seronegative. The virus infection produced a mild patchy pneumonia in infected animals which was resolving at time of sacrifice.

Serum biochemical studies showed that toxin alone and viral-toxin animals did not appreciably differ from corn oil or virus alone animals in levels of alkaline phosphatase, SGOT, or SGPT. Only selected sera were tested for cholinesterase, and these also showed control and test animals to be comparable.

As shown in Table 2, there were appreciate differences for mean triglyceride levels between controls, both corn oil and virus-alone groups, and toxin-alone groups. All but one toxin alone (654 solvent or HAN) showed increased mean triglycerides, and the highest triglyceride level was in the emulsifier group (Toximul S, 414 mg/dl, $p < .005$). Most influenza B plus toxin groups also showed increased triglyceride levels. Influenza A plus toxins (data not shown) had subnormal triglyceride levels in five of the six groups tested. Glucose levels were elevated over corn oil controls in all toxin alone groups and most toxin-influenza B groups. Influenza A plus toxin (data not shown) lowered the glucose levels of 3 groups or were similar to controls in 3 groups (only 6 groups were tested).

TABLE 2

Summary of Triglyceride (TG) and Glucose Studies of Animal Sera

Corn oil, virus, or toxin alone categories	Mean values mg/dl		Toxin plus influenza B	Mean values mg/dl	
	TG	Glucose		TG	Glucose
Corn oil alone	200	122	---	---	---
Influenza A alone	150	136	---	---	---
Influenza B alone	264 *	159	---	---	---
Brush killers alone	238-296	180-266	Brush killers	239-283	176-208
Insecticides alone	239-282	127-168	Insecticides	198-247	108-185
Solvents alone	198-246	149-235	Solvents	230-283	162-182
Emulsifiers alone	241-414	167-202	Emulsifiers	235-346	127-204

*Mean values for individual agents in group, lowest-highest (e.g. Amdon 101
was 238; Esteron was 296; Daconate 6 was 254).

Histologic studies on H and E stained sections of
paraffin imbedded portions of liver showed no apparent
abnormalities. Results of all Oil red O fat stains are
shown in Table 3. Grade 0 represents no fat droplets
whereas grade 4+ stands for diffuse fine droplet fat,
with grades 1+ to 3+ of intermediate degree. Slides
were coded and read without knowledge of the code.
Five of six animals (83%) given corn oil alone showed
no fat, differing from the collective group given toxin
or virus alone in which eight of thirty (27%) showed no
fat (p<.05), and also differing from the group given
toxin plus influenza B where only one of sixteen animals (6%) showed no fat (p<.01). The toxin plus virus
group was not significantly different from the virus or
toxin alone groups. Of note is the striking fatty
involvement occurring with influenza B alone and with
Toximul R alone.

TABLE 3.   Presence of Oil Red O Fat in Liver Tissue

| Animal Group | Grade*: | No. Animals With | | | | |
		0	1^+	2^+	3^+	4^+
Corn oil alone		5	1	0	0	0
Influenza B alone		3	4	3	0	4
Dylox 4 alone		0	2	1	1	0
Toximul R alone		0	0	0	4	0
Toximul S alone		3	0	1	0	0
Sevin 4 alone		2	1	0	1	0
Dylox 4 + Infl. B		0	3	0	0	1
Toximul R + Infl. B.		0	2	0	2	0
Toximul S + Infl. B		0	2	2	0	0
Sevin 4 + Infl. B		1	1	2	0	0

*Range of intensity reckoned on a scale of 0 to 4+

DISCUSSION

These studies in baby hamsters of influenza viruses and selected environmental toxins suggest that
either viruses or toxins alone are capable of producing
metabolic and histologic alterations. The metabolic

alterations found were of a significant but mild degree
revealing abnormalities of serum lipids and of glucose
utilization, both of which are consistent with RS. The
presence of hepatocellular lipid inclusions, not evident using standard H and E staining, was revealed in
the oil red O stained sections. Such accumulation is
compatible with that seen in RS patients, realizing of
course that the exact characterization of the lipid
inclusions in this model by histochemical, ultrastructural, biochemical and/or chromatographic means has yet
to be performed.

We did not show any combined or synergistic
effects of toxin plus virus as others have shown (7,8).
Until we modify our protocol for time of exposure and
sacrifice of animals in a variety of ways, we hesitate
to conclude that combined or synergistic effects are
unlikely. Furthermore, since human studies are conclusive that RS produces characteristic mitochondrial
lesions (9,10), we are anxious to study the mitochondrial ultrastructure of livers and renal tissues of
various groups in our model.

A potentially limiting factor in the model we
have studied is the use of non-adapted influenza
viruses. Since death is an unbiased endpoint for
animal studies, results might be significantly altered
when using hamster adapted virus strains of influenza
A or B.

We conclude from our hamster studies that
exposure to a variety of environmental toxins and to
influenza viruses, separately or together, is capable
of inducing biochemical and histologic alterations
compatible with RS as seen in patients.

The only published report by another investi-
gator looking for influenza-induced findings in animals
compatible with RS is that of Pierson et al (11).
These investigators followed up on the observations of
Thaler et al (12) and Brown et al (13) who found
reductions in serum enzyme activity for ornithine transcarbamylase (OTC) and carbamyl phosphate synthetase
(CPS) in RS patients and related these enzyme reductions

to their hyperammonemia. Pierson infected mice with
adapted influenza A/PR/8/34 or influenza B/Lee/40
given intranasally. Such infections regularly induced
death, however, animals were sacrificed at 5 to 6 days,
shortly before death was expected. After sacrifice,
liver homogenates were studied for OTC and CPS activity,
along with control mice and control human liver homogenates from persons dying without liver disease.
Their results showed that OTC and CPS activity of
influenza infected mice was 83 to 98% of that found in
normal control mice. Normal human liver enzyme activities were comparable to other published results. The
reductions in infected animals were not of the
magnitude (80% reduction) cited by Thaler in RS
patients, however. Their conclusion was that the reduction of OTC and CPS activity reported in RS in man
is not a general manifestation of the severity of the
associated influenza infection.

Thus far I have cited two studies, one failing to
indicate an additive effect of mild influenza infection
to the toxin induced abnormalities of a hamster model,
and a second study failing to show that severe influenza
infection could contribute significantly to urea cycle
enzyme depression in a rat model. There is published
a wide experience in studying influenza A viruses in
laboratory and domestic animals (14); indeed,
influenza is a naturally acquired infection in many
such animals (15). It seems unlikely but admit-
tedly is possible that a RS-like picture would have
been missed. Most virus studies in animals have not
concentrated on biochemical derangements or on special
histologic studies for fat or for ultrastructural
changes.

Partin has suggested that RS may be an epiphen-
omena of influenza (3). Animal studies, to date,
fail to produce compelling evidence to support or re-
fute this hypothesis. Until more studies are done,
using animal models with adapted influenza viruses and
looking specifically for histologic and biochemical
derangements seen in RS, the question remains open.

REFERENCES

1. Johnson, G., Scurletis, T., and Carroll, N. 1963.
    A study of 16 fatal cases of encephalitis-like
    disease in North Carolina. *N.C. Med. J. 24:*464.
2. Corey, L., Rubin, R.J., Hattwick, M.A.W., Noble,
    G.R., and Cassidy, E., 1976. A nationwide outbreak
    of Reye's syndrome. *Am.J.Med. 61:*615.
3. Partin, J.C., Partin, J.S., Schubert, W.K., Jacobs,
    R. and Saalfeld, K. 1976. Isolation of influenza
    virus from liver and muscle biopsy specimens from
    a surviving case of Reye's syndrome. *Lancet. 2:*599.
4. Ruben, F.L. and Michaels, R.H. 1975. Reye's
    syndrome with associated influenza A and B infection.
    *J.A.M.A. 234:*410.
5. Ruben, F.L., Streiff, E.J., Neal, M. and Michaels,
    R.H. 1976. Epidemiologic studies of Reye's syndrome:
    cases seen in Pittsburgh, October 1973 - April
    1975. *Am. J. Publ. Hlth. 66:*1096.
6. Crocker, J.F.S., Ozere, R.L., Safe, S.H., Digout,
    S.C., Rozee, K.R. and Hutzinger, O. 1976. Lethal
    interaction of ubiquitious insecticide carriers
    with virus. *Science 192:*1351.
7. Friend, M. and Trainer, D.O. 1970. Polychlorinated
    biphenyl: interaction with duck hepatitis virus.
    *Science 170:*1315.
8. Crocker, J.F.S., Ozere, R.L., Rozee, K.R., Digout,
    S.C. and Hutzinger, O. 1974. Insecticide and viral
    interaction as a cause of fatty visceral changes
    and encephalopathy in the mouse. *Lancet 2:*22.
9. Partin, J.C., Schubert, W.K., and Partin, J.S.
    1971. Mitochondrial ultrastructure in Reye's
    syndrome. *New Eng.J.Med. 285:*1339.
10. Bove, K.E., McAdams, A.J., Partin, J.C., Partin, J.
    S., Hug, G., and Schubert, W.K. 1975. The hepatic
    lesion in Reye's syndrome. *Gastroenterol 69:*685.
11. Pierson, D., Knight, V., Hansard, P., and Chan, E.
    1976. Hepatic carbamyl phosphate synthetase and
    ornithine transcarbamylase in mouse influenza A and
    influenza B infection. *Proc.Soc.Exp.Biol.Med.*
    152·67.
12. Thaler, M.M., Hoogenraad, N.J., and Boxwell, M.
    1974. Reye's syndrome due to a novel protein-

tolerant variant of ornithine-transcarbamylase
deficiency. *Lancet* 2:438.

13. Brown, T., Hug, G., Lansky, L., Bove, K., Scheve,
     A., Ryan, M., Brown, H., Schubert, W.K., Partin,
     J.C., and Lloyd-Still, J. 1976. Transiently re-
     duced activity of carbamyl phosphate synthetase
     and ornithine transcarbamylase in liver of child-
     ren with Reye's syndrome. *New Eng.J.Med.* 294:861.

14. Hoyle, L. Experimental influenza in animals.
     pp. 243. In L. Hoyle, The influenza viruses.
     Virology monographs, Springer-Verlag, New York.

15. Hoyle, L. Natural infection with influenza virus-
     es in animals. pp. 244. Ibid.

Support in part by a grant from the Health Research
and Services Foundation of Allegheny County. The
excellent technical assistance of L. Heilman and
patient clerical help of S. Bales are acknowledged.

DISCUSSION

J.F.S. Crocker   -   Have you innoculated the full
     range of virus concentrations to lethality?
     Then, does the chemical in small dose increase
     the lethality of your virus?

F.L. Ruben   -   No. In order to do this, it is ne-
     cessary to passage the virus in animals 20 to 30
     times.

D.B. Tower   -   I would like to make a plea for at-
     tention to comparative biochemistry and physiology
     here. If you go back and look at some studies
     that Brodie and his colleagues did many years ago
     on the sleeping times of barbiturates, which de-
     pends upon the rate at which the liver metabolizes
     and detoxifies the barbiturates, you'll find a
     very marked difference between rodents and man.
     This has to do with the difference in the relative
     sizes of the liver and the brain and how much of

the circulation perfuses these two organs in different species. I think that this is a factor
which has to be taken into account in trying to
compare a human syndrome, such as Reye's, with
animal models in which you are going to have very
different ways in which rodents, particularly,
respond. The other aspect of this is the rate at
which animals mature; I have some problem with
visualizing two-week-old hamsters as babies because they are really quite mature at three weeks
and I would think you would have to go down to at
least a week or a week-and-a-half to get any sort
of equivalence to human infants and young children.

L.E. Davis -   I'm not sure you want to go to adapted
    strains, because adapted strains will cause over-
    whelming pneumonia in your animal and change your
    model completely.

J.C. Partin -   That essentially was what I was going
    to comment. I think one of the reasons why we
    have such great ignorance about Influenza B is
    that Influenza B doesn't grow well on the con-
    ventional systems that really were originally in-
    tended for Influenza A. I think most of the
    strains that have been studied extensively have
    been quite far adapted away from their human
    host. If we really are looking at an unconven-
    tional effect of a conventional virus, we proba-
    bly ought to be trying to find a system that is
    much more closely related to the human host to
    work with.

F.L. Ruben -   Could you be more specific about the
    system that you had in mind?

J.C. Partin -   I think that we need to develop either
    a human-derived cell line that would support the
    growth of Influenza B, or we need more studies in
    the basic biology of this virus as it works in
    humans. For example, it's quite unclear to me
    why Influenza B so frequently is associated with

two syndromes, Reye's syndrome and influenza myopathy. In influenza myopathy, unlike Reye's, there is no clinical or biochemical evidence of liver injury. There seems to be quite a bit of organ specificity occurring in an unpredictable fashion. Work has been done at C.D.C., trying to demonstrate some of these effects with tissue culture adapted strains, but it has not been very successful. They use highly selected viruses, since many of the primary isolates just don't grow to a sufficient titre.

M.M. Thaler -   Did you mention whether your animals became ill at all?

F.L. Ruben -   They did not become ill. Rarely, an animal would die but death was certainly random. It took place even with healthy young animals.

M.M. Thaler -   It was very interesting that you found the opposite effect of Influenza A versus Influenza B as far as the triglyceride levels were concerned. In fact, you mention that A was lower than the control -- that could mean that tissue staining might actually show higher triglyceride in your liver. Did you do any?

F.L. Ruben -   We didn't do any tissue studies for triglycerides.

J.V. Baublis-   I wonder if you have had any experience with the model that Henle described some years ago. He was able to document varied toxicity as a characteristic of Influenza A. If one gave mice intranasal doses of Influenza A virus, some got pneumonia, some became deaf, and one was never sure whether this was toxicity or whether this was pneumonia. Inoculation of a large dose of virus intraperitoneally would not replicate, and it had an entirely different effect. These animals died a toxic death and,at the time of death, only rare animals showed dissemination of virus so that lungs were only occasionally involved. On the other hand, most of

them showed a fatty degeneration of the liver and
had evidence of gastric and intestinal hemorrhage.
They also had a tendency to convulse and die. Essentially, it sounds as if he had created an influenza toxicity syndrome which mimicked,clinical-
ly, the picture of Reye's syndrome. I wonder if
anyone has tried to duplicate that, or is familiar
with it at the present time.

L.E. Davis - Yes; I think that work has a bearing on
Reye's syndrome. The thing about that system was
that he used very high titres of virus. Studies
by Mimm suggest that, under those circumstances,
most of the virus is taken up by the reticuloendothelial system of the liver and doesn't get into
the liver cells. Histologically, the system looks
a little bit different, in that there is more inflammation. This is a model which, I think, should
be revitalized and pursued in this context.

J.V. Baublis- Yes; I think specifically the infection
of the reticuloendothelial system could be very
central to the issue. The lack of an intact reticuloendothelial system could be important during
the course of a massive infection like influenza.
We are talking about biochemical changes, in
Reye's syndrome. This should be appreciated in the
context of information on the biochemical alterations of human subjects during chicken pox and
other virus infections. There is a dramatic shift
in the metabolic activities of the body. The deviation of protein synthesis, for example; instead
of going to the continued protein maintenance including enzymes, it seems to be directed toward
the production of acute phase reactants. Now,
whether these are just incomplete proteins or represent something more profound is hard to say.It
may indeed be that Reye's syndrome is really an
exaggeration of what is but a normal response to
severe infection. The influenza A model may, I
think, give us an opportunity to look at the metabolism of severe infection and determine what kind
of factors will predispose humans to central ner-

vous system complications following these metabolic reactions.

S.H. Lee   -   Doctor Ruben, is there any specific
reason why you chose the hamster as your model?

F.L. Ruben   -   Yes; I happened to be working with
hamsters in other studies, and they were convenient.

S.H. Lee   -   This raises a point. Hamsters are a
good model for studying carcinogenesis, but are
relatively poor for studying viral pathogenesis.

VIRUS LIPID INTERACTION AND REYE'S SYNDROME

Roger M. Loria, M.D., and Gordon E.Madge, M.D.

INTRODUCTION

A clinical and pathological entity which consisted of visceral fatty degeneration and encephalopathy was described by Reye, Morgan, and Baral in 1963
(1). With the increase in number of cases examined,
some of the initial pathological findings described to
be characteristic have been somewhat modified.
Presently, it is accepted that the major liver pathology
consists of fatty degeneration of hepatocyte cytoplasm,
without marked inflammation or cellular necrosis.
However, both inflammation and necrosis have been reported to occur (3,7). Fat accumulation is mostly
triglycerides. Alteration in mitochondria, with
swelling and reduction in the number of mitochondrial
dense bodies, and reduction in cellular glycogen
content which is proportional to the severity of the
disease have been documented (2,3,4).

Brain pathology consists of cerebral edema and
anoxic neuronal degeneration with no evidence of gross
inflammation (2,4). In addition, fatty degeneration of
the kidney, fatty infiltration of the heart (2,5) and,
more recently, of the coronary and aortic arteries,
and juvenile atherosclerosis have also been demonstrated
in this syndrome (6,7). Of the initial 21 cases
described by Reye et al. (1), 16 were found to have an
antecedent viral infection (8). Subsequent reports
demonstrate that an association with a viral infection
could be proven in up to 81% of all cases when intensive virological studies were performed (9).

Numerous viral agents have been reported to be associated with Reye's syndrome (RS) and it is now recognized that an antecedent viral episode is one of the several etiological factors in this disease (2).

Some of the many viral agents associated with Reye's syndrome were tabulated by Corey and Rubin (1975) (10) and are listed in table 1. The prevalence of influenza B and varicella virus in association with Reye's was made evident by Noble, Corey and Rubin (11) in their epidemiological studies. Nevertheless, Partin et al.(14) reported the isolation of influenza A (Ohio, 7/76), and an association of Reye's syndrome with adenovirus type 3 was also demonstrated by Brown (12). Other studies showed that a mixed viral infection consisting of herpes virus and a myxo or paramyxovirus was also implicated in this disease (7). Finally, coxsackievirus A crystalline arrays were observed by Alvira and Mendoza (13) in the muscle of two patients with RS and were closely associated with the mitochondria which has been suggested to be the site of pathobolism in this syndrome.

TABLE 1. Viruses Associated with Reye's Syndrome

VIRUS	REFERENCE
Adenovirus Type 3	Dvorackova,I., et al., 1966
Coxsackievirus A	Utian, H., et al., 1964
Coxsackievirus A_9	Barr, R., et al., 1968
Coxsackie B_1 & B_4	Barr, R., et al., 1968
	Johnson, G., 1963
Epstein-Barr	Rahal, T., 1970
Echo 8	Johnson, G., 1963
Echo 11	Golden, G., 1965
Herpes Simplex	Becroft, D.M.O., 1972
Influenza A	Hall, B.D., et al., 1969
Influenza B	Norman, M.G., et al., 1968
Parainfluenza	Powell, H., et al., 1973
Polio Type 1	Bell, W.E., 1974
Reovirus	Joske, R., et al., 1964
	Utian, H.L., et al., 1964
Rubella	Sherman, F.E., et al., 1965
Rubeola	Ferraro, A., 1932

Varicella	Blair, A.W., et al., 1965
	Breen, G. E., 1954
	Glick, T., et al., 1970

Modified from Corey, L., and Rubin, R.J., 1975 and
MWWR <u>20</u>: 101, 1971.

Many investigators in this field suggest that
Reye's syndrome may be caused by the interaction of
viruses, environmental factors, and host genetic
factors (11,12,16-18). Our own experimental results
have shown that viral infection in the hyperlipemic
host leads to a synergistic interaction between
viruses and lipids, resulting in a drastic increase in
lethality and a divergent pathology (19). Many of
the environmental factors implicated in Reye's
syndrome i.e., emulsifiers (16), pesticides, aflatoxins (20), and pentenoic acid (18) are recognized
for their ability to damage the liver or induce liver
fatty changes. Consequently, our findings on virus
lipid interaction suggest a possible mechanism of
action of different viral agents in a Reye's-like
syndrome. This hypothesis has further support from the
fact that most viruses associated with this syndrome,
like influenza, parainfluenza and herpes, are either
enveloped viruses containing lipid and/or fusion factor
or have a lipotropic character like the enteroviruses,
specifically group B coxsackieviruses. This increased
affinity and ability to interact in a hydrophobic environment appears to be the common denominator to most
of the viruses associated with Reye's syndrome. We
propose that a better understanding of the mode of
virus-lipid interaction may provide a rationale for
some of the pathobiological observations seen in Reye's
syndrome of Reye's syndrome-like cases. This report
presents some of our findings on virus-lipid interaction using coxsackievirus B_5 and the hypercholesteremic
mouse as our experimental system.

MATERIALS AND METHODS

Animals: adult outbred male CD-1 (Crl:(ICR) Br),
Charles River Breeding Laboratories, Wilmington, Mass.

and inbred male C57BL/6J mice from Jackson Laboratories
Bar Harbour, Maine, were used in these studies. Hypercholesteremia was induced by nutritional means as described elsewhere(19,21). A 3 to 4-fold elevation in
plasma cholesterol levels was measured within 2 to 4
weeks after initiation of this diet. Three months
later, animals were inoculated intraperitoneally with
0.5 ml of coxsackievirus B5 from a virus pool containing 6×10^9 PFU/ml or dilutions thereof. All experiments involved the following groups: 1) virus infected,
normal animals; 2) hyperlipemic,non-infected animals;
3) hyperlipemic,virus-infected animals; and 4) normal,
non-infected controls.

RESULTS

Table 2 demonstrates the effect of hypercholesteremia on the susceptibility to coxsackievirus B5 infection.

TABLE 2.   Coxsackievirus B5 Infection in CD-1 Male Mice
           on the Test (Hypercholesteremic) Diet *

DAYS POST IN-FECTION	Test Diet Infected	NO. OF ANIMALS DYING	
		Test Diet Non-Infected	ControlDiet Infected
3	3**	0	0
7	5	0	0
8	4	0	0
9	3	0	0
10	4	0	0
12	4	0	0
13	4	0	0
14	2	0	0
Survivors	1/30***	8/8	8/8

*   Animals were 5 mo. old and 3 mo. on the test diet
    when infected.
** Sacrificed at 3 days after infection; the remaining
    animals did not succumb until day 7 or more after
    infection.
*** Equivalent to 96.7% lethality.

It is clear that the combination of hypercholesteremia and infection with this dose of virus was fatal
for the adult mouse. In contrast, normal animals
infected with the same dose of virus and sham infected
hypercholesteremic mice survived without overt signs
of illness.

PATHOLOGICAL FINDINGS

The regular pathological changes associated with
dietary hypercholesteremia were observed in the non-
infected animal on this regime. These included a
marked enlargement of the liver with the appearance
of fatty changes around the central blood vessels without evidence of cellular infiltrates. Despite the
high level of blood cholesterol no evidence of
atherogenic changes were seen in either the heart or
aorta.

Examination of coxsackievirus B5 infected hypercholesteremic mice liver tissues revealed severe fatty
metamorphosis which involved almost all hepatic cells
with cellular necrosis but a conspicuous absence of
an inflammatory infiltrate. Since a cellular infiltration is one of the pathologic hallmarks for recognition of a viral infection, this observation is highly
relevant. Furthermore, hearts of coxsackievirus B5-
infected hypercholesteremic mice revealed a disparate
pathology from the one observed in normal animals
infected with this virus or from the one seen in uninfected hypercholesteremic animals. These consisted
of discrete areas of myocytolysis, muscle bundle degeneration and loss of striation, and loss of nuclei.
Again, cellular infiltrates were conspicuously absent.

Johannsson and Robertson (6) recently reported
the occurrence of juvenile atherosclerosis in Reye's
syndrome, while Tang et al. (7) observed the occurrence of atherosclerotic plaques on the mitral valves
of their Reye's syndrome cases. These observations
are of particular interest since an interaction of
viruses and lipids has been implicated as a possible
mechanism in the initiation of atherogenesis (19). The

etiological role of group B coxsackieviruses in human
heart diseases has been well documented (22) but
relatively little information is available on their
potential as vascular pathogens. From investigations
in our laboratory it is apparent that these human
viruses replicate in the mouse aorta and localize in
this tissue (23) as evident from fluorescent antibody staining, indicating their affinity for this
vascular tissue. In the mouse, no evidence of pathological changes in the aorta was seen by light microscopy during the acute stages of infection. Nevertheless, atherogenic changes were observed later in
coxsackievirus B5-infected hypercholesteremic mice and
were not seen in uninfected hypercholesteremic or
infected normal mice.

Finally, evidence obtained by Kos et al. (24) in
our laboratory showed that hyperlipemia per se
suppressed the host immune response. Hypercholesteremic animals infected with syngeneic methylcholanthrene
induced fibrosarcoma cells (MCA 2182) had a significant
reduction in mean survival time, i.e., from 37.2 days
to 27.6 days ($p \geq 0.05$). Furthermore, the intralesional
injection of the macrophage activating agent,
Corynebacterium parvum, three days after tumor inoculation, protected 50% of the normal mice but did not
protect any hypercholesteremic mice against tumor
death. Similarly hypercholesteremic mice had a 38%
reduction in IgM antibodies to sheep RBC and a 3-fold
decrease in neutralizing antibodies against coxsackievirus B, 14 days after infection (25). These observations demonstrate that hypercholesteremia independently may significantly impair macrophage function
leading to inhibition of both inflammatory response
and antibody formation.

DISCUSSION

Our findings demonstrate that virus infection of
the hyperlipemic host results in greater susceptibility
and fatality, and that the pathological response is
significantly altered under these conditions. Also,
evidence that hyperlipemia independently may suppress

the host immune response leading to increased susceptibility to infections was presented. Tang et al. (7)
showed that "viral injuries seem unable to invoke the
usual inflammatory response" in Reye's syndrome cases
they investigated; while Crocker et al. (16) exposed
mice to emulsifiers and pesticides and infected them
with encephalomyocarditis (a picornavirus of animals)
and noted an increase in mortality and the absence of
an inflammatory response. Bove et al. (3) in their
extensive studies using liver biopsies, noted that
liver samples early in the course of illness were
invariably pale yellow and had a high lipid content
which apparently was present prior to appearance of
cytoplasmic vacuolization.

Finally, significant differences between viruses
and virus strains in lipid content have been reported
by Blough and Tiffany (26). These investigators
measured considerable differences in the phospholipid
content and the phospholipid types of influenza
A/PR8/34 and Influenza B/Lee/40. These differences
in lipids may possibly provide a selective advantage
to one specific strain over the other.

Based on the evidence presented in this report
the following rationale is being proposed. A large
number of environmental substances have been implicated
in the initiation of Reye's disease and are known for
their ability to cause either liver injury and/or fatty
changes. This effect may be dependent on a specific
genetic predisposition. Such hepatic changes would
lead to a greater susceptibility to infection by
enveloped or lipotropic viruses which in turn would
result in a divergent and aggravated pathology due to
a synergistic interaction between viruses and lipid.
The inability to cope with this aggravated pathology
may also be dependent on a specific genetic predisposition which would result in a Reye's-like disease.

REFERENCES

1. Reye, R.D.K., Morgan, G. and Baral, J. 1963.
    Encephalopathy and fatty degeneration of the

viscera. A disease entity in childhood. *Lancet 2:* 749-752.

2. Schiff, G.M. 1976. Reye's Syndrome. *Ann.Rev. of Med.* 27:447-452.

3. Bove, K.E., McAdams,J.A., Partin, J.C., Partin,J.S., Hug,G.,Schubert, W.K. 1975. The hepatic lesion in Reye's syndrome. *Gastroenterol.69:*685-697.

4. Brown,R.E. and Madge, G.E. 1975. The pathology of Reye's syndrome:An overview. In Reye's Syndrome Pollack, J.D.,ed., Grune & Stratton, N.Y. pp 77-92.

5. Brown,R.E. and Madge,G.E. 1971. Cardiac findings in Reye's syndrome.*Arch.Path.92:*244-274.

6. Johannsson, H.J. and Robertson, A.L.,Jr. 1978. Juvenile atherosclerosis and Reye's syndrome. *Arterial Wall 2:*79-87.

7. Tang,T.T., Siegesmund,K.A., Sedmak, G.V., Casper, J.T., Varna,R.R.,McCreadle,S.R. 1975 Reye's syndrome: A correlated electron microscopic viral and biochemical observation.*Jama 232:*1339-1346.

8. Haller.J.S. 1975. Clinical experience with Reye's syndrome. In Reye's Syndrome, Pollack,J.D. ed., Grune & Stratton, N.Y., pp. 3-14.

9. Linnemann,Jr.,C.C., Shea,L., Partin, J.C., Schubert, W.K. and Schiff, G.M. 1975. Reye's syndrome:Epidemiology and Viral Studies 1963-74.*Am.J.Epidemiol. 101:*517-526.

10. Corey,L., and Rubin,J. 1975. Reye's syndrome 1974: an epidemiological assessment. In Reye's Syndrome, Pollack,J.D.,ed., N.Y., Grunne & Stratton,pp. 179-187.

11. Noble,G.R.,Corey,L.,and Rubin,R.J. Virologic components of Reye's syndrome. In Reye's Syndrome Ibid, pp. 189-197.

12. Brown,J.M. 1974. Reye's syndrome associated with adenovirus type 3 infection.*Med.J.Aust.2:*873-875.

13. Alvira,N.M. and Mendoza, M. 1975. Reye's syndrome: a viral myopathy? *N.Eng.J.Med.292:*1297.

14.   Partin, J.C., Schubert, W.K., Partin, J.S.,
      Jacobs, R., and Saalfeld K. 1976. Isolation
      of influenza virus from liver and muscle biopsy
      specimens from surviving case of Reye's syndrome.
      Lancet 1: 594-602.
15.   Randolph, M., Kranwinkel, R., Johnson, R., and
      Gelfman, N.A. 1965. Encephalopathy hepatitis
      and fat accumulation in viscera. *Amer. J. Dis.
      Child. 110:* 95.
16.   Crocker, J.F.S., Ozere, R.L., Safe, S.H.,
      Digout, S.C., Rozee, K.R., and Hutzinger, O.
      1976. Lethal interaction of ubiquitous insecti-
      cide carriers with virus. *Science 192:* 1351-
      1353.
17.   Morens, D.M. and Noble, G.R. 1977. Reye's
      Syndrome and Influenza. *Lancet 2:* 807-808.
18.   Colon, A.R., Ledesma, F., Pardo, B.S.V. and
      Sandberg, D.H. 1974. Viral potentiation of
      chemical toxins in the experimental syndrome
      of hypoglycemia, encephalopathy, and visceral
      fatty degeneration. *Digest. Dis. 19:* 1091-1101.
19.   Loria, R.M., Kibrick, S. and Madge, G.E. 1976.
      Coxsackievirus B infection in the hypercholester-
      emic mouse. *J. Inf. Dis. 133:* 655-662.
20.   Lin, J.J., Liu, C., Svoboda, D.J. 1974. Long
      term effects of aflatoxin B1 and viral hepatitis
      on marmoset liver. *J. Lab Invest. 30:* 267-278.
21.   Loria, R.M., Kibrick, S., Downing, D., Madge,
      G.E., and Fillios, L.C. 1976. Effects of
      prolonged hypercholesteremia in the mouse.
      Nutrition Rev. International 13: 509 .
22.   Ableman, W.H. Clinical aspects of viral cardio-
      myopathy in Myocardial Diseases,Fowler, N.O.,
      ed. Grunne & Stratton, N.Y., 1973.
23.   Campbell, A.E., Loria, R.M. and Madge, G.E.
      Coxsackievirus B cardiopathy and angiopathy in
      the hypercholesteremic host. Atherosclerosis
      1978, in press.
24.   Kos, W.L., Loria, R.M., and Kaplan, A. 1978.
      Effect of hyperlipemia on tumor growth in mice.
      Am Soc. Microbiol. 78th Ann. Meeting, p. 52,
      E59, 1978 (Abstract)

25. Loria, R.M., Kos, W.L., and Kaplan, A.M.
     Suppression of host immunity by dietary hyper-
     cholesteremia. 8th Internat'l. Cong. of the
     RES Soc. 1978.
26. Blough, H.A. and Tiffany, J.M. 1973. Lipids in
     Viruses. *Adv. Lipid Res. 11:* 267-339.

DISCUSSION

J.D. Pollack - We've examined the serum from 22 patients
     with Reye's Syndrome and compared them to a larger
     number of controls. We reported a hypopanlipidemia
     in the Reye's Syndrome patients while assaying for
     total lipid. We also found in these patients a re-
     duced hypocholesterolemia, reduced cholesterol,not
     a hypercholesterolemia. We did, however, find ele-
     vated levels of cholesterol esters, as well as el-
     evated levels of phospholipids. My question is,
     did you examine your animals for phospholipids
     and cholesterol esters and,if so, what was the
     data?

R.M. Loria - We are not contending that our animals
     have Reye's Syndrome. We are only suggesting that
     the mechanism of interaction between viruses and
     lipids is a concept which could apply to this syn-
     drome. The fact that your patients have a hypolip-
     emic serum does not preclude high concentration of
     fat,triglycerides or cholesterol esters in the
     hepatic cell. Also, we can not preclude the pos-
     sibility of lipid-induced cellular injury. In our
     animals,concentration of cholesterol esters in
     the liver are drastically elevated.

D.B. Tower - I'm very much interested in your obser-
     vations about the aorta,and presumably other ves-
     sels. Are we seeing in patients,like those with
     Reye's Syndrome who recover, potential victims of
     early atherosclerosis later on?

R.M. Loria - We obviously are of the same opinion. A
        recent report by Johannsson and Robertson indi-
        cates that juvenile atherosclerosis is more pre-
        valent in Reye's patients. Viruses and lipids
        have also been implicated as having a possible
        role in atherosclerosis. Increased deposition of
        lipid at the site of viral injury might be ex-
        pected.

C.B. Reiner - You pointed out that you are getting cel-
        lular changes with the Coxsackie virus in choles-
        terolemic animals without cellular reactivity,and
        this is actually what we see commonly with Cox-
        sackie virus myopathy and hepatitis. Do you find
        that this is due to the lipid that was given to
        these animals?

R.M. Loria - Yes. In our experiments, infection of
        CD-1 mice with Coxsackie Virus B is uneventful,
        there is no mortality and there is a significant
        lymphocytic infiltration in the tissues. This is
        a classic response to enterovirus infection. The
        absence of an inflammatory infiltrate was thought
        to indicate that virus infection was not implica-
        ted. Our results demonstrate that this is not so,
        since we injected virus into these mice and re-
        covered Coxsackie virus from the tissues which
        have no inflammatory response. We emphasize this
        point to illustrate the possibility of an aber-
        rant response.

HYPERAMMONEMIA IN REYE'S SYNDROME

J.S. Juggi,M.D., N.Iyngkaran, M. D.,

and K. Prathap, M.D.

INTRODUCTION

Ammonium ion has long been known to be an extremely toxic substance and its concentration is sustained
within close limits by hemeostatic control mechanisms
which equilibrate it with glutamate, aspartate and
their derivatives (1). Under varying physiological
and pathological conditions, a tissue or an organ may
be in positive or negative net balance with respect to
ammonia nitrogen turnover. A rise in hepatic ammonia
(and consequently blood ammonia), occurs when the rate
of supply of ammonia is more rapid than the rate of
ammonia removal by the synthesis of urea. The resultant hyperammonemia causes acceleration of cerebral uptake of ammonia, glutamine formation and its release
into blood and cerebrospinal fluid (CSF). Even if
brain ammonia-nitrogen turnover is thus equilibrated
eventually the higher cerebral ammonia concentration
will exceed tolerable levels thereby precipitating coma.
Such a situation is uniformly present in Reye's
syndrome (2) but its patho-physiological effects are
not clearly defined. We have examined the role of
ammonia with respect to the intermediary metabolism in
Reye's syndrome as reflected by a sequential pattern of
changes in concentration of metabolic intermediates in
blood and cerebrospinal fluid. An attempt has been
made to correlate the blood and CSF ammonia levels with
other biochemical abnormalities in order to develop a
non-histologic diagnosis of Reye's syndrome.

MATERIALS AND METHODS

Case Material. Twenty seven patients of Reye's
syndrome admitted into the pediatrics wards of the
University Hospital, Kuala Lumpur, between March 1977
and May 1978 were included in this study.

Epidemiological Observations. Figure 1 shows
the monthly distribution of Reye's syndrome patients
and, as seen, the majority of the patients occurred
between the months of February and May. The age of the
patients ranged from 4 months to 6 years with peak
incidence at less than one year (Fig. 1). Table 1
shows that 15 out of 27 patients were males. One
patient occurred in association with pneumonia and another patient occurred after an attack of measles. All
the patients studied were from the urban or semiurban
areas of the federal territory of Kuala Lumpur.

TABLE 1

REYE'S SYNDROME

Total Number of Cases	27
Number of Males	15
Number of Females	12
Cases associated with Measles	1
Cases associated with Pneumonia	1

Staging Criteria. The clinical state of all the
patients on admission was defined by the "staging
criteria" of Huttenlocher (3) as shown in Table II and
Figure 1.

Histological Methods. Representative pieces of the
liver biopsy tissue were fixed in 10% formaldehyde for
preparation of frozen and paraffin sections. Tissue
for electron microscopy was fixed in cold 4% gluter-
aldehyde in cacodylate buffer, postfixed in osmium
tetroxide, dehydrated in ethanol and embedded in Epon.
Sections were cut at 1 μm on an LKB Ultratome III with

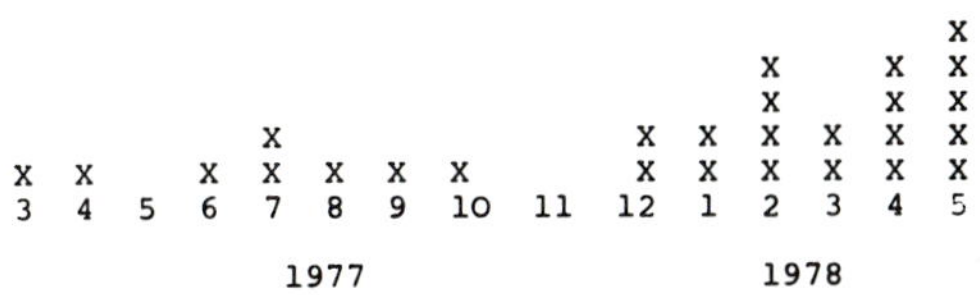

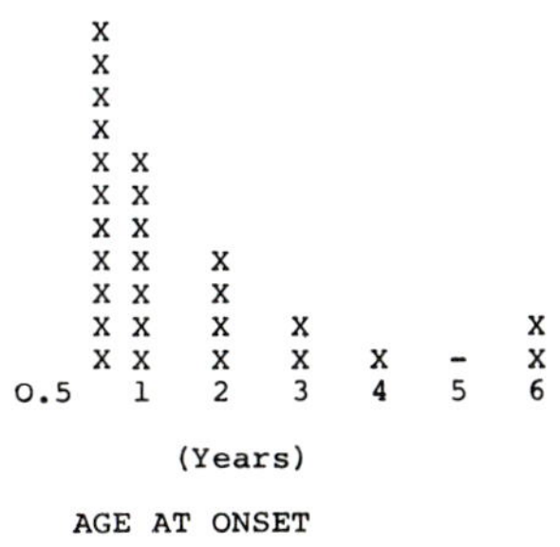

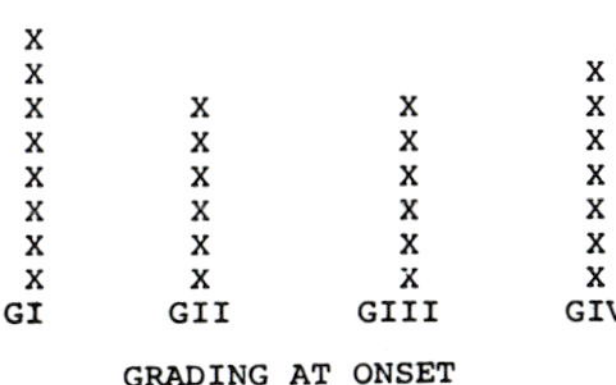

Figure 1. Monthly distribution, age at onset and
grading at onset of patients with Reye's syndrome.
Each x represents one patient

glass knives and stained with uranyl acetate and lead
hydroxide and examined in a Hitachi HS 8 electron
microscope operating at 50 KV. Paraffin sections were
stained with haematoxylin and eosin and frozen sections
were stained with Oil red O.

<u>Biochemical Methods</u>. Blood and CSF ammonia levels
were measured by the enzymatic method using glutamic
dehydrogenase reaction (4). CSF a-ketoglutaramate/
levels (a-KGM) were estimated by the method described

by Duffy et al (5). Glutamate, glutamine, 2-oxoglutar-
ate, aspartate, alanine, malate, lactate, pyruvate,
citrate, adenosine triphosphate, acetoacetate and
β-hydroxybutyrate levels, in the clear and neutralized
perchloric acid extracts of blood and CSF, were
measured by the standard enzymatic methods (6).

TABLE II

GRADING CRITERIA OF PATIENTS

Grade O:	Normal, conscious, rational
Grade I:	Lethargic, drowsy, vomiting
Grade II:	Disorientated, irrational, obtunded or stuporous
Grade III:	Coma, decerebrate - rigidity
Grade IV:	Profound coma, flaccid, apneic

RESULTS

The diagnosis of the patients studied was confirmed by the histopathological examination of the
liver biopsy tissue. A diffuse fatty change, more prominent in the centrilobular areas of the parenchymal
cells, was seen (Fig. 2). Electron microscopy confirmed
the presence of lipids which generally had well defined
membranes and sometimes contained myelin figures
(Fig. 3, Fig. 4). Mitochondria were enlarged and distorted and sometimes had disorientated cristae (Fig. 5).
Smooth endoplasmic reticulum was increased in amount,
swollen and vesiculated (Fig. 3).

The results of the biochemical studies are shown
in Figures 6 to 15 and Tables 3 and 4. In order to
simplify the format, biochemical data of coma Grade I
and Grade II patients were pooled together and each
open circle in the figures represent the mean values
of at least five such patients. Similarly, biochemical
data of coma Grade III and Grade IV patients were

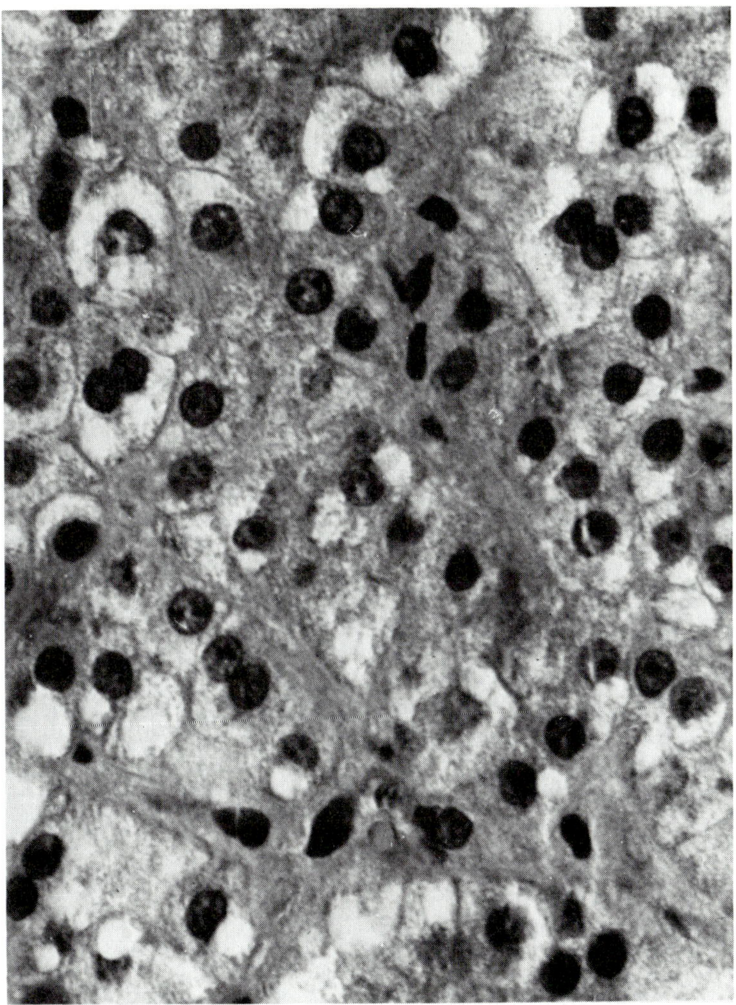

Figure 2. Light micrograph of liver showing
swelling and vacuolation of hepatocytes. Haematoxylin
and Eosin x 800.

pooled together and each closed circle in the diagrams
represents the mean values of at least five such patients.
On the ordinate, the normal range is represented by the
letter "N" and on the abscissa the consciousness level

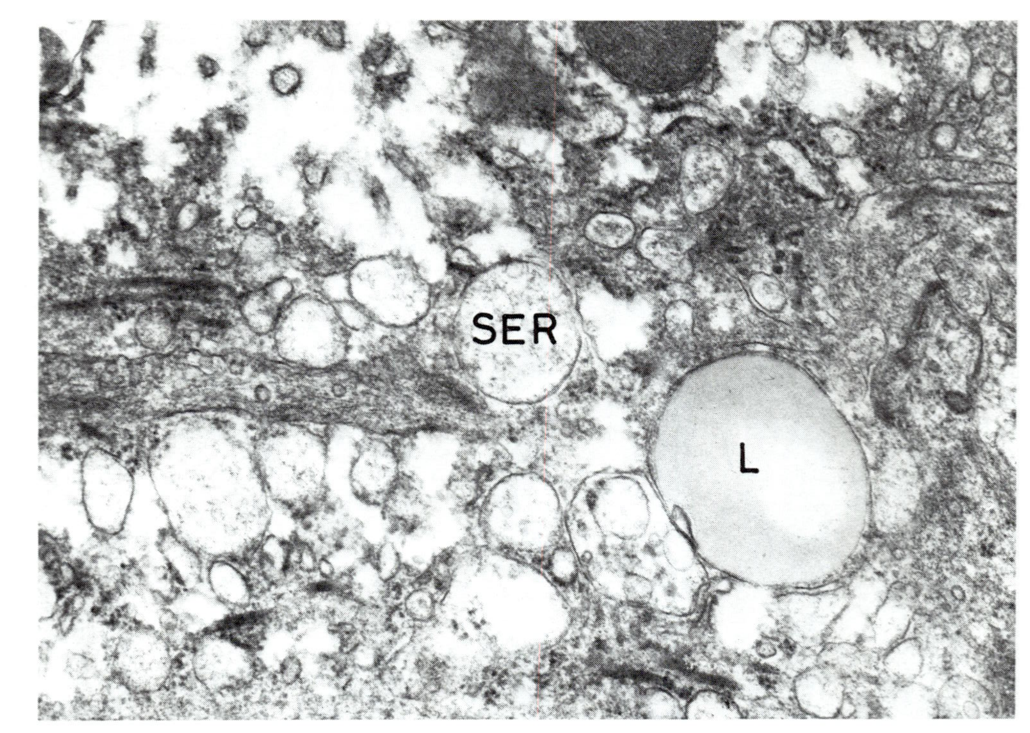

Figure 3. Electron micrograph of hepatocyte showing a membrane-bound lipid (L) and swollen smooth endoplasmic reticulum (SER) x 27,500

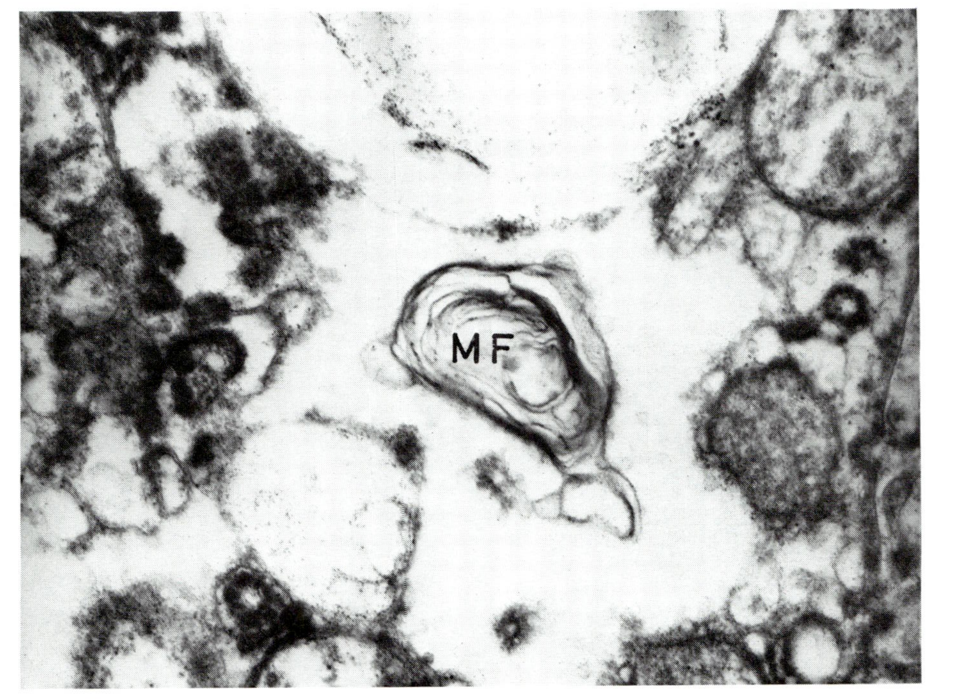

Figure 4. Electron micrograph of hepatocyte showing a
myelin figure (MF) in cytoplasmic lipid (L) x 37,500

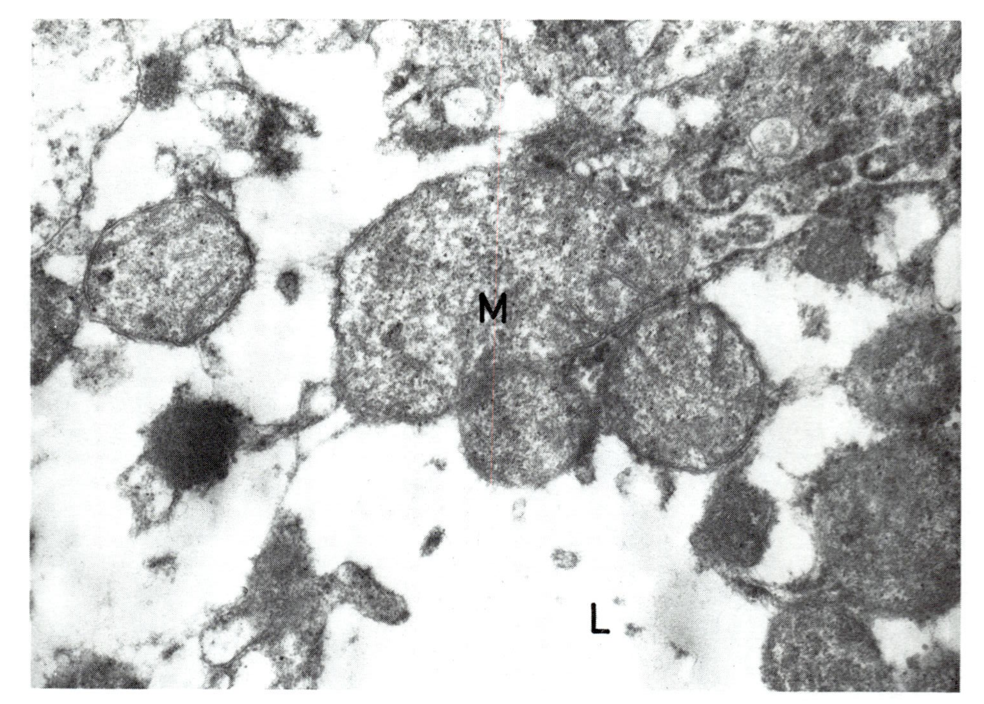

Figure 5.   Electron micrograph of hepatocyte showing enlarged
mitochondria (M) with distorted cristae and non-
membrane bound cytoplasmic lipid (L) x 27,500

of the patients is shown. Patients with coma Grades
I and II recovered and regained full consciousness
(rational) level between 4th and 7th day of the start
of treatment, whereas patients with coma Grade III and
Grade IV recovered and became rational between 7th and
14th day of the start of treatment.

Figures 6 and 7 show the sequential pattern of
changes in the blood and CSF ammonia levels over a
two weeks period of study. As seen, the blood ammonia
is very much elevated on the first two days of hospitalization particularly in coma Grade III and Grade IV
patients. Highest blood ammonia levels recorded were
231.5 μg% and 421.3 μg% in coma Grades I and II and
in coma Grades III and IV patients respectively. As
the patients were regaining consciousness, blood
ammonia levels returned to within normal limits, showing a very good correlation between blood ammonia
levels and the state of consciousness. On the other
hand, no correlation was found between the CSF ammonia
levels and the state of consciousness. CSF ammonia
levels continued to be elevated even though the patients
were showing recovery and had regained consciousness.
The highest CSF ammonia levels recorded were 139.4 μg%
and 218.5 μg% in coma Grades I and II and in coma
Grades III and IV patients respectively. Similarly, no
correlation was found between the elevated blood and
CSF glutamine levels and the state of consciousness
(Fig. 8). Highest blood and CSF glutamine levels recorded were 1.93 mM/L and 1.67 mM/L respectively in
coma Grade III and Grade IV patients.

Unlike ammonia, glutamine has no direct toxic effect on the nervous tissue. Recently, Duffy and associates (7,8) from Cornell University Medical College,
New York and Kardel and Gips (9) from S. Gentofte
Hospital, Copenhagen, have identified a direct neurotoxic metabolite of glutamine called a-ketoglutaramate
(a-KGM) occurring in the CSF of patients with ammonia-
genic encephalopathy. We estimated the level of a-KGM
in the cerebrospinal fluid of four patients of Reye's
syndrome in Grade III and Grade IV coma. There was
an initial 11-fold increase in the levels of a-KGM
which subsequently returned back to near normal values

BLOOD AMMONIA

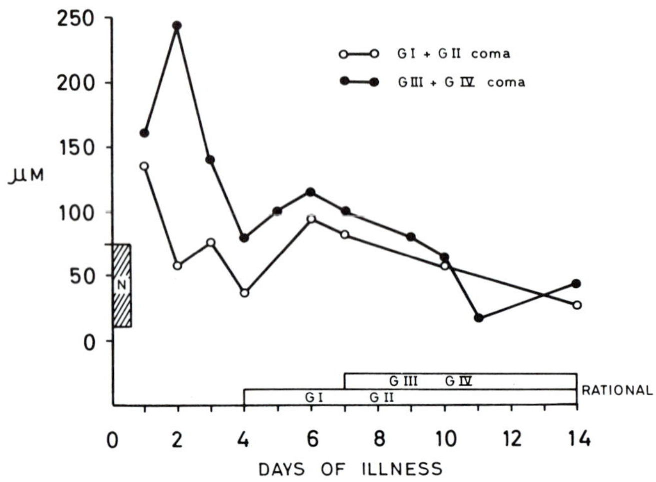

Figure 6.

C.S.F. AMMONIA

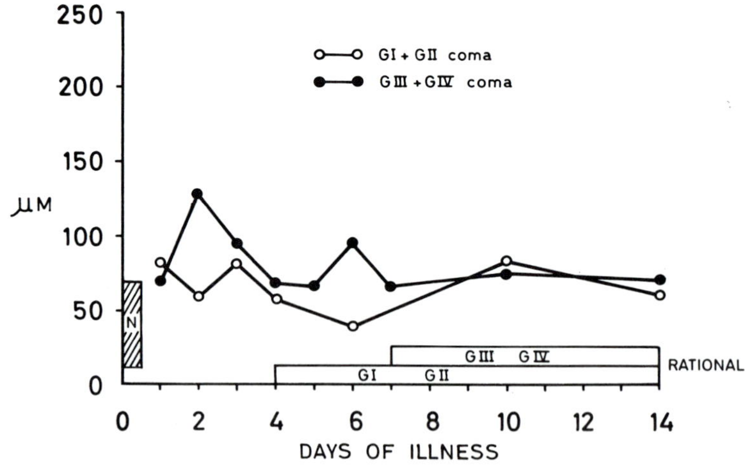

Figure 7.

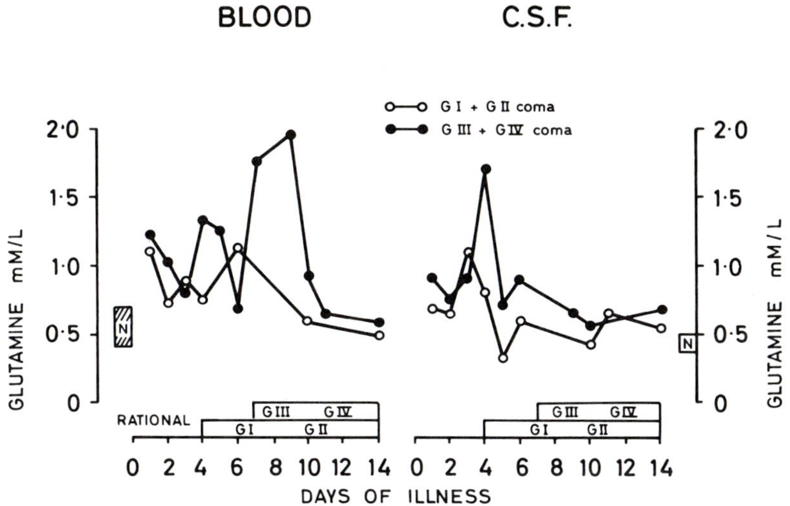

Figure 8.

when the patients recovered completely from the coma,
thereby showing a good correlation between the CSF
a-KGM levels and the severity of coma (Fig. 9).

No significant change was seen in the blood glutamate levels (Fig. 10). CSF glutamate levels were
elevated initially and showed good correlation with the
severity of coma in the subsequent period.

Blood alanine levels showed a 2-fold increase in
patients with Grade III and Grade IV coma and remained
at a higher than normal value even though the patients
were recovering and regaining consciousness. CSF
alanine was markedly elevated in the initial stages of
coma, and showed good correlation with the level of
consciousness subsequently (Fig. 11).

Blood and CSF aspartate levels (Fig. 12) were
found to be within the normal range during the initial
stages of coma. However, as the patients were regaining consciousness and showing improvement in their

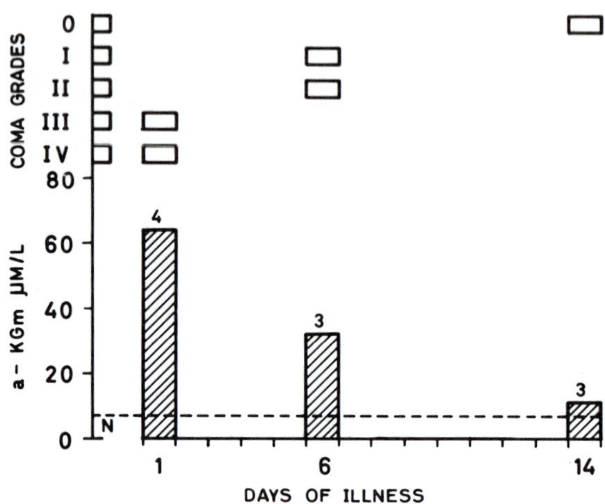

Figure 9.

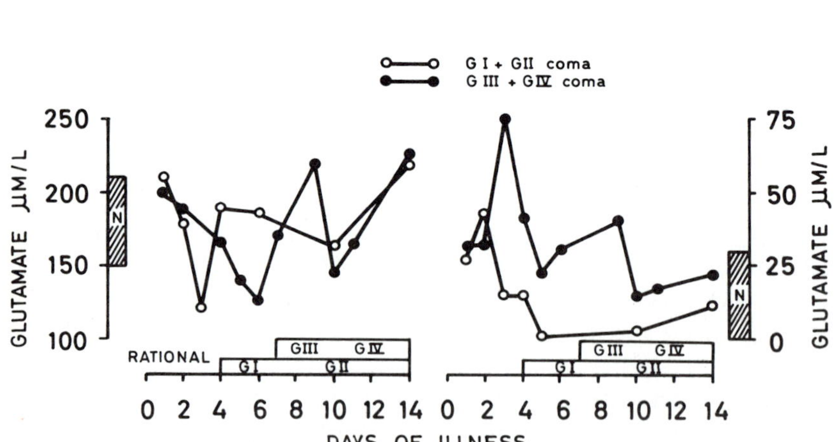

Figure 10.

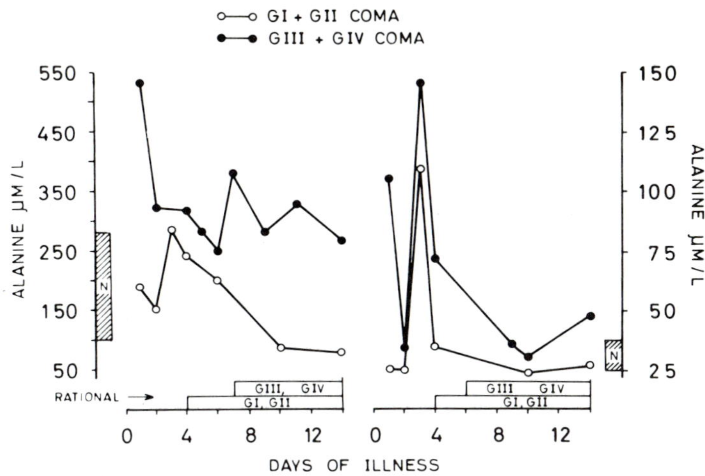

Figure 11.

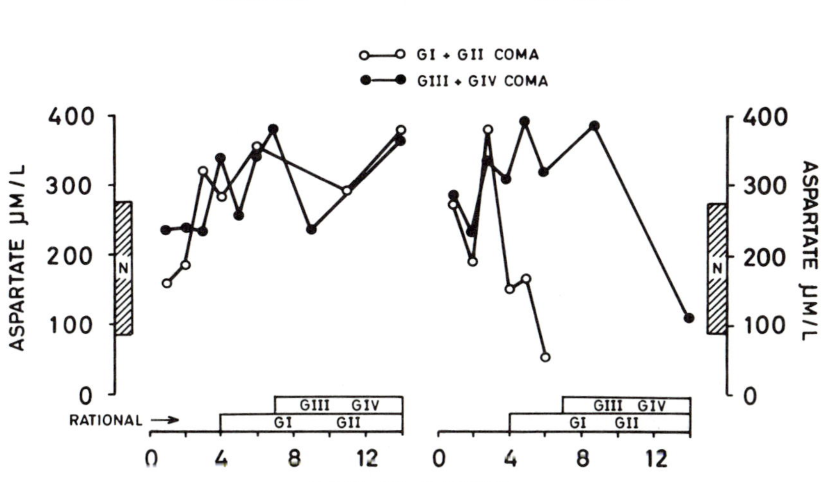

Figure 12.

clinical status, blood and CSF aspartate levels were
found to be very much elevated.

Blood and CSF lactate and pyruvate levels are shown
in Figures 13 and 14. During the first four days of
coma, lactate and pyruvate showed 3-4 fold increase and
the corresponding calculated Lactate/Pyruvate ratios
were 28 and 14 respectively in the blood and CSF. However, during the period of recovery, both lactate and
pyruvate levels and Lactate/Pyruvate ratios gradually
came down to within normal limits.

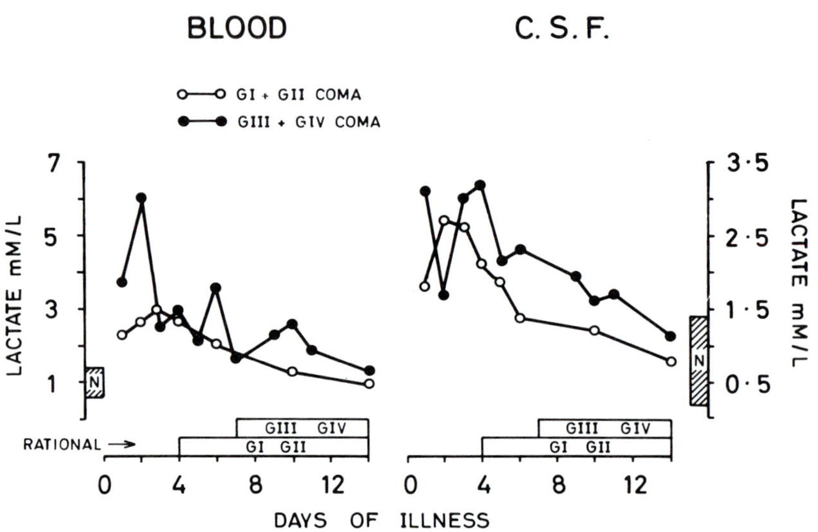

Figure 13.

Table 3 summarizes the blood and CSF levels of
citrate, 2-oxoglutarate and malate. As seen, elevated
levels of all these metabolites, with the exception of
blood citrate and malate, returned back to normal within
10 to 14 days of treatment. Blood adenosine triphosphate
(ATP) levels decreased during the first two days of
coma.

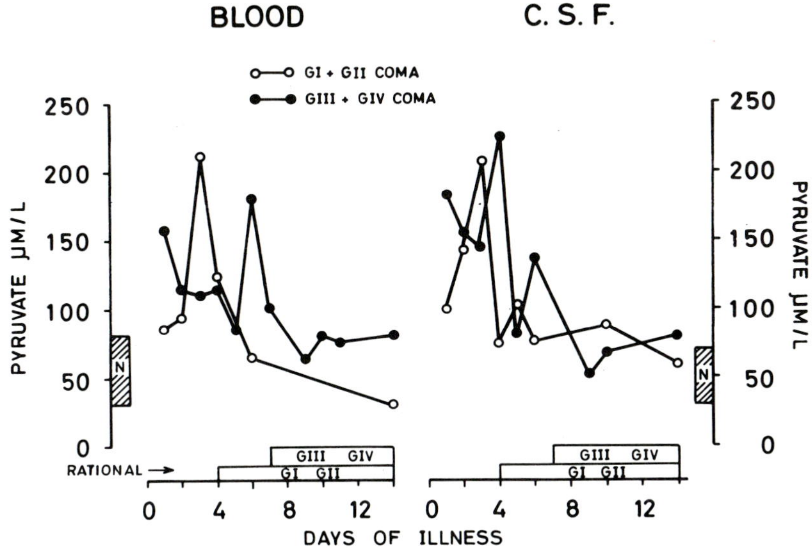

Figure 14.

Levels of acetoacetate and β-hydroxybutyrate were
found to be elevated during the first two days of coma
and subsequently returning back to within normal range
when the patients were regaining consciousness.

Terminal liver biopsy was performed in one patient
of Reye's syndrome in Grade IV coma and liver metabolites
were studied and compared with an otherwise normal liver
biopsy tissue. As seen in Figure 15, there was a tremendous increase in the hepatic ammonia, aspartate,
lactate and citrate levels and a moderate increase in
the glutamine, alanine, pyruvate and malate levels.
The levels of glutamate and 2-oxoglutarate decreased.
The Lactate/Pyruvate ratios showed a 10-fold increase
over the control values.

DISCUSSION

Ammonium ion was incriminated for the first time

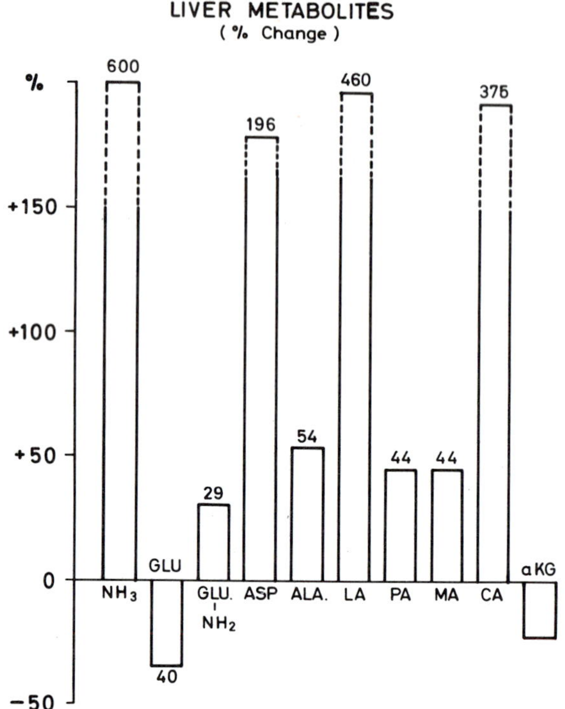

Figure 15. Liver metabolites (% change) in a patient
with Reye's syndrome.

as the toxic agent in Reye's syndrome by Huttenlocher
et al (10) in 1969. In the subsequent years there was
some controversy about the upper level of blood ammonia
which could be considered as toxic (11, 12). The observations that uptake and release of ammonia by the
brain tissue may not correlate with coma (13) are not
difficult to understand. Intracellular toxicity of
ammonia is dependent upon the entry of ammonia into
the cells which is the function of pH. Tissue cells
are relatively impermeable to ammonium ion (NH_4^+) while
being readily permeable to gaseous ammonia (NH_3).
With alkaline pH, NH_4^+ ion dissociates into NH_3 gas
and in alkalosis, intracellular concentration of brain
and muscle ammonia increases whereas in acidosis it
decreases (14, 15). Lactic acidosis is present in
Reye's syndrome patients and this combined with

TABLE III.

Blood and CSF Metabolites in Reye's Syndrome
(µM/L, Mean Values)

Days of Illness

	Blood					CSF				
	Control	1	2	10	14	Control	1	2	10	14
A		105.0	87.0	78.5	116.0		198.0	113.5	148.0	126.4
Citrate	42.4					145.0				
B		115.6	87.0	86.0	92.7		207.0	191.0	232.6	137.0
A		54.6	50.0	30.5	32.0		38.0	42.5	28.0	18.5
2-Oxoglutarate	33.7					22.8				
B		37.9	67.0	78.0	31.0		49.4	209.0	49.0	25.4
A		12.7	21.0	37.5	24.4		17.7	18.0	21.5	20.0
Malate	21.5					17.7				
B		38.7	62.5	42.3	56.0		35.5	4.0	20.4	11.6
A		435	380	410	410					
ATP	435									
B		431	250	360	395					

A = GI + GII COMA   B = GIII + G IV COMA

elevated brain ammonia levels produce central neurogen-
ic hyperventilation (2) which,if unchecked,precipitates
respiratory alkalosis.Reye's syndrome patients' acid-
base status,therefore,may not remain static for a sufficiently long period of time,and such a situation may
produce wide fluctuations in the extra-cellular fluid
ammonia levels. Single determinations of blood ammonia,
therefore,may not reflect the true state of ammonia metabolism in the body. Sequential pattern of changes in
the blood ammonia levels,on the other hand,correlated
very well with the state of consciousness.Identical observations have been made by Aoki et al(16). However,we
could not find any correlation between CSF ammonia levels and the state of consciousness. The brain tissue
takes up ammonia in patients with Reye's syndrome and
the amount of ammonia fixed correlates better with increased cerebral lactate production(17). ATP depletion,
secondary to large amounts of ammonia fixation,occurs
with the resultant lactic acidosis(18) as reflected by
the elevated levels of lactic acid in the cerebrospinal
fluid.

Hepatic levels of glucogenic amino acids;i.e.,ala-
nine,aspartate and glutamine,were very much elevated.In
addition, there were significant changes in the various
citric acid cycle intermediates. Changes in the blood
metabolites generally moved parallel with the changes
in the liver metabolites. Similarly,it could be assumed
that the magnitude of the changes in CSF metabolites reflected,at least in part,hyperammonemia-induced changes
in the brain tissue.A rise of hepatic ammonia occurs
when the rate of supply of ammonia is more rapid than
the rate of removal of ammonia by the synthesis of urea.
In Reye's syndrome,such a situation is created by a
transient and usually reversible mitochondrial injury
which results in decoupling of oxidative phosphorylation, a reduced rate of ammonia detoxification,and interference with many other intramitochondrial functions
(19). The increased formation of alanine and aspartate
through the mediation of glutamate dehydrogenase and
alanine and aspartate amino-transferases and increased
synthesis of glutamine,has been shown to represent alternative pathways for the removal of ammonia as a result of diminished urea synthesis (1).

These reactions may be looked on as a metabolic buffer system that can keep ammonia approximately constant in hyperammonemic situations.

Glucogenic amino acids once formed can either be used in the protein synthesis or enter in metabolic pathways concerned with gluconeogenesis. In the liver, alanine is transaminated with 2-oxoglutarate to form pyruvate and glutamate. Pyruvate generated from both alanine and lactate is converted to oxaloacetate by the carbon dioxide fixing mitochondrial enzyme, pyruvate carboxylase,in the presence of ATP. Limitations of energy supply or a defect in pyruvate carboxylase or in any other rate-limiting enzyme involved in gluconeogenesis, could lead to an accumulation of lactate, pyruvate and alanine. Lowered rates of gluconeogenesis have been found to be associated with lower rates of utilization of precursors, i.e., alanine and lactate,a lower rate of oxygen consumption, and a reduced activity of Krebs cycle (20). Changes in blood and liver metabolites of the present study confirm these conclusions. In addition, marked elevation in the blood and liver lactate and pyruvate levels and a significant increase in the lactate/pyruvate ratios, reflect a shift in the intracellular redox potential to a more reduced state. Identical changes have been found in the cerebrospinal fluid and could be explained in the same way. However,the major buffer mechanism available to the brain tissue for the removal of ammonia is by reductive amination of 2-oxogluterate and amidation of glutamate to form glutamine, an ATP-dependent reaction (21). Glutamine thus formed can diffuse readily into the CSF. Glutamine can be further metabolised in the brain by hydrolysis to glutamic acid and ammonia, a reaction catalyzed by the enzyme glutaminase. Recent studies of Duffy et al (7,8)and Kardel and Gips(9) have confirmed an alternative pathway of glutamine metabolism.Transamination of glutamine with an appropriate a-keto acid occurs in the brain,with the resultant formation of a-KGM and the corresponding a-amino acid. a-KGM can subsequently break down in the presence of enzyme w-amidase to yield 2-oxoglutarate and ammonia, thereby completing the cycle.Elevated levels of a-KGM in the CSF have been found in patients with hepatic encephalo-

pathy (7,8,9) and in the present study it has been
shown to occur in Reye's syndrome patients also. The
exact mechanism by which a-KGM produces neurotoxicity
has not been determined; however, Vergara et al (7)
have postulated that a-KGM might impair neurologic
functions in liver disease by competing for glutamic
acid receptors in the brain.

SUMMARY AND CONCLUSIONS

Sequential pattern of changes in the concentrations
of blood and CSF metabolites was studied in 27 patients
of Reye's syndrome. From the results of these studies,
it was concluded that at least three sets of biochemical investigations are indicated in patients suffering
from Reye's syndrome: (i) Study of the direct neurotoxic metabolites; i.e., blood and CSF ammonia and CSF
a-ketoglutaramate levels (ii) Study of indicators of
alternative pathways for the removal of ammonia; i.e.,
blood and CSF alanine, aspartate and glutamine levels,
and (iii) indicators of the intracellular redox state
of the liver and brain tissue; i.e., blood and CSF
lactate and pyruvate levels.

We conclude that these three sets of investigations, when studied collectively with the clinical and
routine laboratory findings, could provide a useful indicator for the non-histologic diagnosis of Reye's syndrome.

REFERENCES

1.   Brosnan,J.T. and Williamson, D.H. 1974. Mechanism
     of formation of alanine and aspartate on rat liver
     in vivo after administration of ammonium chloride.
     Biochem.J. 138:453-462.
2.   Shannon,D.C.,Delong,R.,Bercu,B.,Glick,T. et al 1975
     Studies on the pathophysiology of encephalopathy in
     Reye's syndrome:Hyperammonemia in Reye's syndrome.
     Pediatrics 56:999-1004.
3.   Huttenlocher,P.R. 1972. Reye's syndrome:relation
     of outcome of therapy.*J.Pediatr.80*:845-850.

4. Kun, E. and Kearney, E.B. 1974. In "Methods of enzymatic analysis" 2nd ed. *Academic Press, New York*.

5. Duffy,T.E., Cooper,A.J.L. and Meister,A. 1974. Identification of a-ketoglutaramate in rat liver, kidney and brain. *J.Biol.Chem. 149*:7603-7606.

6. Bergmeyer, H.U. 1974. In "Methods of enzymatic analysis" 2nd ed.*Academic Press,New York*.

7. Vergara,F.,Duffy,T.E. and Plum, F. 1974. a-ketoglutaramate, A neurotoxic agent in hepatic coma.*Trans.Assoc.American Physicians 86*:255-263.

8. Duffy,T.E.,Vergara, F. and Plum, F. a-ketoglutaramate in hepatic encephalopathy. *Res.Publ.Assoc.Neur. Ment.Dis.53*:39-52.

9. Kardel,T. and Gips, C.H. 1974. a-ketoglutaramate, glutamate antagonism and GABA depletion-clues to the pathogenesis of hepatic encephalopathy. *Neth.Med.J. 17*:37-41.

10. Huttenlocher, P.R., Schwartz, A.D. and Klatskin,G. 1969. Reye's syndrome: ammonia intoxication as a possible factor in the encephalopathy. *Pediatrics 43*:443-454.

11. Glasgow,A.M., Cotton, R.B. and Dhiensiri, K. 1972. Reye's syndrome I. Blood ammonia and consideration of non-histologic diagnosis. *Am.J.Dis.Chid.124*:827-833.

12. Lovejoy,F.H.,Smith,A.L.,Bresman,M.J.,Wood,J.N., Victor,D.I. and Adams, P.C. 1974. Clinical staging in Reye's syndrome. *Am.J.Dis.Child.128*:36-41.

13. Walker,C.O. and Schenker, S. 1970. Pathogenesis of hepatic encephalopathy - with special reference to the role of ammonia. *Am.J.Clin.Nutr.23*:619-632.

14. Stabenau,J.R.,Warren,K.S. and Rall,D.P. 1959. The role of pH-gradient in the distribution of ammonia between blood and cerebrospinal fluid,brain and muscle.*J.Clin.Invest.38*:373-383.

15. Moore,E.W.,Strohmeyer,G.W. and Chalmers,T.C.1963. Distribution of ammonia across the blood cerebro-spinal fluid barrier in patients with hepatic failure. *Am.J.Med. 35*:350-362.

16. Aoki,Y., and Lombroso, T. 1973. Prognostic value of electroencephalography in Reye's syndrome. *Neurology 23*:333-343.

17.   Smith, A.L. 1976.   Ammonia disposal in Reye's
      syndrome. *New England J.Med. 294:897-898.*
18.   Hindfelt, B. and Siesjo, B.K. 1971. Cerebral
      effects of acute ammonia intoxication II. The
      effect on energy metabolism. *Scand.J.Clin.Lab.
      Invest. 28:365-374.*
19.   Bove, K.E. 1974.   The character and specificity
      of hepatic lesion in Reye's Syndrome. In "Reye's
      syndrome" Edited by J.D.Pollack. Grune & Stratton
      New York pp.93-116.
20.   Henley,K.S.,Laughrey,E.C. and Clancy,P.E.   1974
      Gluconeogenesis in the fatty liver and cirrhotic
      liver of rat. The effect of Oleate and Ethanol.
      In "Regulation of hepatic metabolism" Edited by
      F.Lungguist and N.Tygstrup. Munksgaard, Copen-
      hagen p.401.
21.   Weil-Malherbe, H. 1958. The metabolism of ammonia
      in brain. In "Consciousness and chemical environ-
      ment of the brain" Ross Laboratories, Columbus,
      Ohio p.50.

ANTECEDENT MITOCHONDRIAL CHANGES TO THE
APPEARANCE OF FATTY DROPLETS AND ATP
CONCENTRATIONS IN RAT LIVER TREATED WITH
4-PENTENOIC ACID

Ichiro Yoshida,M.D., Fumio Yamashita,M.D.,
Makoto Yoshino,M.D. and Shojiro Okada,M.D.

INTRODUCTION

In Reye's syndrome, it has been said that increased
concentrations of short-chain fatty acids act as toxic
substances to liver, central nervous system and other
organs. 4-pentenoic acid is one of these short-chain
fatty acids. Recently Glasgow showed experimentally
that 4-pentenoic acid produced the clinical features of
Reye's syndrome (1). The purpose of this study is to
elucidate the mechanisms of hepatic lesions caused by
4-pentenoic acid, as an experimental model of Reye's
syndrome.

MATERIALS AND METHODS

Male Wister strain rats, weighing 200-270 g were
used. Methods of administration of 4-pentenoic acid
were generally followed according to Glasgow (1). Food,
except water, was removed during the time of the experiment. For electronmicroscopic studies, rats were
injected intraperitoneally every 4 hours with 50 mg/kg
body weight of 4-pentenoic acid for 10 doses and in
another group for 21 doses. Two hours after the last
50 mg/kg dose, a 200 mg/kg dose was given intraperitoneally. Samples were collected 25-45 minutes later for
electronmicroscopic studies. For ATP measurements, a-
cute experimental rats were killed 30 minutes after
the injection of 200 mg/kg of 4-pentenoic acid and

chronic experimental rats were killed after 72 hours
(every 4 hours for 19 doses of 50 mg/kg dose)`. ATP
measurement was done after Bucher's method using GAPDH
(Figure 1). The number of specimens for morphological
and biochemical studies was 19 and 14 respectively.

```
LIVER
 |
GRIND IN LIQUID NITROGEN
 |
DEPROTEINIZATION(6% PERCHLORIC ACID)
 |
HOMOGENIZE IN ICE-WATER
 |
CENTRIFUGE(3000-5000G 15 MINUTES)
 |
NEUTRALIZATION OF SUPERNATE( KOH)
 |
SAMPLE + 0.5M TRIETHANOLAMINE BUFFER
 |        4mM MgSO₄
 |        2.5mM NADH ------------(A)
 |
(A) + GLYCELALDEHYDE-3-PHOSPHATE DEHYDROGENASE
 |     3-PHOSPHOGLYCERATE KINASE
 |     GLYCEROL-1-PHOSPHATE DEHYDROGENASE
 |
 |   (—NADH)
 |

SPECTROPHOTOMETETRY(340Mμ)
```

BÜCHER, TH.;BIOCHEM.BIOPHYS.ACTA,1947.

Figure 1.

RESULTS

     In electronmicroscopic studies, we found that the
appearance of abnormal mitochondria predominated with
a few fatty droplets in the early phase. The degree of
fatty change gradually increased in the later phase
following the appearance of abnormal mitochondria.
For example, Figure 2 shows hepatic changes about 38
hours after the initial treatment. There were few
fatty droplets at this stage and mitochondria were of
apparently abnormal appearance. In this picture, mitochondrial changes were prominent compared with other
cell organelles. Figure 3 is a picture of a later phase
which shows changes 86 hours after the initial treatment. In this picture, we recognized the appearance of

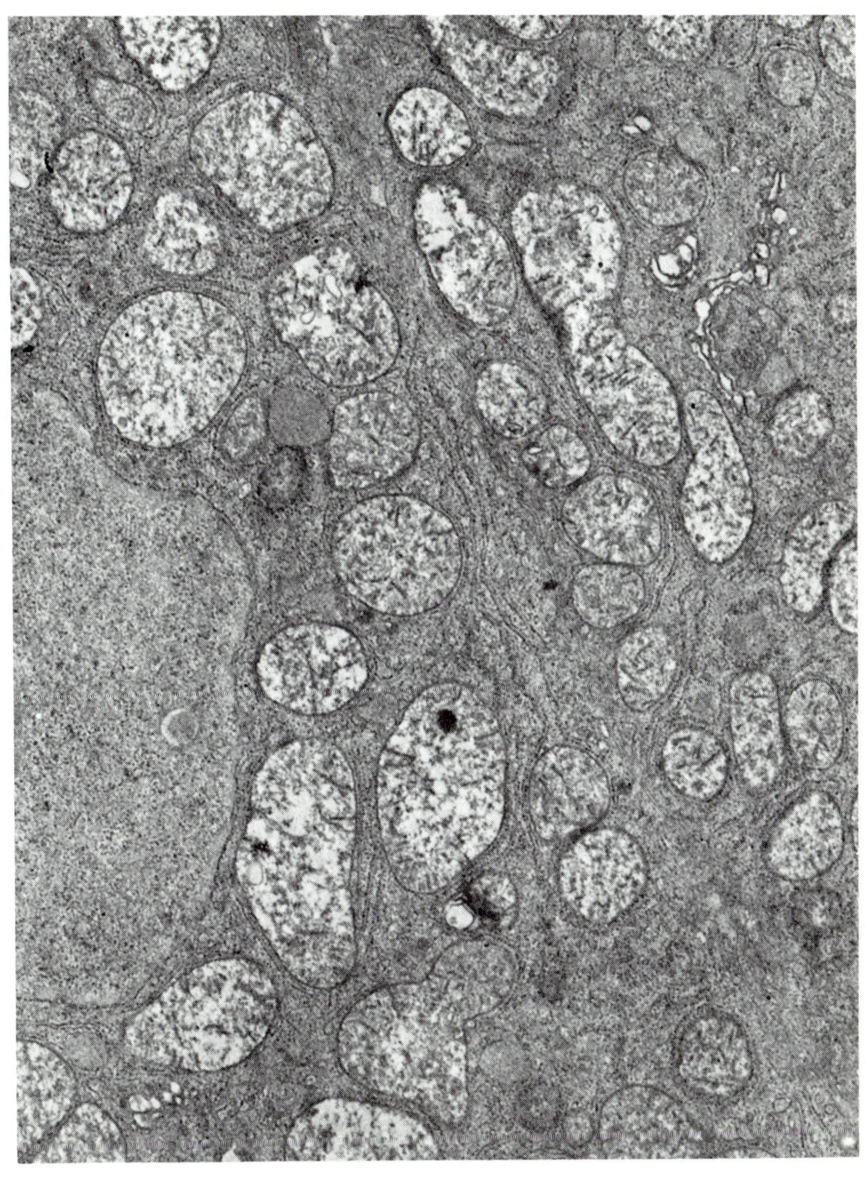

Figure 2.   In abnormal mitochondria, derangement
of cristae, low density of matrix are
seen with few fatty droplets.

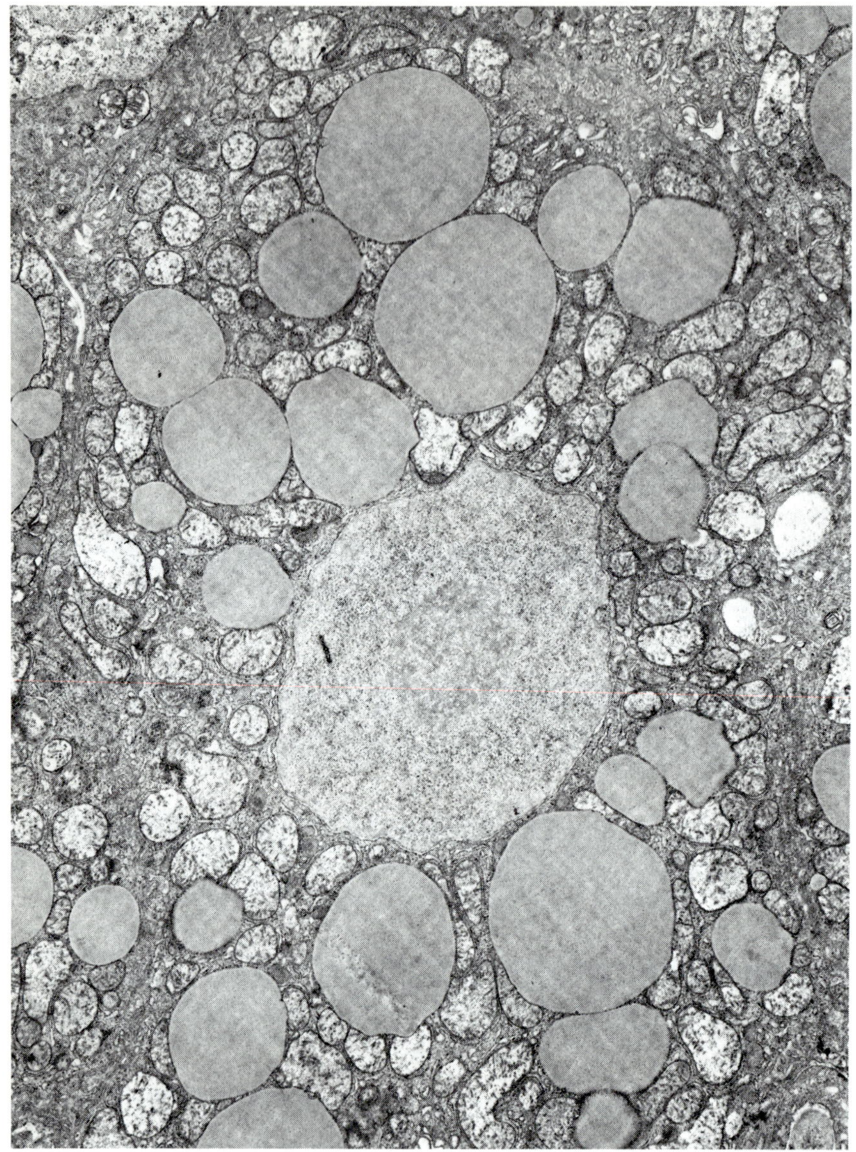

Figure 3. Fatty droplets are seen around the nucleus
following the appearance of abnormal mitochondria.

fatty droplets around the nucleus and also abnormal
mitochondria. Chronological hepatic changes as seen
by the electronmicroscope are shown in Figure 4.

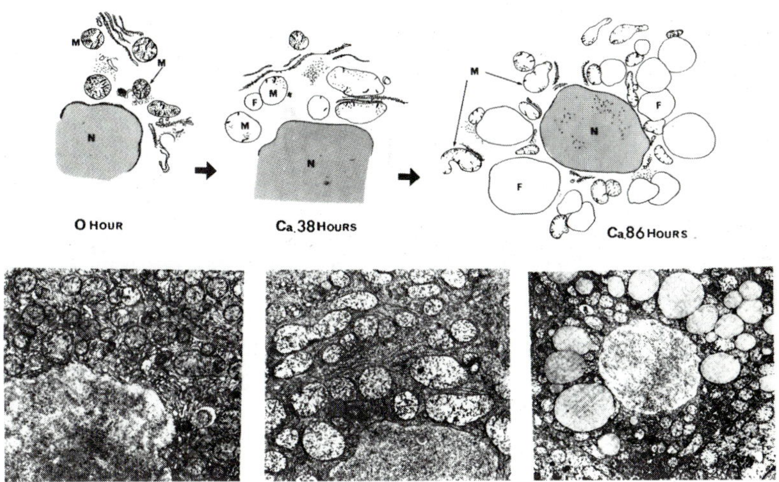

Figure 4.   Hepatic lesions in rats treated with
            4-pentenoic acid (every 4 hour)

     Hepatic ATP concentrations were measured in two
situations. One was in the acute experiment and the
other the chronic experiment. Hepatic ATP levels in
acute and chronic experiments were 4.7mM ± 0.9SE and
4.2mM ± 0.2SE per g of wet tissue, respectively. There
was no significant ATP reduction compared with controls
in either the acute or chronic experiments. In the
chronic experiment, however, further studies will be
required to confirm these results, because the number
of specimens was not sufficient. (Figure 5.)

DISCUSSION

     In these morphological studies, we showed that
only mitochondrial changes predominated in the initial
phases and these were prominent compared with other
cell organelles and many fatty droplets were prominent.
in the later phase. The fatty liver in Reye's syndrome
is histologically characterized by the following two
features. One is emergence of markedly abnormal mito-

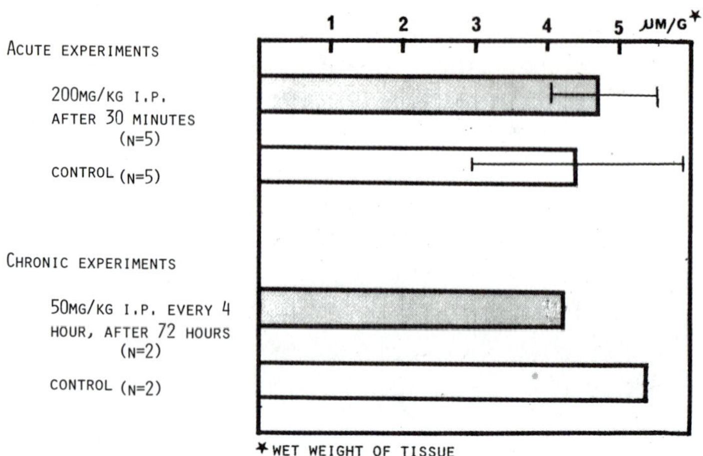

Figure 5.   Hepatic ATP concentrations in rats treated
            with 4-pentenoic acid.

chondria and the other is centrinucleated fatty degeneration of hepatocytes. It was reported that these
were the same pathological changes seen in hepatic
lesions caused by treatment with 4-pentenoic acid.

In Reye's syndrome, no reduction of hepatic ATP
concentration has been reported, although there existed
markedly abnormal mitochondrial changes (2). We have
found these results in 4-pentenoic acid induced fatty
liver, both with respect to the histological aspects and
ATP levels. In conclusion, 4-pentenoic acid induced
fatty liver is consistent to the fatty liver in Reye's
syndrome in both morphological and energic aspects.

In Japan, there exists a famous disease named
"Ekiri". This disease is a fulminant type of dysentry
infection and it has the same clinico-pathologic features
of Reye's syndrome except for an enterocolitis (3,4,5,6).

Recently, Yoshino et al succeeded in producing the
biological and histological features of Reye's syndrome,
such as elevated SGOT and SGPT, hyperammonemia, decreased blood glucose level and fatty liver, using Shigella
flexneri endotoxin in rabbits (7). No hepatic ATP re-

duction in this liver was found. There are common
histological and pathogenic features, such as appearance of abnormal mitochondria, fatty droplets and no hepatic ATP reduction among these three fatty livers,
namely Reye's syndrome, 4-pentenoic acid induced fatty
liver and fatty liver by Shigella flexneri endotoxin.
These three fatty livers are different from the fatty
liver with ATP reduction, without abnormal mitochondrial
changes, such as orotic acid induced fatty liver. We
could therefore, call these three fatty livers, "Fatty
Liver of the Reye's Syndrome Type", although further
studies will be required to elucidate the pathogenesis
of this fatty liver.

CONCLUSION

    These reports suggest that antecedent mitochondrial
changes may play a primary role in the pathogenesis of
fatty liver induced by 4-pentenoic acid, although ATP
changes in concentration did not accompany the mitochondrial damage.

REFERENCES

1. Glasgow, A.M. and Chase, H.P. 1975. Production of
    features of Reye's syndrome in rats with 4-pentenoic
    acid. *Pediatr. Res. 9:* 133-138.
2. Green, H.L., Wilson, F.A., Glick, A.D., Dunn, G.D.,
    and Kilroy, A.W. 1976. Hepatic ATP Concentrations
    and Glycolytic enzyme activities in Reye syndrome.
    J. Pediat. 89: 777.
3. Kobayashi, N. 1970. Ekiri, The Ekiri-like Syndrome
    and Acute Encephalopathy of Obscure Origin.
    Paediatria Universitatis Tokyo 18: 88-98.
4. Chin, I. Clinical studies on the pathogenesis of
    the so called Ekiri-like syndrome. Advance in the
    study of Ekiri in Japan, 1955.
5. Funatsu, I. 1962. The pathogenesis of so-called
    Ekiri-like syndrome and consideration of treatment
    of the bacillary dysentery. *J. Formosan Med.
    Assoc. 61:* 913.
6. Suwa, N. Pathologische Anatomie der Ekiri. Advance
    in the Study of Ekiri in Japan. 1955.

7. Yoshino, M. Effect of experimental endotoxemia
    on ureagenesis, unpublished.

ACKNOWLEDGEMENT

     We would like to thank Dr. Kyuichi Tanikawa,
Naoki Ikejiri for his good advice on the morphological
studies and acknowledge the assistance of Miss Masako
Sakai and Miss Takeko Matsuda.

     This study was supported by a grant for research
on the prevention of handicapped children by the
Japanese Ministry of Health and Welfare.

DISCUSSION

C. Solomons   -   Which method did you use for determi-
        ning ATP? I am amazed that one didn't find any-
        thing in ATP.

I. Yoshida   -   We used Bucher's method.

E. S. Kang   -   The phenomenon of the effect of endo-
        toxin of shigella is reminiscent of abnormali-
        ties due to cholera toxin. Cholera toxins bind
        to the surface of cells,stimulate the cyclic nu-
        cleotide system, and cholera toxin apparently
        doesn't get systemically circulated because it
        is to large that it is localized to the intes-
        tinal compartment. I just wondered about your
        shigella toxin; whether or not you know the cy-
        clic AMP levels of the patients or the animals
        that you have studied?

I. Yoshida   -   Unfortunately, I don't know.

J.V. Baublis   -   In the absence of Doctor Cooperstock
        who was, as far as I know, the first to utilize

the limulus assay in an imaginative way and demonstrate the presence of an endotoxin-like substance in the cerebral spinal fluid and in the plasma of patients with Reye's syndrome, I think it is important to retain the designation "endotoxin-like substance". There were some characteristics of the substance which were a little bit different from the conventional E Coli types of endotoxin. It could not be neutralized or blocked with polymyxin B. Many of the endotoxins can be blocked with polymyxin B. We considered the prospect that this was perhaps not E Coli endotoxins but one created by some of the anaerobic flora of the gut.

We have been focusing upon the hepatocyte as the site of action for many things in Reye's syndrome, but there are also the macrophages whose function it is to inactivate and process endotoxin. If we have an overwhelming infection, and it is made overwhelming by substances which are going to enhance infectivity of the body, then we are also going to lose a defense against the body's own endotoxin. It is unusual, in our cases with Reye's syndrome, that the patient enters hospital with an intact gastrointestinal tract. Most of them had at least hematemesis, suggesting some disruption of the barrier which could predispose to absorption of greater quantities of endotoxin than might normally be seen. With regard to endotoxin as a punitative factor in producing some of the metabolic effects, I was pleased to see the work which did show an impaired urea cycle function on the basis of endotoxin.

EMULSIFIERS AS ENHANCEMENT FACTORS IN VIRUS VIRULENCE

Kenneth R. Rozee, PHD, Mary Laltoo, MSc
Spencer H.S. Lee, PhD, John F.S. Crocker, M.D.
and Stephen Safe, PhD

INTRODUCTION

Many popular insecticides are immiscible with
water and require organic solvents and/or emulsifiers to
aid in their dispersal as aqueous sprays. Earlier we
showed (1,2) the enhancing action of certain fenitrothion
(FT) spray components on virus infections in mice. We
noted that the increased incidence of mortality of FT
spray-intoxicated mice after infection with encephalomyocarditis (EMC) virus was probably due largely to
emulsifiers (3). A number of these emulsifying chemicals
have now been shown by us to enhance the sensitivity of
several cultured mammalian cells to virus infections,
and this is the subject of this report.

A variety of commercial emulsifiers such as Toximul
MP8 were capable of enhancing the sensitivity of cultured
cells to infection with several viruses. Some emulsifiers
were not active as enhancers, and those viruses that
responded to the enhancing emulsifiers were single-stranded ribonucleic acid viruses. The double-stranded viruses
that were tested were nonresponders.

When the mechanism of Toximul MP8 enhancement was
investigated it was found that the increased ability of
cells to replicate virus was associated with an enhanced
uptake of virus from the media.

We further showed that the ability of interferon
to protect cells from virus infection was impaired if

these cells were first pre-treated with Toximul MP8.

We propose a mechanism of action of Toximul MP8 and other emulsifiers based on their ability to effectively increase the multiplicity of infection when treated cells are compared to controls at similar levels of virus exposure. This may have the effect of increasing the challenge dose of virus per cell and consequently reducing the effectiveness of interferon in treated cultures.

MATERIALS AND METHODS

Cells. The continuously cultured cell lines of African green monkey kidney cells (VERO) and mouse L-929 cells used in this study were originally obtained from Dr. K. MacCarthy, University of Liverpool, U.K. and Dr. R. Stewart, Queen's University, Ontario respectively. HeLa cells were obtained from our own culture bank and originally from the American Type Culture Collection. They were passaged and stored in vials in liquid nitrogen. All cultures were grown in Eagles minimum essential medium (MEM) containing 10% fetal bovine serum (FBS, Flow). The medium used to maintain mature monolayer cultures during and following treatment was MEM containing 0.5% FBS. Dilutions of virus or emulsifiers were made in MEM alone.

Viruses. Stocks of Vesicular Stomatitis virus (VSV; Indiana strain), Encephalomyocarditis virus (EMC), Vaccinia virus, Herpesvirus hominis type 1 (Herpes 1) and Reovirus type 2 (Reo 2) were grown in L-929 cells, titered and stored at -70°C in sealed vials. Poliovirus type 1 (Polio 1) stocks were grown in VERO cells and similarly stored.

Insecticide and emulsifiers. Fenitrothion (FT), confirmed by us as >98% pure by gas chromatographic analysis; a solvent used to solubilize FT (Aerotex 3470, Texaco of Canada) and two emulsifiers used in FT dispersal as an aerial spray (Toximul MP8, Chas. Tennant & Co. Ltd.; Atlox 3409, Atlas Chemical Industry Ltd.) were obtained from commercial sources. Other emulsifiers mentioned were obtained either commercially or as gifts from the manufacturers.

RESULTS

Enhancement Assay. Cells were first grown to monolayer culture in 60 mm Petri dishes (Falcon) as previously described (4). They were then exposed for 18 hours
at 37°C to dilutions of a commercial FT spray or to
emulsifiers or other component of the spray. When different emulsifiers were applied to the cell cultures,
all applications had MEM as a diluent. Following this,
the responses of the treated cell cultures and their
controls to virus infection were evaluated.

Treated and control cultures were first washed and
triplicates were inoculated with 0.3 ml of MEM containing an amount of virus calculated to form a countable
number of plaques in the control cultures. Adsorption
was allowed to proceed, with occasional tilting to mix,
for 90 minutes. At this time the cultures were over-
layed with 5 ml of 0.6% agarose in MEM containing 1%
FBS and incubated for 2 days at 37°C. Virus plaques
developing in the cultures were then identified, counted
and recorded. The average number of plaques in treated
cultures were compared to those found in control cultures
as an "enhancement index". An outline of this assay is
given in Figure 1.

Sensitivity of Various Cells. Using the assay
method as described, experiments with mouse L-929,
primary human kidney (HK), VERO, LLC-MK$_2$ and HeLa cell
cultures were performed. These cells were exposed in
triplicate for 18 hours at 37°C to MEM or to various
concentrations of Toximul MP8 in MEM. They were then
washed and inoculated with 0.3 ml of MEM containing an
amount of VSV which was calculated to produce a countable number of plaques on control cultures. The
cultures were then incubated at 37°C for 2-3 days for
plaques to develop. The results are given in Table 1.

Table 2 shows that all of the cells are rendered
more permissive to VSV. This was particularly true of
HeLa cells; they proved to be especially susceptible to
Toximul MP8 enhancement.

__MAMMALIAN CELL__

MONOLAYER CULTURES

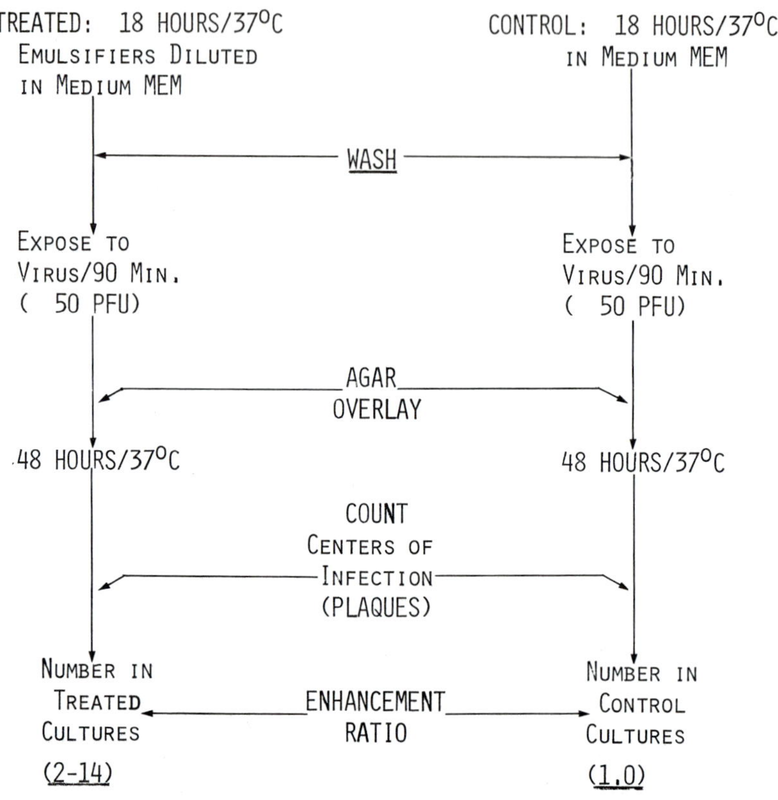

Figure 1.   The protocol used for enhancement assays of
            emulsifiers.

__The Response of Different Viruses to Toximul MP8.__
We next determined whether different viruses could participate in the enhancement phenomenon. The experimental protocol was as described for VSV with the exception
that other virus inocula, containing a countable number
of plaque-forming units, replaced VSV. L-929 cell
monolayer cultures were exposed to 10 PPM of Toximul MP8
in MEM overnight before infection with VSV, EMC, Vaccinia, Herpes 1 or Reo 2. VERO cells were similarly
exposed prior to infection with Polio 1 since L-929 cells
will not support the growth of poliovirus.

TABLE 1. The enhancing effect of the emulsifier,
          Toximul MP8, on the ability of mammalian
          cell cultures to support vesicular stomatitis
          virus(VSV) replication.

| | VSV PLAQUES PER CULTURE[a] | | | | |
| CELL | CONCENTRATION OF TOXIMUL PPM | | | | |
TYPE	0	0.25	1.0	2.5	10.0
L-929	50 ± 0.6	51 ± 4.5	65 ± 4.4	111 ± 7.2	218 ± 10
LLC-MK$_2$	21 ± 1.8	20 ± 2.6	23 ± 2.4	35 ± 3.2	54 ± 3.8
VERO	69 ± 1.8	72 ± 4.3	76 ± 3.0	99 ± 3.1	110 ± 5.3
HeLa	68 ± 2.8	196 ± 6.6	$490^b\pm10$	$380^b\pm40$	-
HK	27 ± 2.4	32 ± 2.3	41 ± 2.3	79 ± 4.9	73 ± 2.8

[a] The values are the mean $\pm$ standard error.
[b] Estimate: cultures had too many plaques for accurate
    counting.

     Following a wash in MEM, triplicate cultures were
infected with a dose of appropriate virus which was
calculated to produce a countable number of plaques in
control cultures. They were then incubated for the
time required for plaques to develop; 2 days for VSV,
Polio 1 and EMC; 4 days for Vaccinia and Herpes 1; and
7 days for Reo 2. Average plaque counts were recorded
for both Toximul-treated and untreated control cultures
and the ratio of these plaque numbers was calculated as
an index of enhancement. The data of one such experiment
is given in Table 2 where it can be seen that the
infectivity of single-stranded RNA viruses (VSV, EMC
and Polio 1) is enhanced while the infectivity of
double-stranded RNA virus (Reo 2) is not enhanced.

     Effect of Emulsifiers other than Toximul MP8. We
next ascertained if the enhancing activity of Toximul MP8

TABLE 2.   The effect of exposure of L-929 cells to
           10 PPM Toximul MP8 on the plaque efficiency
           of various viruses.

| | PLAQUES PER CULTURE[a] | | | (RATIO) ENHANCEMENT |
VIRUS	TREATED	/ CONTROL =	INDEX
VSV	218.7±19.0	50.0±1.0	4.37
EMC	36.3±5.5	10.7±1.2	3.39
POLIO 1[b]	62.3±1.5	36.3±6.6	1.72
HERPES 1	42.3±2.9	40.7±4.5	1.04
VACCINIA	112.0±16.0	106.7±11.5	1.05
REO 2	16.7±3.8	16.0±4.0	1.04

[a]Mean ± standard deviation.
[b]Experiment performed in VERO cells.

was shared by others of a wide variety of emulsifiers.
An attempt was also made to compare the chemical com-
positions of enhancing emulsifiers to see whether any
similarities were present.

These emulsifiers were evaluated in a similar
manner to that employed for Toximul MP8. A change was
made, however, in the type of cell culture. We observed,
above, that HeLa cells appeared more sensitive to the
effects of Toximul MP8 than other cells. Consequently
HeLa cells were used in these experiments. They were
grown in monolayer culture and exposed to various
dilutions of each emulsifier for 18 hours at 37°C.
They were washed and infected with an amount of VSV
calculated to produce a countable number of plaques.
Average plaque numbers were calculated on the basis of
three cultures per dilution. Untreated control cultures
were exposed to diluent and similarly infected. The

ratio of the average number of plaques found in emulsifier treated cultures divided by the average number
found in control, untreated HeLa cell cultures,was calculated as an index of enhancement. The results are
given in Table 3 in which enhancement was shown to occur
following exposure of cells to the Toximul series, Plur-
onic L64, Brij 56, Atlox 3409, Polytergent FL62, Marl-
ophen 810 and Sodium dodecyl sulphate. Eight other
assorted emulsifiers did not cause enhancement.

   Figure 2 presents a summary of the characteristics
of this phenomenon as determined by these and other
experiments reported elsewhere (1,2,3). There is a
requirement that cells be exposed for some 4-6 hours at
37^OC before they become sensitized by the emulsifier.
Exposure at 4^OC is not effective and the effect is
reversed in 4-6 hours if the emulsifier is removed. The
active emulsifiers have no measurable effect on viruses
alone. Various cells are differentially sensitive to
this effect with the most responsive cell being HeLa.
Single stranded viruses are enhanced but those viruses
having double stranded nucleic acid as their genome are
not. The enhancing emulsifiers appear to be non-ionic
polymers of polyoxyethylene ethers.

   <u>Mechanism of Action of Toximul MP8.</u> We began our
investigation into the mechanism(s) by which emulsifiers
render cells more permissive to virus infection by de-
termining the amount of virus taken up by treated as
compared to control cells.

   L-929 cells, grown to confluent monolayer cultures
in petri dishes, were treated with 10 PPM Toximul MP8,
in MEM, at 37^OC for 18 hours. Identical cultures were
kept in MEM alone under similar conditions as control
cells.

   Following treatment, both groups of cultures were
infected with an amount of EMC equivalent to 0.1 plaque
forming unit per cell. The infected cultures were then
incubated at 37^OC for 90 minutes at which time the
supernatant fluid was removed and assayed for its virus
content. The cells were trypsinized and monodispersed

RATIO OF TREATED:CONTROL PLAQUE NUMBERS

EMULSIFIER (PPM)	100	10	5	1	0.1	CHEMICAL NATURE
Toximul MP8	-	14.5	2.0	1.0	1.0	anionic-nonionic blend of dodecyl-benzene sulphonate and polyoxy-ethylene ethers
Marlophen 810	-	toxic	toxic	12.7	0.9	surfactant (composition unknown)
Polytergent FL62	-	11.1	11.0	1.4	0.8	polyalcoxyether indeterminant composition
Pluronic L64	-	toxic	toxic	11.0	0.5	polyoxypropylene/polyoxyethylene copolymer
Brij 56	-	toxic	toxic	9.9	1.6	polyoxyethylene cetyl ether
Toximul D	-	toxic	8.0	1.8	1.0	anionic-nonionic blend of dodecyl-benzene sulphonate and polyoxy-ethylene ethers
Toximul R	-	toxic	7.1	1.6	1.3	anionic-nonionic blend of dodecyl-benzene sulphonate and polyoxy-ethylene ethers
Atlox 3409	-	3.6	1.9	1.1	0.8	anionic-nonionic blend of dodecyl-benzene sulphonate and polyoxy-ethylene ethers

Sodium dodecyl sulphate	toxic	2.1	-	0.8	-	anionic detergent - $C_{12}H_{25}NaO_4S$
Varine 17	toxic	1.7	1.3	1.4	0.7	sodium dodecylbenzene sulphonate anionic detergent
Plurafac RA30	toxic	1.6	0.8	1.0	0.8	polyoxyethylene alcohol
Nonidet P40	toxic	1.5	-	1.3	1.1	nonionic detergent $C_8H_{17}C_6H_4O(CH_2CH_2O)_9H$
Richonate 40B	toxic	1.4	1.4	0.7	1.1	sodium dodecylbenzene sulphonate anionic detergent
Toximul MP10	toxic	1.4	1.1	0.8	0.9	anionic-nonionic blend of dodecyl-benzene sulphonate and polyoxy-ethylene ethers
Triton X-100	toxic	1.2	-	1.1	1.0	nonionic detergent $C_8H_{17}C_6H_4O(CH_2CH_2O)_{9-10}H$
Sterox SL	toxic	toxic	-	0.8	1.0	nonionic detergent $C_{14-15}O(CH_2CH_2O)_{12}H$
Pluronic L31	toxic	0.8	0.8	0.7	0.7	nonionic polyalcoxyether polymer

TABLE 3.   The effect on HeLa cells exposed to different concentrations of various emulsifiers and subsequently infected with VSV.

451

FIGURE 2.

CHARACTERISTICS OF TOXIMUL MP8
ENHANCEMENT OF VIRUS INFECTIVITY

1. Exposure time required - 4-6 hours.

2. Temperature required - $37^{\circ}C$, Neg. at $4^{\circ}C$.

3. Reversible in 4-6 hours following washing at $37^{\circ}C$.

4. Pre-exposure of virus is not effective, nor is
    virus titer lowered.

5. Spectrum of cell sensitivities

    Marginally Sensitive ___________ Highly Sensitive
         (VERO)   (HeLa)

6. Spectrum of virus types affected

    No Effect   _______________ 4-6 X Enhancement
    (HERPES, REO)   (EMC, VSV)

7. Enhancing emulsifiers seem to be non-ionic polymers
    of polyoxyethylene ethers.

---

in MEM and then assayed for infectious centers. The
data from these assays are recorded in Table 4 which
shows that 3.13 times the number of infectious centers
were found in Toximul-treated cultures as compared to
controls. In addition, the treated cultures had only
0.64 the amount of virus remaining in the supernatant
as was found in the controls. The obvious conclusion
is that Toximul treated cells absorbed significantly
larger amounts of virus than did untreated cells.

   Toximul MP8 and the Interferon Response. The
efficacy of applied homologous interferon varies inversely with the amount of challenge virus used to
infect interferon-treated cells. In interferon assays,
the higher the challenge dose of virus (the higher the
multiplicity of infection {MOI}) the lower is the
determined titer of interferon (5). Bearing this
relationship in mind, we investigated whether or not
certain emulsifiers, capable of increasing the MOI of
an infective inoculum when treated cells are used,

TABLE 4.   The number of infectious centers in cultures
           and plaque forming units in supernatants of
           cells treated with 10 PPM of Toximul MP8 for
           18 hours at 37°C in comparison to untreated
           control cultures.

	# INFECTIOUS CENTERS		# pfu REMAINING IN s/n	
	+ Tox	− Tox	+ Tox	− Tox
	800	290	1000	1600
	800	240	1000	1800
	1300	280	1500	1800
	600	310	800	1500
Total	3500	1120	4300	6700
Average	875±298	280±29	1075±299	1675±150
Ratio:	3.13		0.64	

could diminish the ability of cells to respond to interferon.

Three groups of L-929 monolayer cultures in Petri
dishes were set up. One group was exposed for 18 hours
at 37°C to 25 PPM Toximul; another group to 25 PPM Atlox
and a third group to the MEM diluent alone.

Following exposure each group was divided into
triplicate cultures and each triplicate was exposed to
a dilution of mouse interferon for 6 hours at 37°C.
The triplicates of all three groups were then infected
with an amount of VSV challenge virus precalculated to
develop about 50 plaques on the untreated control cultures. 90 minutes with occasional shaking were allowed
for adsorption and then a nutrient overlay containing
agar was placed over each culture. Following a three
day incubation at 37°C, plaques were counted in each of

the groups. The data is plotted in Figure 3 which
shows a substantial and significant loss of potency of
interferon when assayed in Toximul or Atlox treated
cells.

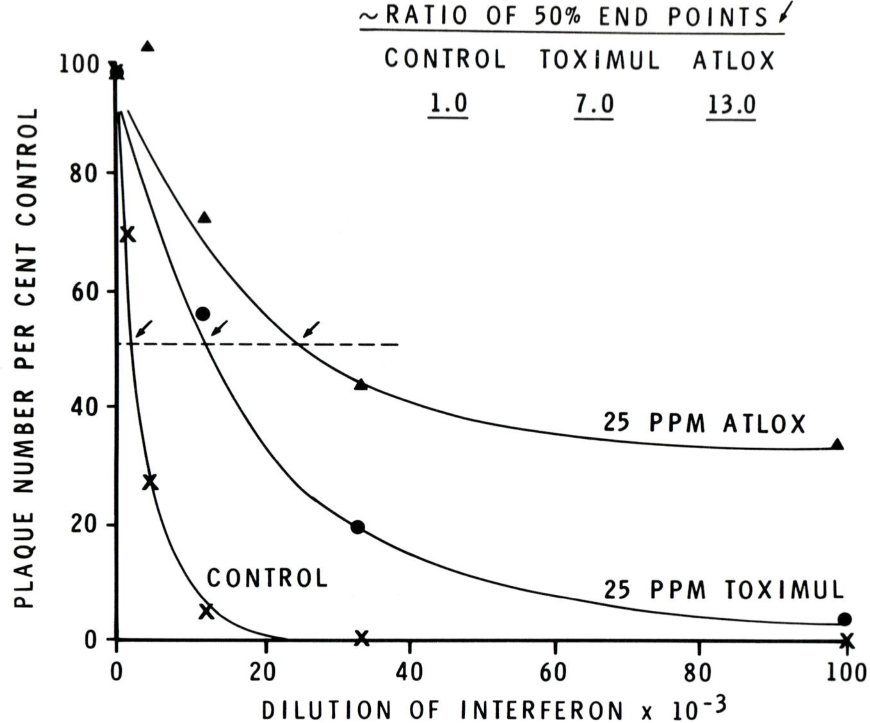

DISCUSSION

There can be no doubt that certain emulsifiers
induce cells to a higher level of permissiveness with
respect to virus infection. It would appear that sub-
stantially more virus is taken up by cells treated with
these emulsifiers. As a consequence of this greater
virus uptake the effective MOI for treated as compared
to untreated cells, with any particular virus inoculum,
is at least several fold higher. This has the effect
of reducing the efficacy of the interferon response,
since this is directly dependent upon the amount of
infective virus available in the environment of the cell.

We propose that this mechanism may be operational

in the up-to-now inexplicably severe response of
Reye's syndrome patients to infection with certain
viruses. Perhaps small amounts of emulsifiers or like
chemicals, in the environment are sufficient to reduce
the interferon response of exposed individuals. On
infection with one of several suitable viruses these
compromised persons may suffer a profoundly overwhelming
infection which manifests itself as Reye's syndrome.

REFERENCES

1. Crocker, J.F.S., Rozee, K.R., Ozere, R.L., Digout,
    S.C., and Hutzinger, O. 1974. *Lancet 1974 II*:22.
2. Crocker, J.F.S., Ozere, R.L., Safe, S.H., Digout,
    S.C., Rozee, K.R., and Hutzinger, O. 1976. *Science
    192:* 1351.
3. Rozee, K.R., Lee, S.H.S., Crocker, J.F.S., and
    Safe, S.H. 1978. *Appl. Environ. Microbiol. 35*:297.
4. Lee, S.H.S., O'Shaughnessy, M.V., and Rozee, K.R.
    1972. *Proc. Soc. Exp. Biol. Med. 139:* 1438.
5. Rozee, K.R. and Lee, S.H.S., in Interferons and
    Their Actions, W.E. Stewart II (ed.), C.R.C.
    Publications, 1977.

DISCUSSION

Unidentified -   Have you tried the myxoviruses in
    this system, Influenza A or B or C?

K.R. Rozee   -   No; we haven't tried any myxovirus-
    es in this system at all. We plan to.

Same Speaker -   You noticed the most pronounced ef-
    fect with VSV, which is a notorious virus that ag-
    gregates. Is it possible that what you are obser-
    ving is really a disaggregation of the virus by
    the emulsifier,giving you an increased efficiency
    of placquing?

K.R. Rozee   -   No; when we put the virus in the
        emulsifier and then placque subsequently, we
        see no difference in the placquing.

Same Speaker   -   So you have to pre-treat the cell?

K.R. Rozee   -   You have to pre-treat the cell.

D.B. Tower   -   I don't know about your EMC virus,
        but VSV is very prone to produce defective in-
        fectious particles. In some cell preparations,
        these DI particles are a very excellent stimu-
        lus for the production of interferon. I just
        wonder whether you have examined the possibili-
        ty of there being some alteration in this cha-
        racteristic of a VSV virus in your particular
        experimental condition?

K.R. Rozee   -   No; we haven't examined that,even
        though we are aware of the phenomenon of de-
        fective interfering viruses. The other inter-
        esting thing about VSV, of course, is that
        it's a membranous virus. I was interested in
        the comments that were made this morning,par-
        ticularly related to that.

Unidentified   -   I think that the ability to dilute
        to get this sort of an effect with parts per
        million is very interesting. Doctor Halstead,
        in his studies of Dengi in Thailand, has point-
        ed out the role of presumably an enhancing
        antibody in that an antiserum to Dengi, dilu-
        ted beyond its neutralizing ability,began to
        show an enhancing effect on the cells of the
        system. I wonder if, in the case of some chil-
        dren with Reye's syndrome who have been ex-
        posed to some of these products, one might not
        see a similar effect if one goes beyond the
        neutralizing effect. Let's say for influenza
        one might find that an enhancing effect due to
        some of these emulsifiers might be detected.
        Have you looked at any Reye's serum to see if
        there is an enhancing effect?

K.R. Rozee   -   No; we haven't looked at any Reye's
          serum yet. I should point out that the concen-
          trations that are operational here in our cul-
          tures are just sub-toxic concentrations. What
          we do ordinarily when we are assaying an emul-
          sifier is to run it up to its level of toxici-
          ty,and then back off; we find that this is ap-
          proximately the level where it is actively en-
          hancing.

J.D. Pollack   -   Ken, very interesting results in
          view of the reversibility of the effect..this
          suggests an interesting mechanism of exposure
          of receptors and then, somehow, covering up
          the receptors as an effect of the solvent.

K.R. Rozee   -   The reversibility of this phenomenon
          is interesting in that it may be important if
          these emulsifiers find a place in the etiology
          of Reye's. Exposed people will be intermit-
          tently susceptible, depending on the time of
          exposure to the ingredient.

INTRACELLULAR CHANGES INDUCED BY
EMULSIFIER-VIRUS INTERACTION IN
VIVO AND IN VITRO IN THE MOUSE.

Dugald A. Taylor, Ph D., Philip
C.Bagnell, M.D., Kenneth Renton,
Ph D., and J.F.S.Crocker, M. D.

INTRODUCTION

The use of insecticides in forest spray programs
requires the use of one or more solvents and a blend of
emulsifiers for aerial dispersal. Observations on the
increased incidence of Reye's syndrome in a group of
Canadian children living contiguous to the area of a
forest spray program, have led to our investigations of
a hypothesized interaction between insecticide carriers,
emulsifiers and viruses, as reported elsewhere.(1,2).

One of the emulsifiers, Toximul MP8 (Charles Tennant & Co. Ltd.) has been shown to enhance the lethality of encephalomyocarditis virus in newborn mice, and
virus infectivity in cultured cell lines (3). The present study concerns morphologic evidence of a direct
toxic effect of this emulsifier alone, in mice IN VIVO

and in embryonic mouse liver cultures at concentrations
of 10-100 ppm. Preliminary observations of an effect on
cultured human embryonic liver are also reported.

METHODS

(1) IN VITRO embryonic mouse liver: liver lobes
were obtained from mouse embryos at approximately 10
days gestational age and maintained in culture for 19,
42 or 72 hours by a modified Grobstein method (3) with
10, 20 or 100ppm of Toximul MP8 added to the medium.
Control tissues were obtained and cultured in an identical fashion, but with no emulsifier added. At the end
of the culture period, the tissues were removed and
placed in fixative.

(2) IN VIVO mouse studies: young suckling mice,48
hours of age, were maintained in the laboratory from 2
to 11 days and were daily exposed to a 7% solution of
Toximul MP8 (in council) by dermal application. Then
mice were sacrificed at age 17, liver tissue was removed and placed in a fixative. Control mice were maintained in the same facilities, but were exposed dermal-
ly to corn oil.

(3) IN VITRO human embryonic liver: slices of liver tissue from vacuum currettage therapeutic abortions
were obtained and maintained in culture as for the mouse
liver tissue. One portion of each specimen was exposed
to emulsifier (Toximul MP8) and another portion of the
same liver served as a control.

(4) Specimen preparation and examination: tissues
were fixed in 2% glutaraldehyde in cacodylate buffer,
toxicity adjusted to 300 mOsm/l for 4 hours, washed in
buffer, post-fixed in OsO_4 and embedded in TAAB resin.
Sections cut at 0.5μ were stained with Toluidine blue.
Selected blocks were trimmed and thin sections cut and
stained with Uranyl and Lead. Grids were examined on a
Phillips EM300 electron microscope.

(5) Benzo(a)pyrene hydroxylase was determined in
tissue homogenates as described by Wattenberg and Leong
(4).

RESULTS

Controls in all series showed orthodox mitochondrial configuration, with normal electron density of the matrix and the presence of matrix granules. Some culture artifact was noted in the controls, with occasional large empty cytoplasmic vacuoles noted at 19 hours inoculation (Figure 1) and very occasional necrotic cells present by 42 hours of culturing (Figure 4). However, mitochondria in preserved cells maintained normal appearance. The number of autophagic vacuoles increased with time in culture.

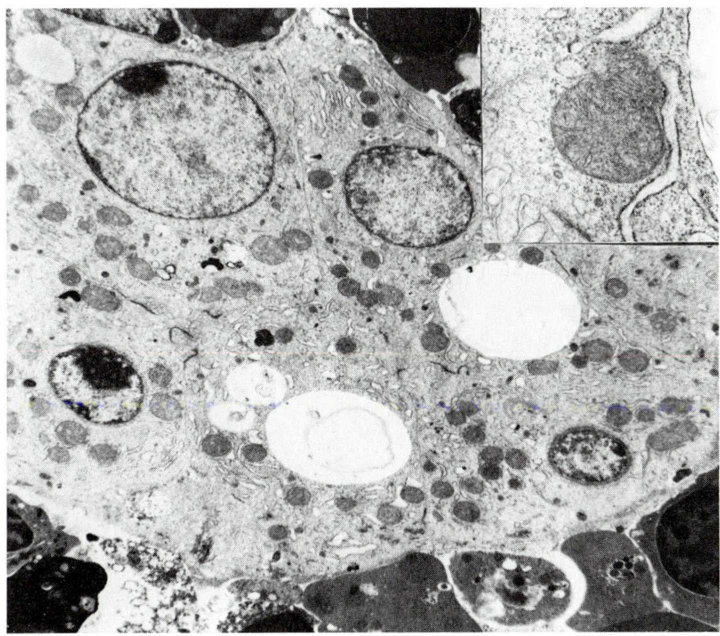

Fig.1.   Mouse <u>in vitro</u> control (19 hours); magnification x3306.5. Hepatocytes in center show normal configuration with mitochondria of normal size and density.(Insert: mitochondrion x 16,575).The large empty cytoplasmic vacuoles are artifacts of culture. Numerous small dark hematopoietic cells are present at the periphery.

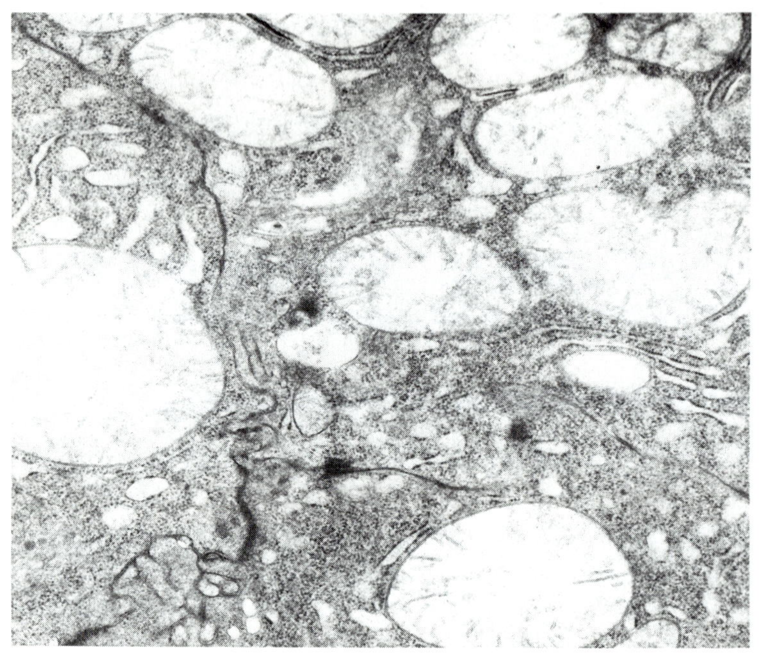

Fig.2. Mouse <u>in vitro</u>, 10 ppm Toximul MP8 (19 hours);
        magnification x 15,600. Mitochondria are swollen
        and pale,with margination of cristae and loss of
        matrical densities.

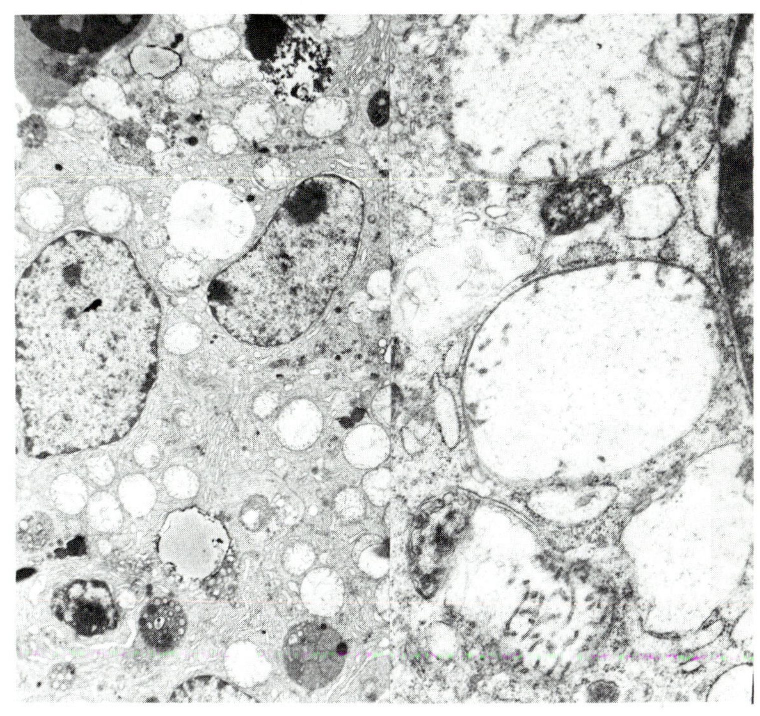

Fig.3. Mouse <u>in vitro</u>, 100 ppm Toximul MP8 (19
       hours); magnifications x 3,112 (left) and
       x 15,600 (right). Mitochondria are swollen
       with disruption of cristae. Autophagic and
       fat vacuoles are prominent in cytoplasm.

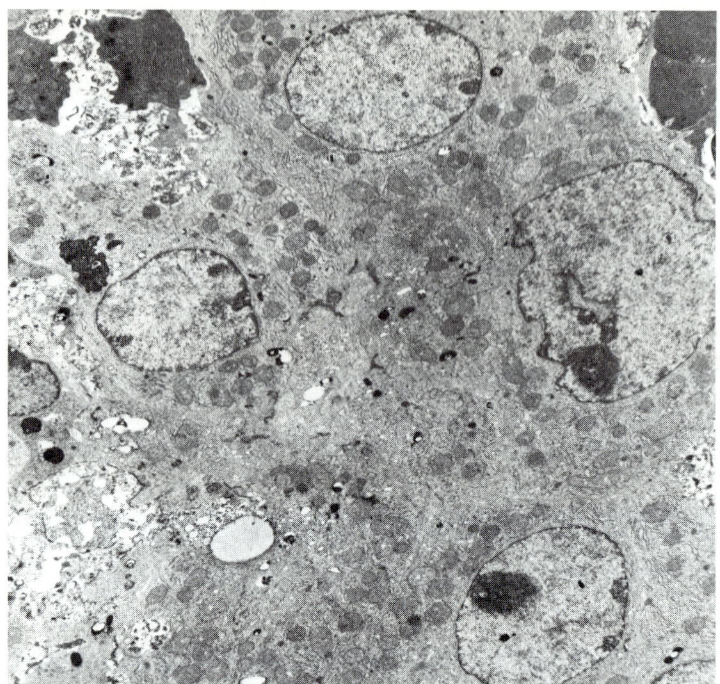

Fig.4.   Mouse _in vitro_ control (42 hours); magni-
         fication x 3,112. Hepatocytes show normally
         dense small mitochondria. Autophagic vacuoles
         are increased,and occasional necrotic cells are
         present, at left.

     IN VITRO cultured mouse liver tissue showed pro-
gressive mitochondrial damage, generally increasing
with the concentration of Toximul MP8 and with the time
in culture. Figures 2 and 5 of cultures at 19 hours in
10 ppm Toximul MP8 and at 42 hours in 20 ppm Toximul MP8
show marked mitochondrial swelling with margination and
disruption of cristae, and a striking rarefaction of the
matrix.   Changes by 19 hours at 100 ppm were more marked,with degenerating mitochondria and occasional cytoplasmic lipid vacuoles and increased autophagy (Fig.3).
By 42 hours in 100 ppm Toximul MP8, there was also
marked dilation of endoplasmic reticulum, and many cells
were necrotic (Fig. 6).   The changes in endoplasmic reticulum were also reflected in benzo(a)pyrene hydroxylase activity which was decreased by 70% compared to
control cultures.

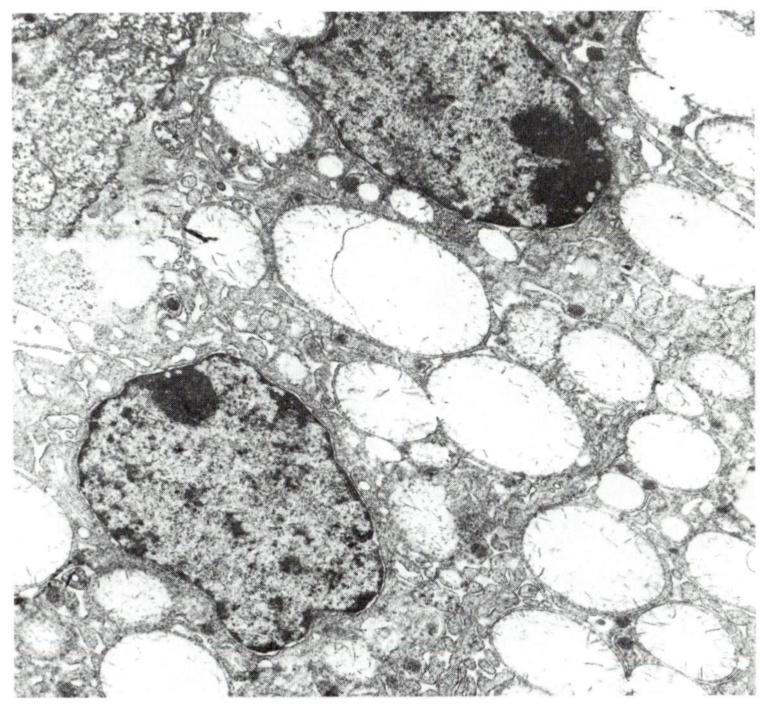

Fig.5. Mouse _in vitro_, 20 ppm Toximul MP8
   (42 hours); magnification x 6,672. Mitochondria
   are markedly swollen, with size approaching that
   of the nuclei.

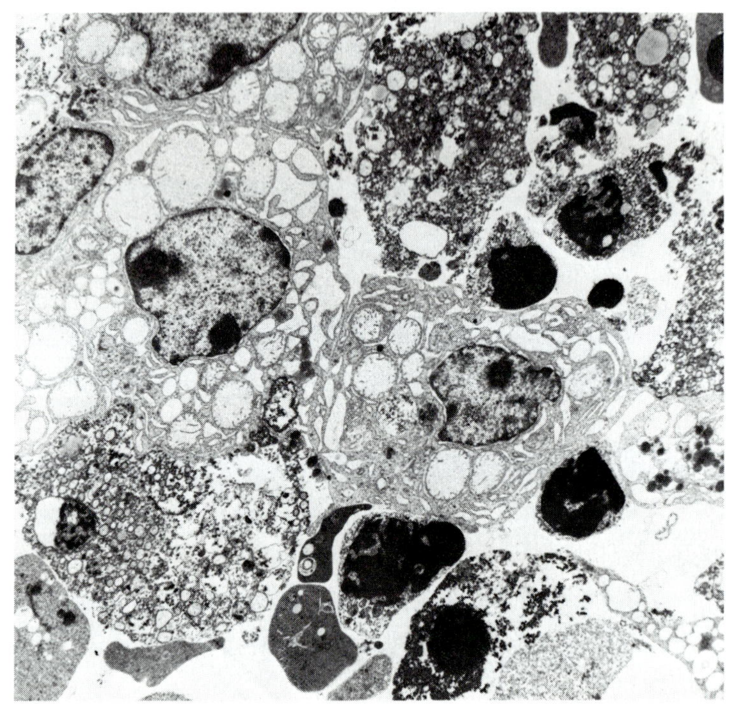

Fig. 6. Mouse <u>in vitro</u>, 100 ppm Toximul MP8
(42 hours); magnification x 3,112. Many
necrotic cells are present; viable cells show
prominent swelling and pallor of mitochondria,
and dilation of endoplasmic reticulum.

TABLE I.

CYTOCHROME P-450 DEPENDENT BENZO(A)PYRENE
HYDROXYLATION IN FETAL MOUSE LIVER ORGAN CULTURE

Treatment	Benzo(a)pyrene hydroxylation (% of corresponding control)
Control	100 ± 13.4 (N=6)
Toximul MP8 (100ppm)	29.6 ± 4.3 *(N=9)

*Significantly different from control (P<0.01)

In the Toximul MP8 - treated liver IN VIVO, mitochondrial enlargement and pallor of the matrix but well-
preserved cristae, were observed (Fig.7).

Preliminary observations on IN VITRO human liver,
cultured for 72 hours with and without 100 ppm Toximul
MP8, are demonstrated in Figures 8 and 9. The control
shows general good preservation of cytoarchitecture with
normal mitochondria, and the treated sample shows necrosis with total destruction of membranous structures,
and pyknotic nuclei and fat globules.

DISCUSSION

These studies are preliminary, but there appears
to be a demonstratable toxic effect of the emulsifier
Toximul MP8 with ultrastructural alterations and, particularly, mitochondrial changes both IN VIVO and more
markedly IN VITRO. While fatty changes are not marked
nor consistent in these tissues, we have reported fatty change previously in our mouse model, when both emulsifier and virus were used (5). The present observations
could be considered in the context of a suggested pathogenic sequence in the evaluation of the lesion of Reye's
syndrome, with mitochondrial abnormalities preceding the
fatty change (6).

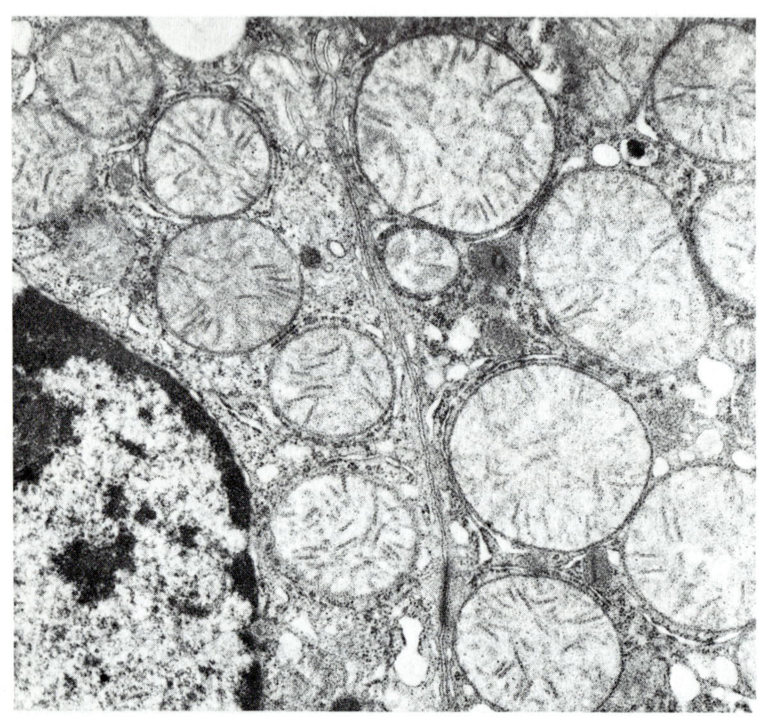

Fig.7. Mouse _in_ _vivo_, Toximul MP8 treated;
    magnification x 15,600. Mitochondria are
    mildly enlarged and pale, with near-normal
    pattern of cristae.

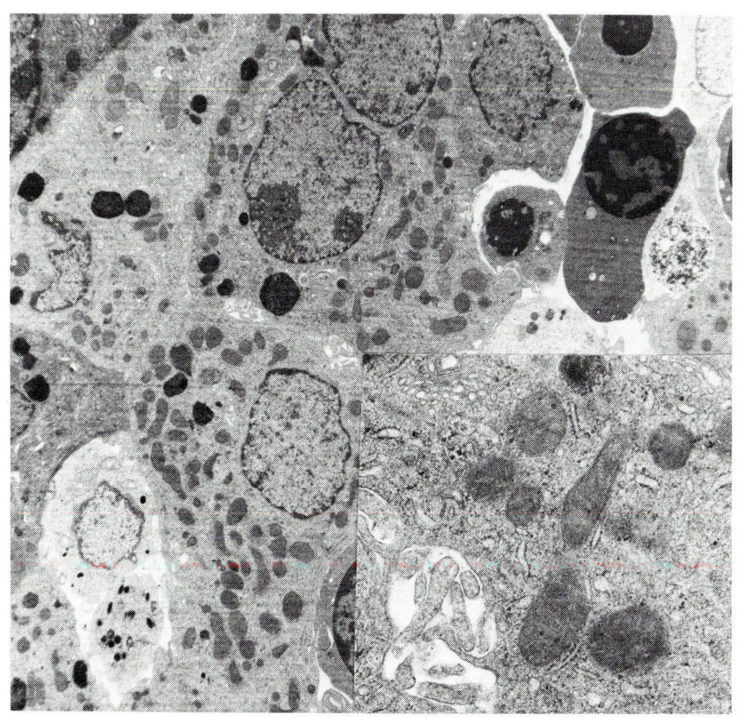

Fig. 8. Human _in vitro_ control (72 hours);
magnification x 3,112. Hepatocytes show
near normal morphology,with increased autophagic vacuoles but normally dense small
mitochondria (Insert:mitochondria x 15,600).
The small dark cells are hematopoietic cells.

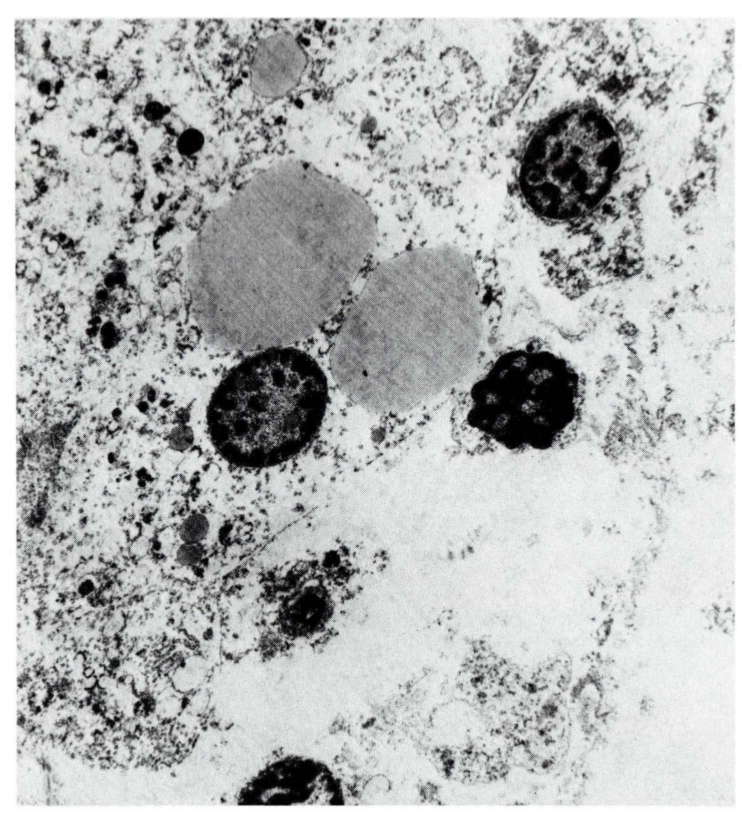

Fig.9. Human _in vitro_, 100 ppm Toximul MP8
        (72 hours); magnification x 3,501. Necrotic
        debris with membranous fragments, pykotic
        nuclei, and grey globules of lipid.

The decrease in benzo(a)pyrene hydroxylase (which is a cytochrome P-450 dependent enzyme located in the endoplasmic reticulum) demonstrates that the effects of Toximul MP8 are not confined to the mitochondria. Dilation of endoplasmic reticulum membranes was also noted in some electron micrographs of Toximul MP8-treated cultures (Fig.6) and by Juggi and Iyngkaran in patients with Reye's syndrome (7).

Further morphologic studies are intended, and work has recently begun on changes in cytoplasmic and mito-chondrial enzyme levels in response to challenge by emulsifier.

REFERENCES

1. Reye,R.D.K.,Morgan,G.,and Baral,T. 1963. Encepha-lopathy and fatty degeneration of the viscera: a disease entity in childhood. *Lancet II:*749.

2. Crocker,J.F.S.,Ozere,R.L.,Safe,S.H.,Digout,S.C., Rozee,K.R.,Hutzinger,O. 1976. Lethal Interaction of Ubiquitous Insecticide Carriers with Virus. *Science: 192:*1351.

3. Rozee,K.R.,Lee,S.H.S.,Crocker,J.F.S.,Safe,S.H., 1978. Enhanced Virus Replication in Mammalian Cells exposed to Commercial Emulsifiers. *Appl.Environm. Microbiol. 35(2):*297.

4. Grobstein,C., 1957. Some transmission characteris-tics of the tubule inducing influence on mouse me-tanephrogenic mesenchyme.*Exp.Cell Res.13:*575.

5.   Wattenburg, L.W. and Leong,J.L. 1962. Benzo(a)pyrene hydroxylation action in G.I. tract. *Cancer Research* 22:1120.

6.   Crocker,J.F.S.,Ozere,R.L.,Rozee,K.R.,Digout,S.C., Hutzinger,O. 1974. Insecticide and Viral Interaction as a Cause of Fatty Visceral Changes and Encephalopathy in the Mouse. *Lancet* :22.

7.   Yoshida,I.,Yamashita,F.,Yoshino,M. and Okada,S., 1978. Antecedent Mitochondrial Changes to the Appearance of Fatty Droplets and ATP Concentration in Rat Liver treated with 4-Pentenoic Acid. *Int'l Conf. Reye's Syndrome, Halifax, N.S.*

8.   Juggi,J.S, Iyngkaran,N., Prathap, K. 1978. Hyperammonemia in Reye's syndrome. *Int'l Conference on Reye's Syndrome, Halifax, N. S.*

DISCUSSION

J.R. Aprille   -   I was wondering; are the concentrations you're using concentrations that you would expect to find naturally acquired, or are these really excessive that you need to produce the effects that you are seeing?

D.A. Taylor   -   I don't know what results of assays in tissues have been, and we have not analyzed concentrations produced by the skin painting.

B.C. Reiner   -   I couldn't really make out dense granules. Does your test animal normally have dense granules in the mitohypochondria like the human does,and what happens to the dense granules?

D.A. Taylor -   The control animals normally do
have dense granules and these disappear with the
onset of swelling. They are absent in the mild
swelling.

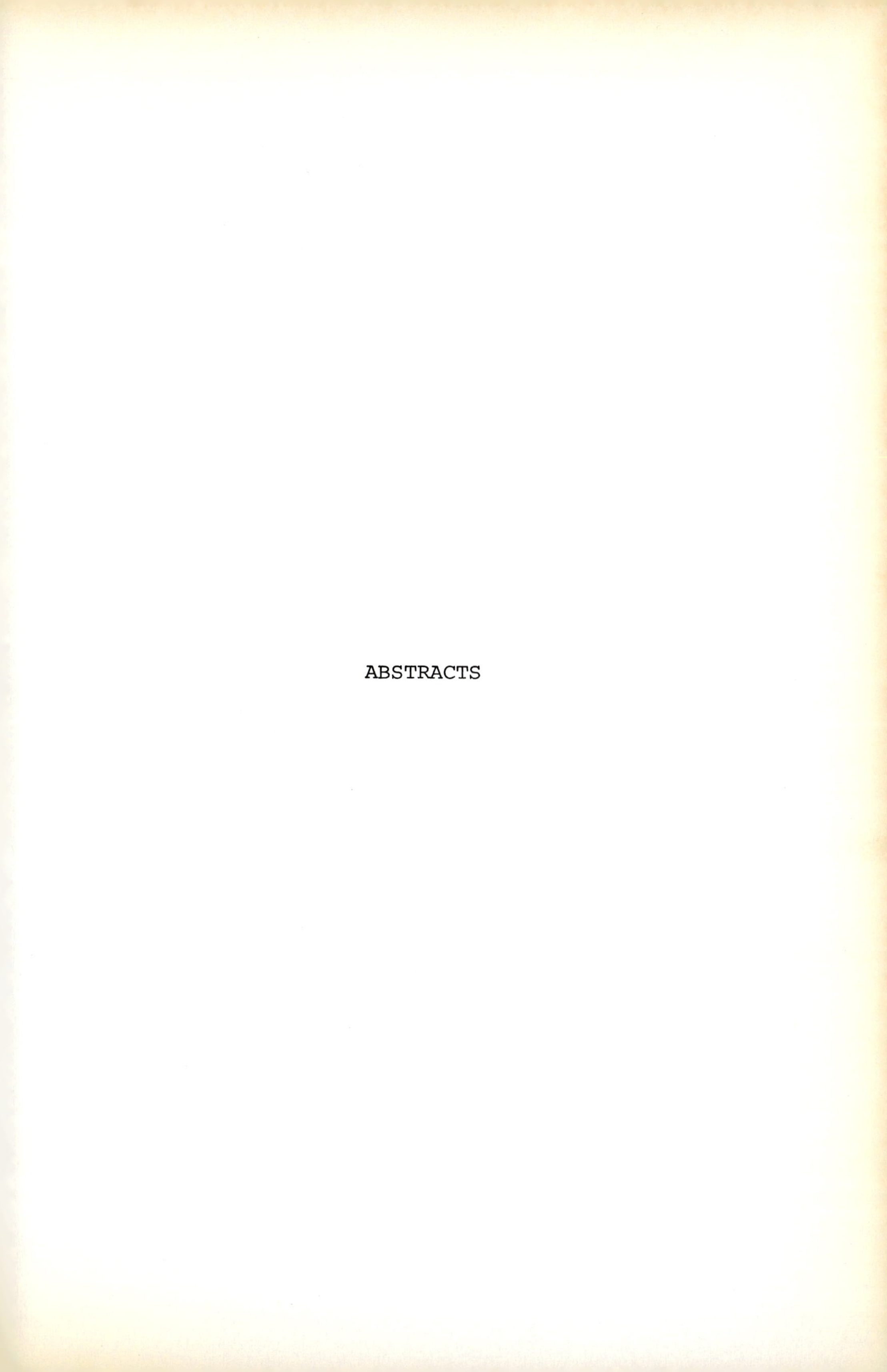

ABSTRACTS

REYE'S SYNDROME IN ADULTS

L.E. Davis, M.D. and M. Kornfeld, M.D.

Although Reye's syndrome primarily occurs in children, the age spectrum of this disease is increasing. Cases have been described in infants, and we report here two cases in adults. A 57-year-old man and an 18-year-old woman developed a mild influenza illness followed by the abrupt onset of vomiting, delirium, seizures, coma and death. Serum glutamic-oxaloacetic transaminase levels were elevated in both. At autopsy, both cases demonstrated brain edema without inflammation, and fatty degeneration of the liver. Influenza A/Victoria/3/75 virus was isolated from the trachea and spinal cord of one case, and serological evidence of an acute infection with Influenza A virus was demonstrated in the second. Reye's syndrome should be considered in anyone who presents with a mild upper respiratory illness followed by vomiting, seizures, and coma.

(Supported in part by Research Service, Veterans' Administration.)

URINARY AND PLASMA TYRAMINE IN PATIENTS

WITH REYE'S SYNDROME

B.A. Faraj, M.D., D.B. Caplan, M. D.,
S.L. Newman, M.D., P. A. Ahmann, M. D.,
and F.M. Ali, M. D.

Some of the neurological manifestations of hepatic encephalopathy may be due to the accumulation of
false neurotransmitters such as tyramine (T). Normally
T and other aromatic amines are largely metabolized by
the liver; but when hepatic function is impaired, they
may flood the nervous system and probably affect brain
function by replacing normal transmitters. In support
of this hypothesis, Faraj et al (N. Engl. J. Med. 294:
1360, 1976) found that plasma T levels were significantly higher in encephalopathic cirrhotics than in
non-encephalopathic cirrhotics, hospitalized patients
without hepatic disorders and normal controls. With the
availability of a sensitive and specific radioimmuno-
assay for T (Faraj et al, Proc. Soc. Exptl. Biol. Med.
149:664, 1975), we were able to evaluate the role of T
in Reye's syndrome. Plasma levels and 24 hr urinary
excretion of T were compared in 12 patients (age 1/2 -
14 yrs) with Reye's syndrome at time of admission and
following their treatment and discharge from the hos-
piral and 4 healthy control subjects (age 2-6 yrs).
The results indicated that in patients with Reye's
syndrome there was a significant (p<0.02) elevation of
average plasma (3.6, range 2.50-5.40 ng/ml) and 24 hr
urinary excretion of T (0.85, range 0.52-2.85 mg/24hr)
as compared to normal controls (0.75 ng/ml, 0.30mg/
24 hr), respectively. The hypertyraminemia seen in
these patients appeared to correlate with their comatose state since following treatment and discharge
there was an appreciable drop in their average plasma
T (1.5, range, 1.22-2.07 ng/ml). Furthermore, the
majority of the patients also exhibited abnormal average plasma tyrosine levels (15, range 37-5; normal
range 3.1-7.1mmoles/100 ml). These preliminary studies

suggest that major disturbances exist in the hepatic
degradation of tyrosine and T as demonstrated by an
increased proportion of circulatory tyrosine and T in
children with Reye's syndrome. These metabolic abnormalities may contribute to the pathogenesis of this
syndrome and that the measurement of T in plasma may
be used as specific marker for the development of hepatic coma in these patients.

DECREASED SERUM VLDL-TRIGLYCERIDES AND

HDL-CHOLESTEROL IN REYE'S SYNDROME

E.Chaves-Carballo, M.D. and G. A. Carter,M.D.

Lipoprotein triglyceride (TG) and cholesterol
(CHOL) concentration were measured serially, after pre-
parative ultracentrifugation, in five patients with
Reye's syndrome. Very-low-density lipoprotein triglyceride (VLDL-TG) concentrations on the day of admission
averaged 33% (range, 17 to 77%) of VLDL-TG concentrations found at the time of recovery or death (mean±SEM,
18.8±5.1 versus 52.4±12.4 mg/dl; $p<0.05$). However,
initial VLDL-TG concentrations in Reye's syndrome patients were not significantly different from mean control
values (28.2±1.3 mg/dl). There was a compensatory increase of TG transport by low-density lipoproteins
(LDL) (34.4±2.2 versus 19.9±0.4 mg/dl; $p<0.01$) and by
high-density lipoproteins (HDL) (19.8±2.7 versus 5.8 ±
0.3 mg/dl; $p<0.01$) in Reye's syndrome patients. Cholesterol concentrations were low on the day of admission
in HDL fractions (35.6±4.9 versus 50.6±6.5 mg/dl;
$p<0.05$) and in LDL fractions (75.6±8.5 versus 103±1.3
mg/dl; $p<0.05$). HDL-CHOL concentrations decreased
further during hospitalization (23.8±6.9 versus 50.6±
6.5 mg/dl; $p<0.02$) in Reye's syndrome patients. Of
particular interest was the lipoprotein pattern found
in one Reye's syndrome patient who died: VDLD-TG

concentrations increased progressively during hospitalization and reached the highest value (88 mg/dl) of any
patient studied, while HDL-CHOL concentrations decreased until none were detected on the last day of hospitalization. These results suggest that decreased TG
transport by VLDL may not be an important factor in the
development of fatty liver in Reye's syndrome, and that
metabolism of HDL particles may be impaired in patients
with Reye's syndrome.

AMINO ACID STUDIES IN REYE'S SYNDROME

C.A. Romshe, M.D., M.D. Hilty, M.D.,
H.J. McClung,M.D., B. Kerzner, M.D.,
and C.B. Reiner, M.D.

We have studied the quantitative serum amino
acids (aa) in 51 patients with Reye's syndrome (RS) and
have compared the results with the clinical course of
the illness with liver biopsies, including light and
electron microscopy, and with other illness in children
that might be confused with RS. All specimens were
drawn at the time of admission when the patients were
in Stage I or early Stage II. There is marked elevation of several amino acids, but those most elevated
are glutamine, proline, alanine, α-amino-N-butyrate and
lysine with normal or near normal levels of methionine,
phenylalanine and tyrosine. There is a significant
difference $p < 0.001$ noted in the mean of those who survived versus those who expired.

AMINO ACID	(normal)	EXPIRED (m)	SURVIVED (m)	p
Threonine	(8-24)	23±4	11.7±1	<.001
Serine	(7-19)	25±4	15±1	<.001
Glutamine	(6-47)	378±47	180±19	<.001
Proline	(5-20)	179±36	68±12	<.001
Glycine	(14-27)	59±9	29±2	<.001
Alanine	(17-38)	291±77	83±10	<.001
α-amino-N-butyrate	(1-3)	16±5	4.7±1	<.001
Lysine	(11-27)	162±28	83±8	<.001

Liver biopsy tissue was available for examination in 31
of the 51 patients and all showed changes characteristic of RS, microvesicular fat and mitochondrial injury.
To estimate, the specificity of the amino acid pattern
to RS, quantitative aa were compared on patients with
viral hepatitis, chicken pox, salicylism, fructose in-
tolerance, glycogen storage disease (I) and hepatic
necrosis. The amino aicd pattern observed in each of
the conditions was different than that of RS. The
explanation for the unique pattern is probably related
to the acute hepatic mitochondrial injury, inhibition
of mitochondrial enzymes and the release of amino acids
from muscle during the illness with an inability of the
injured liver to clear these aa. In conclusion, we
have shown that the abnormal pattern is present early
in the course of RS and that it is as specific as a
liver biopsy in confirming the diagnosis, with much
less risk to the patient. The correlation with severity is useful in assessing the clinical course of the
patient and in evaluating the efficacy of various
treatment modalities.

A RETROSPECTIVE EPIDEMIOLOGIC STUDY OF

REYE'S SYNDROME IN MICHIGAN

F.A. Luscombe, M.P.H., A. S. Monto,
J. V. Baublis,M.D., Ph D.

Since 1974, an increased number of children with
the diagnosis of Reye's syndrome have been admitted to
major hospitals. This phenomenon may reflect a growing
awareness of the disease or may suggest a true increase
in incidence. Although nationwide incidence has been
estimated during recent epidemic years, little is known
of the extent of the disease prior to 1974. During
that year, Michigan was among the states with the highest incidence of Reye's syndrome. Thus, Michigan was
selected as the site for a retrospective, epidemiologic
study of the disease from 1969-1976. This study, utilizing death certificates as the primary source of data,
was designed to: 1) obtain a consistent tabulation of
Reye's syndrome deaths over this period of time, 2)
determine the temporal relationship of Reye's syndrome
to known influenza outbreaks and 3) examine the geographic distribution of deaths for clustering, urban-
rural differentiation and relation to agricultural
crops and animals. Death certificates for children
less than or equal to 18 years of age were reviewed for
15 Reye's syndrome-related causes of death. To verify
the proportion of these deaths which may actually have
been attributed to Reye's syndrome, hospital records
were examined for a sample with diagnoses of encephalopathy or cerebral edema and encephalitis of viral or
unknown etiology. Based on standard diagnostic criteria, approximately 50% of the deaths in the sample
were probably due to Reye's syndrome, thus increasing
the number of known cases. The temporal analysis of
the death certificate data demonstrates a possible
association of Reye's syndrome with known outbreaks of
influenza. These data further show a higher frequency
of Reye's syndrome in whites than in blacks. On the

basis of residence, deaths due to Reye's syndrome were
significantly more frequent in children from rural
counties than in urban children and clustering of
deaths was noted in certain agricultural crop districts.
An association between this phenomenon and exposure to
petrochemicals is possible.
(Supported by grants from The Upjohn Company, Kalamazoo,
Michigan and the National Reye's Syndrome Foundation.)

REYE'S SYNDROME IN SIBLINGS

M.D. Hilty, M.D., H.J. McClung, M.D.,

R. Haynes, M.D., C.A.Romshe, M.D., and
E.S. Sherard,Jr., M.D.

Reye's syndrome (RS) in siblings was seen in
three of 85 families at Children's Hospital since 1968
and the incidence of RS in these family groups appears
to exceed that of the general population. The intervals between development of RS in the first and second
case siblings was 2-11 days and related to the incubation period of the initial viral infection. In our
patients the index case and the second case siblings
have the same preceding viral illness. In five of the
children the infection was chicken pox and in two, an
unspecified upper respiratory illness. The coma level
of the index case patients was higher, III-V, than it
was in second case siblings, where it was 0-I. In two
siblings, one in stage III coma and the second in stage
0, liver biopsies were performed. The light and electron microscopy indicated the diagnosis of Reye's syndrome. To assess genetic factors HLA typing was performed on all seven children, however a common genetic
marker was not identified. Further HLA typing and
other methods of genetic assessment need to be evaluated to better define this aspect of the illness. All
three families resided in rural and suburban areas and
a common exposure could not be identified. Environmental factors may be etiologically important in the

development of RS and the familial pattern is consistent with an environmental influence. One can hypothesize that the "right" combination of viral illness
and as yet unidentified environmental factor(s) may
precipitate the development of RS. The concept of interaction between viruses and toxins has been generated from both epidemiologic and animal studies. The relationship of genetic and environmental factors in RS
has not been defined and the study of RS in siblings
may clarify their role. The recognition that RS occurs
in family groups may offer opportunities for studies in
clinical management, etiology and pathogenesis. Diagnosis of RS in one family member should suggest the
possible development of RS in other siblings. Serum
transaminase assays in siblings of an affected family
member may identify children with mild disease prior
to the development of encephalopathy.

MANAGEMENT OF REYE'S SYNDROME

A.H. Menezes, M.D., P. G. Kealey, M.D.,

T. Yamada, M.D., and W.E.Bell,M.D.

Thirteen children suffering from Reye's syndrome were aggressively treated in a prospective study over the past two years. All patients started with clinical stage IV (scale I-V) and EEG grade IV (scale I-V) or worse. Our protocol consists of endotracheal intubation, curarization, mechanical ventilation, fluid restriction, and hypothermia to 31° C. In all cases the electroencephalogram (EEG), intracranial pressure, cardiac output and aterial blood gases were constantly monitored. Hepatic,renal, pancreatic and coagulation studies were closely followed. Barbiturate coma was induced only when intracranial hypertension existed despite the above protocol. The pulmonary artery wedge (PAW) pressure was maintained between 3-5 torr although it had a tendency to drop further with deep hypothermia and barbiturate coma. The arterial pCO_2 ranged between 20-25 torr. ICP remained <u>below</u> 20 torr, except in 3 cases (up to 60 torr) who survived using barbiturate coma. Hyperventilation, mannitol boluses,hypothermia and barbiturate coma were used in ascending order to control ICP elevation. The EEG was used for initial staging and later to monitor the progress of the disease. An improving EEG was one of the criteria for discontinuing active therapy. The youngest child was 20 months and the oldest was 15 years. Ten patients made a complete recovery and 3 died. The deaths occurred within 48 hours,and in all 3 cases acute pancreatitis led to acute hypotension and loss of cerebral perfusion. The duration of active intervention as previously outlined was 4 days to 2 weeks. A relapse(clinical and EEG)was documented in two patients without elevation in serum ammonia or other chemistries,after previous definite improvement. The significant complications of Reye's syndrome encountered in this series were:pancreatitis in four patients (three deaths), acute renal failure in two, cardiomyopathy in one, autoimmune response with coagulopathy in one and, in two patients, a Guilliam-Barre picture during recovery. The serum ammonia and SGOT levels did not seem to affect prognosis. We feel that the above treatment protocol has been effective in lowering the mortality of critical cases. Careful intensive monitoring is mandatory. The fatal outcomes were not a direct cause of intracranial hypertension, but pancreatitis.

PATHOLOGIC VASODILATATION AS A CAUSE OF INCREASED INTRACRANIAL PRESSURE IN REYE'S SYNDROME

J.W. Hopkins, M.D., S.L.Giannotta, M.D.,   and
G.W. Kindt, M. D.

Raised intracranial pressure invariably accompanies severe cases of Reye's syndrome with coma. The cause of this increase in intracranial pressure is still subject to investigation. Some studies based on autopsy findings have suggested that the increased intracranial pressure was due to cerebral edema. It is also known that primary pathologic vasodilatation can cause severe increases of intracranial pressure without edema in certain cases of brain trauma. We have reported from our laboratory that massive increases in intracranial pressure can occur in primatēs at serum ammonia levels seen clinically in Reye's syndrome. Specific gravity studies on the animal brains showed no increase in water content. We have recently studied children who present with coma and have Reye's syndrome with serial CT scanning. This report concerns our experience with the use of the CT scanning in Reye's syndrome. The contrast infusion demonstrates marked increases in vascularity suggesting vasodilatation. The vasodilatation decreases as the patient improves. We conclude that a pathologic cerebral vasodilatation may be the cause of increased intracranial pressure in children with Reye's syndrome, and that serial CT scanning is helpful in following these children.

PLATELET ATP METABOLISM IN REYE'S SYNDROME

C.C. Solomons, Ph D., A. Silverman, M.D.

The difficulty of studying the metabolic course of
patients with Reye's syndrome is enhanced by the need
for repeated liver or brain tissue biopsies. However,
information which appears to be meaningful with regard
to the basic mechanism and clinical supportive management can be obtained from the patient's circulating
cells. Red blood cells and platelets are relatively
easy to obtain by venipuncture and allow for individu-
alized evaluation of the glycotic and oxidative aspects
of ATP metabolism. Four male and six female patients
(aged 5 -17 years) with Reye's syndrome were studied
with respect to ATP, ADP, and AMP synthesis from U-C-14
adenine by platelet-rich-plasma. Thin layer chromatography was used to quantitate the nucleotides formed. A
significant decline of C^{14} ATP from a normal level of
60+8% of the (platelet) C^{14} nucleotide pool to below
20% was observed in two patients who died. Patients who
recovered completely or partially also had an initial
decline in platelet ATP, but this was followed by a return toward normal levels. With newer techniques,these
results can be obtained within 30 minutes after venipuncture and appear to be of prognostic value. The
platelets would seem to provide an effective model for
studying the etiological importance of circulating toxins, as well as helping to objectively evaluate the efficacy of drugs and the clinical management protocols
in patients with Reye's syndrome. In addition, the nature of cellular membrane lesions and the possibilities
for their correction can be studied using this model.